Mental Health Policy, Practice, and Service Accessibility in Contemporary Society

Jennifer M. Martin
Swinburne University, Australia

A volume in the Advances in Human Services and Public Health (AHSPH) Book Series

IGI Global
DISSEMINATOR OF KNOWLEDGE

Published in the United States of America by
IGI Global
Medical Information Science Reference (an imprint of IGI Global)
701 E. Chocolate Avenue
Hershey PA, USA 17033
Tel: 717-533-8845
Fax: 717-533-8661
E-mail: cust@igi-global.com
Web site: http://www.igi-global.com

Library of Congress Cataloging-in-Publication Data

Names: Martin, Jennifer (Associate professor of social work), editor.
Title: Mental health policy, practice, and service accessibility in contemporary society / Jennifer M. Martin, editor.
Description: Hershey PA : Medical Information Science Reference, [2019] | Includes bibliographical references and index.
Identifiers: LCCN 2018025684| ISBN 9781522574026 (hardcover) | ISBN 9781522574033 (ebook)
Subjects: | MESH: Mental Health Services | Mentally Ill Persons | Health Services Accessibility | Health Policy | Human Rights | Australia | Case Reports
Classification: LCC RA790.5 | NLM WM 30 KA8 | DDC 362.2--dc23 LC record available at https://lccn.loc.gov/2018025684

This book is published in the IGI Global book series Advances in Human Services and Public Health (AHSPH) (ISSN: 2475-6571; eISSN: 2475-658X)

British Cataloguing in Publication Data
A Cataloguing in Publication record for this book is available from the British Library.

Advances in Human Services and Public Health (AHSPH) Book Series

Jennifer Martin
RMIT University, Australia

ISSN:2475-6571
EISSN:2475-658X

Mission

The well-being of the general public should be a primary concern for any modern civilization. Ongoing research in the field of human services and public healthcare is necessary to evaluate, manage, and respond to the health and social needs of the global population.

The **Advances in Human Services and Public Health (AHSPH)** book series aims to publish high-quality reference publications focused on the latest methodologies, tools, issues, and strategies for managing the health and social welfare of the public. The AHSPH book series will be especially relevant for healthcare professionals, policy makers, government officials, and students seeking the latest research in this field.

Coverage

- Social Work
- Health policy
- Healthcare Reform
- Domestic Violence
- Public Welfare
- Public Funding
- Youth Development
- Poverty
- Medicare and Medicaid
- Access to Healthcare Services

IGI Global is currently accepting manuscripts for publication within this series. To submit a proposal for a volume in this series, please contact our Acquisition Editors at Acquisitions@igi-global.com or visit: http://www.igi-global.com/publish/.

The Advances in Human Services and Public Health (AHSPH) Book Series (ISSN 2475-6571) is published by IGI Global, 701 E. Chocolate Avenue, Hershey, PA 17033-1240, USA, www.igi-global.com. This series is composed of titles available for purchase individually; each title is edited to be contextually exclusive from any other title within the series. For pricing and ordering information please visit http://www.igi-global.com/book-series/advances-human-services-public-health/102256. Postmaster: Send all address changes to above address.

Titles in this Series

For a list of additional titles in this series, please visit: www.igi-global.com/book-series

Ethical Issues in Social Work Practice
Antonio Sandu (Ştefan cel Mare University of Suceava, Romania) and Ana Frunza (LUMEN Research Center in Social and Humanistic Sciences, Romania)
Information Science Reference • copyright 2018 • 328pp • H/C (ISBN: 9781522530909) • US $195.00 (our price)

Global Perspectives on Human Migration, Asylum, and Security
Christina M. Akrivopoulou (Hellenic Open University, Greece)
Information Science Reference • copyright 2018 • 268pp • H/C (ISBN: 9781522528173) • US $185.00 (our price)

Nutraceuticals and Innovative Food Products for Healthy Living and Preventive Care
Amit Verma (SDAU, India) Kajal Srivastava (GBPUAT, India) Shivom Singh (ITM University, India) and Hukum Singh (Forest Research Institute, India)
Medical Information Science Reference • copyright 2018 • 462pp • H/C (ISBN: 9781522529705) • US $245.00 (our price)

Health Information Systems and the Advancement of Medical Practice in Developing Countries
Kgomotso H. Moahi (University of Botswana, Botswana) Kelvin Joseph Bwalya (University of Johannesburg, South Africa) and Peter Mazebe II Sebina (University of Botswana, Botswana)
Medical Information Science Reference • copyright 2017 • 350pp • H/C (ISBN: 9781522522621) • US $200.00 (our price)

Examining the Role of Environmental Change on Emerging Infectious Diseases and Pandemics
Maha Bouzid (University of East Anglia, UK)
Information Science Reference • copyright 2017 • 327pp • H/C (ISBN: 9781522505532) • US $200.00 (our price)

Sexual Misconduct in the Education and Human Services Sector
Christopher Schwilk (Shippensburg University, USA) Rachel Stevenson (Shippensburg University, USA) and David Bateman (Shippensburg University, USA)
Information Science Reference • copyright 2017 • 291pp • H/C (ISBN: 9781522506577) • US $190.00 (our price)

Public Health Genomics and International Wealth Creation
E. William Ebomoyi (Chicago State University, USA)
Information Science Reference • copyright 2015 • 463pp • H/C (ISBN: 9781466685598) • US $235.00 (our price)

IGI Global
DISSEMINATOR OF KNOWLEDGE

701 East Chocolate Avenue, Hershey, PA 17033, USA
Tel: 717-533-8845 x100 • Fax: 717-533-8661
E-Mail: cust@igi-global.com • www.igi-global.com

Table of Contents

Detailed Table of Contents

This chapter reflects on the importance of the historical narrative of mental illness, arguing that Western countries have sought new ways to confine the mentally ill in the post-asylum era, namely through the effects of stigma and medicalization. The walls are invisible, when once they were physical. The chapter outlines how health and illness can be understood as socially constructed illustrating how mental health has been constructed uniquely across cultures and over time. To understand this process more fully, it is necessary to consider the history of madness, a story of numerous social flashpoints. The trajectories of two primary mental health narratives are charted in this chapter. The authors argue that these narratives have played, and continue to play, an important role in the social construction of mental illness. These narratives are "confinement" and "individual responsibility." Drawing on the work of Michel Foucault and Roy Porter, the authors describe how Western culture has come to consider the mentally ill as a distinct, abnormal other.

Risk assessment and management are considered core elements of healthcare practice. However, a brief examination of the theoretical literature on risk demonstrates that it is not a fixed concept. This chapter will critically analyze the impact that focusing on risk has on healthcare practice. The authors will join many others in pointing out the many potential negative impacts of viewing healthcare through the lens of risk. One risk type, suicide risk, will be examined closely. It will be shown that health professionals often fear liability when risk is a factor. In order to dissuade these fears, the legal elements of liability will be outlined, and relevant common law judgements will be discussed. Finally, future directions will be discussed.

The aim of this chapter is to explore the factors that health managers adopt when making decisions on how to allocate limited healthcare resources. The objective is to increase knowledge and understanding of decision making processes at the macro, meso, and micro levels and priority setting. An examination of current healthcare decision-making processes used for resource allocation around the world highlights the disparities in models and approaches and the often ad hoc nature of decisions made. A description of the allied health workforce highlights the size and significance of this workforce and why understanding decisions made in regards to allied health resources is of importance. Issues of access and equity are also considered in relation to notions of fairness and efficacy in relation to health outcomes.

The aim of this chapter is to contribute to addressing issues of access and equity in social work education for people with mental health disabilities. The objective is to carefully consider the introduction of inherent requirements in universities, and particularly in relation to social work education, in Australia. A targeted review of relevant literature including legislation, policy, and practice standards frameworks identifies the parameters of inherent requirements and possible areas of discrimination. Consideration of the use of inherent requirements in social work education is from a human rights social justice perspective that acknowledges the strength and resources of people and communities and actively advocates for the protection of disability rights.

This chapter presents a critical discussion on the understanding and access of mental health services by people from diverse refugee backgrounds delivered in a Western cultural setting. Mental health services are heavily influenced by a biomedical approach, but there is a growing understanding of the importance of culture and biopsychosocial approaches. This chapter highlights some of the institutional and cultural issues that need to be addressed for the services to be effective. Practical approaches that have worked in different places are explored and critically discussed. A recovery-oriented model that recognizes that the individual is part of the community and the importance of spirituality are canvassed.

This chapter explores the extent to which journalists draw on long-standing mental health narratives when telling their stories about the "mentally ill" and, in particular, their tendency to depict the mentally ill as violent and dangerous. The chapter is divided into three sub-categories based on the perpetrators of violent crime committed against members of their immediate family. These were "fathers," of which 24 articles were dedicated to the stories of 11 men; "mothers," where 22 articles documented the stories of 24 mothers who harmed their children; and finally, "progeny," where 58 articles presented 17 cases of sons or daughters who killed, or planned to kill, one or both of their parents. Despite differences in the way Australian journalists explain the violence depicted in these stories, particularly when the perpetrator was a female, they continually drew on mental health as an explanatory device to account for how and why these crimes took place. This provides evidence for a continuation of the confinement narrative presented in Chapter 1.

This chapter outlines the key features of the diagnosis of borderline personality disorder. This is a diagnosis that has attracted significant levels of stigma and has generally been viewed as difficult to treat. This has resulted in often inadequate service responses for people experiencing high levels of distress. Increased understanding is facilitated by exploring precipitating factors leading to this diagnosis, including invalidating and often traumatizing environments. Available evidence from Australian and international literature is considered, with main treatments identified to inform improved treatment outcomes. The need for attention to biological, psychological factors is highlighted and in particular acknowledgment of the high prevalence of trauma, particularly childhood sexual assault, amongst the mostly women who are given this diagnosis.

This chapter details some key considerations for health and human services professionals working with lesbian, gay, bisexual, and transgender (LGBT) people in care relationships. Reflecting on the impacts of stigma and discrimination as well as the social, cultural, and political contexts of LGBT communities and carers, this chapter will explore some of ways these factors (as well as heterosexist and cis-genderist assumptions about families and partners) impact the identification, support, and recognition of LGBT people in care relationships. Finally, this chapter will recommend strategies to reduce poor mental health and wellbeing outcomes among people in care relationships where one or all people involved are LGBT, and explore some key actions that may assist health and human services better support and include LGBT people in care relationships.

This chapter will look at the current situation concerning youth mental health in Australia and provide information about youth mental health literacy, which was first coined by Jorm in 1997. A literature review of current Australian mental health promotion and education programs being offered in schools will be conducted as well as examples of some of the better-known ones that have been implemented internationally. The evolution of mental health education in Australian schools will be examined so as to provide a perspective of how some of the current programs came into being or existence. The main aim of this chapter will be to highlight the high prevalence of mental illness that exists amongst young people in Australia and how implementing mental health education in schools can be beneficial and helpful in improving their mental health and wellbeing. Mental health education in schools can help in breaking down the stigma surrounding mental illness. Another benefit is that young people will be able to identify mental health problems earlier amongst their peers and in themselves, which can lead to early help seeking, especially due to young people gaining a higher level of mental health literacy through mental health education programs.

There are many misconceptions about older adults' capabilities and aspirations, and especially their attitudes and approach towards technology. They are often misunderstood and seen as uninterested and unmotivated to engage with use of technology. Due to an absence of an "interest" framework for older adults to learn mobile touch screen technologies, this chapter investigates the role that pre-existing interests play in older adults' adoption of technology. Can a curriculum guided only by pre-existing interests of older adults, rather than a structured curriculum have a positive influence on its adoption for mobile touch screen technologies? The results show that when older adults are taught according to requests based on their pre-existing interests, it encouraged long-term adoption of technology including building up their confidence in usage of mobile touch screen technologies.

This chapter examines the correlation between environmental issues and wellbeing. A broad literature review illustrates that changing climate, increasing populations, and degrading natural environments have negative impacts on health and wellbeing. The focus of this chapter is on conflicts arising from the limited supply of natural resources and competing needs, interests, and demands. This can create high levels of tension and division within communities that erodes community spirit, support, and connectedness as people compete for limited resources. The conflict arising from such disputes has negative impacts on social cohesion and the high levels of stress experienced, without adequate supports, can trigger mental ill health. The example of basin level water conflict in Turkey is used to illustrate this.

Preface

Mental Health Policy, Practice, and Service Accessibility in Contemporary Society is framed by the World Health Organisation's Global Mental Health Action Plan: 2013-2020. According to the World Health Organisation (WHO), one in four people in the world will experience 'a mental or neurological disorder' at some point in their lives. This is within the context of just under half of the countries in the world not having any mental health policy, with a quarter having no mental health legislation and one third not having specific mental health services. Even where treatments are available, nearly two thirds of people diagnosed with a mental health disorder do not seek assistance from a mental health professional (WHO, 2013, p. 8). The six main principles of the WHO Action Plan are: (1) universal health coverage; (2) human rights; (3) evidence-based practice; (4) life course approach; (5) multi-sectoral approach and; (6) empowerment of persons with mental disorders and psychosocial disabilities (WHO, 2013, p. 10). These principles are enacted across policy and law, resource planning, stakeholder collaboration and 'the strengthening and empowerment of people with mental disorders and psychosocial disabilities and their organisations.

In addition to being responsive to the needs of people with mental health issues, a priority is national efforts to develop policies and programs that promote the mental health and wellbeing of the whole population. This includes targeted programs for infants, children, adolescents, adults and older people. The values, principles and objectives of this policy are codified in legislation on mental health, health and capacity to establish oversight mechanisms to protect human rights, tackle stigma and support the development of accessible services in the community. Mental health legislation, policies and plans are also underpinned by obligations under the Convention on the Rights of Persons with Disabilities and other international, regional and national human rights conventions. Actions proposed by WHO include the strengthening of leadership and governance through government working with key stakeholders to identify main areas for action. Central to these actions are respect for the dignity and human rights of people with mental disorders and psychosocial disabilities. This requires empowerment and involvement in all aspects of service design and delivery including the framing of legislation, policy and service plans; mental health advocacy, service provision and monitoring; and research and evaluation.

Decision-making includes consideration of evidence-based approaches, fiscal responsibility, issues of access and equity and protection for the most vulnerable and disadvantaged. This level of governance and strategic planning means that mental health services and interventions are likely to be more effective and responsive to the populations and communities they serve. Such an approach encapsulates a broad range of government and private sector organisations across multiple jurisdictions reflecting the mainstreaming of mental health services within the community. This is reflected in mainstream mental health interventions into health, human rights, disability, education, employment, housing, poverty reduction, children and families, substance misuse and abuse, and criminal justice. Activities are aimed at mental health prevention, early intervention and the promotion of recovery based upon international and regional human rights frameworks. Recovery involves the empowerment of people to live full and productive lives in the community.

Contemporary mainstream service models acknowledge the contributions of a broad range of people with increased collaboration between mental health professionals and families, school teachers, non-government organisations, police, religious leaders, faith healers and traditional healers. Services are required to be sensitive to trauma-related issues and emergency situations that may involve isolated incidents or ongoing conflict, violence and disasters. They need to be responsive to the needs of vulnerable and marginalised groups that include: low income families, people living with HIV/AIDS, women and children living with violence, survivors of violence, Indigenous people, refugees and asylum seekers, immigrants, lesbian, gay, bisexual, transgender and intersex people, those deprived of their liberty and others who are in a minority within a national context.

Service evaluation and research is essential for the generation of new knowledge to inform evidence-based practices and service improvements. The research imbalance between high income and middle and low-income countries needs to be addressed so that cost effective and culturally appropriate service responses can be provided to meet the mental health needs of local communities. This includes the involvement of people with mental health disorders and their organisations in developing and implementing research agendas on a global level to advance 'mental health promotion, prevention, treatment, recovery, care, policy and service evaluation (WHO, 2013, p. 19).

Mental Health Policy, Practice, and Service Accessibility in Contemporary Society covers main areas of mental health policy and practice for contemporary and future mental health service design and delivery. All chapters are concerned with accessibility and innovative practices into the future across a range of populations and topics. The backgrounds of the contributing authors reflects the diversity of mainstream mental health policy and practice and includes journalism, social science, social work, occupational therapy, physiotherapy, bio-medicine, information systems, nursing, community work and engineering. Many of the authors are also mental health practitioners, consumers and carers.

The chapters in this book address the main principles and priority areas of the World Health Organisation's Global Mental Health Action Plan: 2013-2020 (WHO, 2013). For the newcomer, the field of mental health is perplexing, surprising and possibly somewhat disappointing. This book is important as it names and tackles difficult issues in a balanced and informed manner utilising the latest research conducted by authors who are recognised experts on their topic areas. There has been little scientific progress in the diagnosis and treatment of mental health problems at a time when there have been significant advancements made in many areas of health, neuroscience included. There remains a reliance upon the *Diagnostic and Statistical Manual* (DSM) of the American Psychiatry Association and the *International Classification of Diseases* (ICD) of the World Health Organisation. Both manuals are symptom-based and do not reply upon any diagnostic testing beyond the reporting of subjective observed behaviours. With every new edition of the ICD and DSM comes an expanded list of diagnoses, each with an approved medical intervention. Access to mental health treatment, covered by government funding or private insurance, usually requires an "approved" ICD or DSM diagnosis. Worldwide we are witnessing a growth in the diagnosing and prescribing of medications to adults and children for mental health issues. This medicalisation of "human distress" overlooks the environmental contexts within which mental health problems develop and perpetuate. It also takes attention and services away from those with more serious mental health concerns who are often more difficult to work with and not necessarily reliable when it comes to attending appointments. In a policy context of individualised service funding, clients who do not attend scheduled appointments become a liability due to lost income and private practitioners may not want to see them because of this.

Mental Health Policy, Practice, and Service Accessibility in Contemporary Society draws upon the latest knowledge and practice experience in the physical, behavioural and social sciences and is relevant for all students, educators and practitioners in the mental health field who want to improve their understanding of contemporary issues for policy and innovative practice and how to apply these. It is relevant for all disciplines in the health and human services including psychiatrists, nurses, psychologists, social workers and other allied health disciplines including allied health assistants, consumer consultants, carer consultants and peer workers. It is pertinent as a text for courses in health and human services including social work, psychology, medicine, nursing, occupational therapy, criminology, legal studies, youth work, community work and welfare studies. The multidisciplinary nature of the book lends itself to media and communication studies, journalism, planning, engineering and human computer interaction. It is also relevant to health professionals and community workers in mainstream settings due to people living with mental health issues using a wide range of health and community services. Hence, its relevance to anyone in the community who wants to further develop and enhance their knowledge and understanding of contemporary mental health issues and professional skills for innovative ways forward into the future. The chapters presented in this book are based on sound theoretical underpinnings and practice experiences.

In Chapter 1, Samuel Teague and Peter Robinson from Swinburne University in Australia reflect upon the importance of the historical narrative of mental illness, arguing that western countries have sought new ways to confine the mentally ill in the post-asylum era. They argue that confinement now occurs through the effects of stigma and medicalization and that the walls that in the past were physical are now invisible. The chapter outlines how health and illness can be understood as socially constructed illustrating how mental health has been viewed across different cultures over time. They consider the history of "madness" and highlight a number of social flashpoints in this story. The authors argue that the two dominant narratives of "confinement" and "individual responsibility" play an important role in the social construction of mental illness.

In Chapter 2 by Kellie Grant, Jenni White and Terry Haines from Monash University and Jennifer Martin from Swinburne University in Australia, assessment and management of risk are considered as core elements of health care practice. In their examination of the theoretical literature on risk the authors demonstrate that risk is not a fixed concept. They highlight numerous ways that an overemphasis on risk can negatively impact upon mental health service responses particularly in relation to suicide. The perceptions of health professionals when it comes to risk are discussed focusing on the fear of liability. The authors examine the validity of such fears by examining legal aspects and relevant common law judgements.

In Chapter 3, Haylee Lane and Terry Haines from Monash University and Jennifer Martin from Swinburne University in Australia explore factors that health managers take into consideration when making decisions on how to allocate limited healthcare resources. They examine priority setting at the macro, meso, and micro levels. A discussion of current health care decision making processes, used for resource allocation around the world, highlights the disparities in models and approaches and the often ad hoc nature of decisions made. The authors highlight the size and significance of the allied health workforce and the importance of understanding decision making in regards to resource allocation. Issues of access and equity are considered in relation to notions of fairness, efficacy and health outcomes.

Chapter 4 by Steve Boucher from RMIT University in Australia addresses issues of access and equity in post-secondary education for people with mental health disabilities. The author carefully considers the introduction of inherent requirements in universities, and particularly in relation to social work education, in Australia. A targeted review of relevant literature including legislation, policy and practice standards frameworks identifies the parameters of inherent requirements and possible areas of discrimination. The use of inherent requirements in social work education is considered from a human rights and social justice perspective. This approach acknowledges the strength and resources of people and communities and the importance of actively advocating for the protection of disability rights.

In Chapter 5, Ndungi wa Mungai and Ruth (Isobel) Bailey from Charles Sturt University in Australia and Jeanette Ninnis, from the New South Wales Services for Treatment & Rehabilitation of Torture & Trauma Survivors (STARTTS) discuss access issues for people from refugee backgrounds. This includes consideration of different cultural understandings of mental health for people from diverse refugee backgrounds when services are delivered in a western cultural setting. They highlight institutional and cultural issues that need to be addressed for mental health services to be effective including acknowledgment of spirituality. Practical approaches that have worked in different places are explored using a recovery-oriented approach.

Chapter 6 by Christina David, Carmel Laragy and Elizabeth Hudson from RMIT University in Australia outlines the key features of individual funding programs and examines their suitability for people with mental health issues. They highlight how this is a contested area with some arguing that mental illness is different from other types of disability and unsuitable for individual funding. According to this view, the recovery model and the episodic nature of mental illness are seen as conflicting with individual funding eligibility criteria for consistent and permanent disability. The authors focus on the counter view that sees flexible individual funding as ideally suited to meeting the fluctuating needs of people with mental illness and how its key principles of empowerment and self-direction are consistent with the recovery paradigm. Evidence from Australian and international studies is reviewed suggesting that successful outcomes can be achieved if the necessary supports and resources are available to meet people's needs.

Jennifer Martin, Susan Roberts, Zac Haussegger and Emily Greenwood from Swinburne University and Jenni White, Kellie Grant and Terry Haines from Monash University in Australia are concerned with Aboriginal wellbeing and cultural safety in health and mental health services in Chapter 7. The aim of this chapter is to contribute to addressing the gap between policy and practice for the development and implementation of accessible health and wellbeing organisations and practices from a culturally safe, trauma-informed approach. The findings of a targeted literature search identify the main features of a cultural safety trauma-informed framework and implementation plan. The authors argue that to achieve improved health and wellbeing outcomes with Aboriginal people, historical and contemporary political, economic and social contextual factors relating to colonisation must be acknowledged. In the Australian context, particular attention must be given to the impacts of The Stolen Generations across many generations.

In Chapter 8, Samuel Teague and Peter Robinson from Swinburne University in Australia review the extent to which journalists draw on long-standing mental health narratives when telling their stories about the "mentally ill", and in particular, their tendency to depict the mentally ill as violent and dangerous. They consider three sub-categories based on the perpetrators of violent crime committed against members of their immediate family. These are fathers, mothers and progeny. The authors highlight how despite differences in the ways Australian journalists explain the violence depicted in the stories they report, particularly when the perpetrator is a female, they continually draw on mental health as an explanatory device to account for how and why these crimes took place.

Chapter 9, by Peter King from RMIT University and Jennifer Martin from Swinburne University in Australia, considers access to evidence-based services for individuals with borderline personality disorder. The key features of this diagnosis are presented followed by a discussion that highlights the significant levels of stigma attached to it. The authors explore precipitating factors leading to this diagnosis, including invalidating and often traumatising environments, and how service responses, particularly for people experiencing high levels of distress are often inadequate. Available evidence from Australian and international literature is considered, with main treatments identified to inform improved treatment outcomes. The need for attention to biological, psychological and social factors is highlighted and in particular acknowledgment of the high prevalence of trauma, particularly childhood sexual assault, amongst the mostly women who are given this diagnosis.

In Chapter 10, Gabriel Aleksandrs, a senior policy advisor, from Carers Victoria in Australia, introduces key considerations for health and human services professionals when working with lesbian, gay, bisexual, and transgender (LGBT) people in care relationships. The author reflects on the impacts of stigma and discrimination directed toward LGBT communities. Ways in which political, social and cultural factors influence the identification, support, and recognition of LGBT people in care relationships are examined. Strategies are recommended to reduce poor mental health and wellbeing outcomes among people in care relationships where one or all people involved are LGBT. Key actions that may assist health and human services better support and include LGBT people in care relationships are presented.

Chapter 11 by Matthew Dale from Mind Australia examines youth mental health in Australia. The results of a literature review of current mental health promotion and education programs being offered in Australian schools are presented including examples of evidence-based programs that have been implemented internationally such as youth mental health literacy. The author highlights the high prevalence of mental illness that exists amongst young people in Australia and how implementing mental health education in schools can be beneficial in improving mental health and wellbeing outcomes for young people. He discusses how mental health education in schools can help to identify mental health problems early on and reduce stigma.

The authors of Chapter 12, Jeanie Beh, Bruno Mascitelli and Sonja Pedell from Swinburne University in Australia explore the role of ICT in encouraging social inclusion for older adults. They highlight misconceptions of older adults' capabilities and aspirations, and especially their attitudes and approach towards technology. They present an "interest" framework for older adults to learn mobile touch screen technologies. A curriculum guided only by pre-existing interests of older adults, rather than a structured curriculum, is demonstrated to have a positive influence on the adoption of mobile touch screen technologies in this age group. The authors discuss a number of benefits of usage of mobile touch screen technologies for social inclusion and improved wellbeing outcomes for older people.

In Chapter 13, Fatih Bodzemir from RMIT University and Jennifer Martin from Swinburne University in Australia examine the correlation between environmental issues and wellbeing. A broad literature review illustrates how changing climate, increasing populations and degrading natural environments can have negative impacts on health and wellbeing. The focus is on conflicts arising from the limited supply of natural resources and competing needs, interests and demands. The impacts of ongoing tensions and divisions within communities, including the erosion of community spirit, support and connectedness are discussed. The authors argue that conflict arising from such disputes, and the high levels of stress experienced, can trigger mental ill health and impede recovery that is reliant upon community inclusion and support.

People and societies today face a number of critical challenges that require the strengthening of individual and community capacity and humanitarian interventions beyond narrow psychiatric diagnoses and interventions. As the reader you are encouraged to consider the wide ranging views presented in this book and to draw your own conclusions as to the main challenges in mental health policy and service provision and how to best respond into the future. In doing so readers are encouraged to reflect on the priorities set out in the Mental Health Action Plan 2013-2020 of the World Health Organisation that recognise a clear link between health and mental health outcomes:

1. More effective leadership and governance for mental health;
2. The provision of comprehensive, integrated mental health and social care services in community-based settings;
3. The implementation of strategies for promotion and prevention; and
4. Strengthened information systems, evidence and research. (WHO, 2013, p. 10)

REFERENCES

World Health Organisation. (2013). *Mental Health action plan 2013-2020*. Geneva, Switzerland: World Health Organisation.

Chapter 1
The History of Unreason: Social Construction of Mental Illness

Samuel Teague
Swinburne University, Australia

Peter Robinson
Swinburne University, Australia

ABSTRACT

This chapter reflects on the importance of the historical narrative of mental illness, arguing that Western countries have sought new ways to confine the mentally ill in the post-asylum era, namely through the effects of stigma and medicalization. The walls are invisible, when once they were physical. The chapter outlines how health and illness can be understood as socially constructed illustrating how mental health has been constructed uniquely across cultures and over time. To understand this process more fully, it is necessary to consider the history of madness, a story of numerous social flashpoints. The trajectories of two primary mental health narratives are charted in this chapter. The authors argue that these narratives have played, and continue to play, an important role in the social construction of mental illness. These narratives are "confinement" and "individual responsibility." Drawing on the work of Michel Foucault and Roy Porter, the authors describe how Western culture has come to consider the mentally ill as a distinct, abnormal other.

INTRODUCTION

In the years preceding the seventeenth century, the mentally ill were placed on boats, taken to foreign locations, and dumped there, and for European populations, this was the primary method for dealing with a portion of society considered abnormal (Foucault, 1967). Michel Foucault (1967) described this *Ship of Fools* as a vessel for those who had no real connection to time or place, for "as the madman sets sail for the other world, it is from the other world that he comes when he disembarks" (p. 8). This image of the mad as incongruous and lost on the high seas resonates in the imagination of the twenty-first century sociologist, because while the *Ship of Fools* no longer exists, the authors suspect that society's perception of the mentally ill as both deviant and abnormal endures.

DOI: 10.4018/978-1-5225-7402-6.ch001

Even throughout the twentieth century, western civilization continued to perceive and construct mental illness as an abnormality. In the original 1952 edition of the Diagnostic and Statistical Manual of Mental Disorders (American Psychiatric Association, 1952), patients could be diagnosed under one or more of 106 conditions. In 1994, the DSM-IV contained nearly 300 disorders, an increase of close to 300% in just five decades (American Psychiatric Association, 1994). Peter Conrad (2007) included these statistics in his thesis on the problems inherent in modern medicalization, and used them to outline the modern trend within which human beings are increasingly defined as sick rather than healthy, and as abnormal rather than sane. Certainly, the introduction of Prozac in 1987 as a drug for the treatment of depression has signaled the dawn of a new era where antidepressant medication is used to treat "life problems" as well as serious illness (Conrad, 2007, p. 61). In this chapter, we show that from the *Ship of Fools* to the introduction of Prozac, western civilization has sought to understand and develop ways of controlling those being treated for mental illness.

This chapter details the history of mental illness, as portrayed by Roy Porter (1987; 2002), Michel Foucault (1967), Andrew Scull (2015), Erving Goffman (1959; 1963), and Peter Conrad (2007). The authors trace the trajectory of the principal narratives that have characterised this history, and outline how they persist and operate today. Scholars who have sought to interpret present media portrayals of the mentally ill have neglected an appreciation of the history of mental illness. An account of the history of mental illness is critical in interpreting the present socio-cultural media landscape. In constructing this detailed historical account, the chapter is divided into four parts.

The first introduces the notion that the lived experience of mental illness can be understood as socially constructed. Attention is given to the debate between essentialist and constructionist perspectives, and the authors outline how the two can be considered in unison. The section summarizes the biomedical approach to health for the purpose of detailing how social understandings of health and illness are constructed uniquely across cultures. The second section of this chapter describes the history of madness, and drawing predominantly on the work of Michel Foucault, the authors chart the trajectory of two primary mental health narratives which have played, and continue to play, an important role in the social construction of mental illness. These narratives are "confinement" and "individual responsibility". In part three, this historical account continues, addressing the legacy of Sigmund Freud, the closing of asylums in the 1980s, and an account of the breadth and scope of modern medicalization. The chapter concludes with a focus on Australia's mental health history from 1870 to the present.

BACKGROUND

Mental Illness as Socially Constructed

The experience of mental illness can be understood as socially constructed. By considering mental health from this standpoint, emphasis is placed on the importance of historical accounts, the mental health narratives that underpin these, and print media's role in shaping public attitudes towards the mentally ill. It is the social constructionist standpoint that forms the foundation for this chapter. Questions around how mental illness can be understood have long been characterised by the philosophical debate between "constructionists" and "essentialists". Greider and Garkovich (1994) argue that even the physical environment – a wheat field or savannah plain – can be understood as a socially constructed "symbolic landscape" (p. 1). They propose that a real estate developer, a farmer, and a hunter each perceive the environment in distinct ways, making a concrete physical reality a myriad of potentials "grounded in the cultural definitions of those who encounter that place" (p. 2). For these scholars, a rock is not merely a rock, but a sacred stone, a cutting tool, or a wishing pebble, as the world is infinitely constructed and reconstructed.

Latour and Woolgar (1979) expand on this argument, arguing that the scientific study of external phenomena is mostly political and "entirely fabricated out of circumstance" (p. 239). Observing scientists at work in a laboratory, these theorists found that the objective of positivist study was to extend and speed up the credibility cycle for scientists through the creation of work that would grant them a status of higher esteem. In other words, scientists are social creatures first and foremost. Latour and Woolgar (1979) found that the scientists at the center of their research were writers and readers in the business of being convinced and of convincing others, operating within a laboratory that engaged in an organised system of "persuasion through literary inscription" (p. 88). Neurosurgeon and writer Paul Kalanithi (2017) wrote just twelve months before his death in March 2015:

Scientific methodology is the product of human hands and thus cannot reach some permanent truth. We build scientific theories to organise and manipulate the world, to reduce phenomena into manageable units. Science is based on reproducibility and manufactured objectivity (p. 169).

This particular example illustrates the breadth and scope of the constructionist perspective, which suggests that if scientific facts can be understood as socially constructed, then so too can mental illness.

Bury (1986) presents an alternate perspective, arguing that in giving little attention to the existence of a concrete physical reality, constructionists undersell the important role it plays in shaping our understanding of the world. Bury argues that physical reality and human knowledge partake in a fluid relationship, whereby knowledge engages and operates with physical reality, while that physical reality simultaneously imposes itself on human knowledge. He believes that too much emphasis is placed on the human appreciation of a landscape or phenomenon, when the relationship between the two is an interwoven tapestry, and he takes issue with Steven Shapin's (1982) argument that scientific knowledge is routinely constructed to serve the interests of its users. In other words, facts about the origins of a particular disease are "discovered" in the laboratory so as to aid doctors in the treatment of their patients, and Bury argues in response to this that by representing medical knowledge as constructed in the interests of powerful institutions and groups, the sincerity and compassion at the basis of the medical profession is undermined. If facts about illness are constructed, then doctors become mere actors in the constructed play of life.

A balanced view can be a panacea to a philosophical divide. A concrete physical reality can exist, but the construction of attitudes, perceptions, and beliefs around the phenomenon are fluid, malleable, and worthy of study. Barnes (1977) argues that a concrete physical reality and our ideas about it can exist together.

Knowledge is related to activity which consists precisely in men attempting to manipulate, predict and control the real world in which they exist. Hence knowledge is found useful precisely because the world is as it is; and it is to that extent a function of what is real, and not the pure product of thought and imagination. Knowledge rises out of our encounters with reality (p. 110).

This perspective emphasizes the power of social institutions and the human beings who operate within them to construct external phenomena. As a result, social constructions can be liberating because they remove expectations and allow for reconstructions.

A significant amount of social research supports this argument, that an external social world can be constructed around a distinct organic entity. Julie Hepworth's (1999) account of the social construction of anorexia nervosa suggests that the reality of this illness, for many centuries, has involved three common elements: the starving of oneself, weight loss, and the exhibiting of a common mental dullness. In the twelfth and thirteenth centuries, anorexia nervosa was associated with holiness, as those who chose to subsist on minimal nutritional quantities were considered divine, and subsequently revered (Hepworth, 1999, p. 13). Today, the same individuals are defined as unwell, mentally ill. While the three common elements of the illness have not changed significantly, society's understanding of the phenomenon has, and in a cyclical fashion. This shift in understanding and attitude has transformed the lived experience of anorexia nervosa, which we argue is evidence of the power of human beings to construct and re-shape reality.

Michel Foucault (1967) and Roy Porter (2002) base their respective historical accounts on the assumption that the lived experience of mental illness can be understood as dependent on social forces. Foucault's thesis concerns the power and influence of social institutions.

Whether madness is described as a religious or philosophical phenomenon … or as an objective medical essence … these conceptions are not discoveries but historical constructions of meaning (p. xiv).

While Porter questions some aspects of Foucault's argument, he supports the claim that the history of madness is an account "not of disease and its treatment but of questions of freedom and control, knowledge and power" (Porter, 2002, p. 3). Neither Foucault nor Porter claim that psychological anguish is fictitious, but that the social world around the individual being treated for mental illness is a construction.

Thomas Szasz was a significant figure in the anti-psychiatry movement, which was most prominent in the second half of the twentieth century, and he states in his thesis on "the myth of mental illness" that madness is manufactured to serve the interests of psychiatrists with a view to professional advancement, "endorsed by society because it sanctions easy solutions for problem people" (Porter, 2002, p. 2). Szasz contends that the majority of human suffering originates from life circumstances and stress and that the psychiatric profession routinely medicalises these experiences. This chapter acknowledges this claim, but draws more on the accounts of Foucault and Porter because of the attention they give to the significance of historical narratives.

Biomedical Approach

Western culture's construction of health and illness is apparent in the dominance of the biomedical approach. Biomedicine explains illness as a malfunction of the body's biological mechanisms, and it generally ignores the social origins of health and illness (Engel, 1977). It is a model that places medical professionals such as doctors in positions of power based on their status as experts in the field (Wreford, 2005). Like health and illness more broadly, medical practice has been constructed uniquely across cultures and over time. Engel was one of the first scholars to outline biomedicine's fallibility in its failure to account for the psychological, social, and environmental aspects that are so important in understanding health and illness. Engel's (1977) utopia is one where diabetes and schizophrenia are human experiences as well as disease, and he presents the biopsychosocial model as an alternative to biomedicine. Cooper, Stevenson, and Hale (1996) offer support for this approach.

With the biomedical approach, healthy people become manifestations of healthy, cellular activity; ill people become manifestations of dysfunctional cellular activity. The patient becomes a 'problem' to be solved, and the solution to that problem lies in adopting a scientific, mechanistic approach that precludes any consideration of social, psychological, or behavioural influences.

Cooper, Stevenson, and Hale (1996) draw attention to a subtle irony that underpins western medicine in that while biomedicine is itself a cultural construction, illness is considered almost entirely through the framework of biological function or malfunction.

That biomedicine is a social construct is supported by the differences in treatment and medical beliefs that exist cross-culturally. In African cultures, traditional healers are important in providing spiritual assistance to the sick and dying (Wreford, 2005). South American shamans see illness as a force beyond the confines of physical degradation, instead addressing sickness as "inherently socio-political and cosmological" (Greene, 1998, p. 641). In the remote ethnic communities of Peru, physical affliction is considered the product of spirits, natural forces, and even deceased ancestors. This approach is not considered guesswork in this culture, but a legitimate medical practice broadly termed "shamanism" (Bastien, 1992; Mehl; 1988). A comparison of biomedicine and shamanism emphasizes that where the custodians of legitimate medical knowledge differ, human beings forge unique and contrasting models of health and illness.

Even one's definition of mental illness can be problematic. A sociological definition of mental illness must acknowledge health and wellbeing as constructed distinctly across cultures, environments, and historical epochs, while simultaneously accepting the dominance in Western culture of biomedicine, a medical model which assumes mental illness is a disease. The argument underpinning this chapter, that mental illness can be understood as socially constructed, is derived from the work of both historians and sociologists. Thomas Szasz (2007, p. 3) described mental illness as a "metaphorical disease", invented by psychiatrists to legitimate their authority, while Roy Porter (2002) and Michel Foucault (1967) illustrated the construction of madness across specific socio-historical contexts.

Aneshensel, Phelan, and Bierman (2013) describe mental illness as a concept requiring the insights of several disciplines, and in reviewing the literature from the standpoints of psychiatry, psychology, anthropology and sociology, divided opinion prevails in the search for a universal definition of mental illness. Aneshensel and colleagues (2013) argue that mental illness consists of a vast range of behavioural, cognitive and emotional phenomena, including:

Speaking to a companion whom no one else can see; sitting silently in a room, alone, eating little and sleeping less, contemplating death; becoming suddenly overwhelmed with intense anxiety for no apparent reason; consumption of alcohol to such a degree that it becomes difficult to hold a job or maintain friendships; frequent sickness with no identifiable physiological disease; and feeling no remorse when others are injured by one's actions.

The behavioural, cognitive and emotional phenomena included in this description can form part of the lived experience of mental illness. Feelings of intense and overwhelming anxiety are often characteristic of deeper mental health issues, while the use of alcohol and illicit drugs as a form of self-medication to mask underlying mental health concerns is common and can lead to significant upheaval in an individual's life circumstances (Harris & Edlund, 2005).

As a definition, however, the description is inadequate because one could reasonably assume some of these behaviours and emotions are characteristic of the lived experience of the mentally well person. A readiness to associate problematic behaviour with mental illness is at the core of negligent media reporting on mental health topics. And the rush to explain violence through the lens of mental illness offers an explanatory device for every perpetrator of domestic violence.

THE HISTORY OF MENTAL ILLNESS

The history of mental illness is a story of control; a tale of both subtle and transparent confinement. It begins in the early thirteenth century, when according to Michel Foucault (1967), King Louis VIII set in motion the opening of "lazar houses", secure places for the containment of those individuals with leprosy. Such was their effectiveness that by the middle of the thirteenth century, two thousand of these institutions were in operation across France (Foucault, 1967, p. 3). While the mentally ill would not pose a problem requiring state-sanctioned control for at least another three centuries, Foucault argues that the leprosaria are an important institution in the history of madness because they signaled the creation of a specific "fearsome figure" who could be carefully excluded from society "after a sacred circle had been drawn around him" (Foucault, 1967, p. 5). Put simply, madness was leprosy's heir to the throne of otherness.

The lazar houses closed at varying rates across Europe between the fourteenth and eighteenth centuries. In 1348, the leper house at Saint-Alban in France was home to just three inhabitants, and in 1627, the leper house of Saint Bartholomew was closed also. Throughout the decades in which the lazar houses were abandoned, and before the institution of the asylum appeared across Europe, the mentally ill were placed on boats, taken to foreign locations and dumped there (Porter, 2002). This practice was the dominant means for ridding cities of the presence of an undesirable group, and it is in this practice that we find the legacy of the leprosaria. Important are its implications for European attitudes towards abnormality and deviance in the seventeenth and eighteenth centuries. Long after leprosy had vanished along with the fear of its burden, the physical structures, social attitudes, values and images that had been attached to the leper and associated with a fearsome "other", would be attributed to the mad.

In a number of European states, the seventeenth century saw the emergence of a more organised form of social control, what Foucault (1967) calls "The Great Confinement". The year 1656 marks the date, founding in Paris, the first Hôpital-Général. These institutions were not houses created solely for the insane, but for those members of the population that posed a threat to normality and progress. The idle were locked away with the mad; the venereal with the gypsies. Within three years, the Hôpital-Général in Paris became home to more than 6000 people – approximately one per cent of the French population – and just twenty years later, a royal edict decreed that an institution of the sort established in Paris should be built in every city of the Kingdom (Foucault, 1967, p. 54). The rate at which the mad were confined within these institutions differed across most European nations. Britain appears to have followed the trend in Paris. In 1651, the Navigation Act was passed in Britain signaling the formal beginning of a movement which would utilize every member of the 'abnormal' population as part of the broader workforce (Foucault, 1967, p. 67). The structures that formerly housed the lepers became sites for the confinement of vagrants, homeless, gypsies, prostitutes, and the mentally ill.

The process of placing the "abnormal" within structures that had previously been utilized for the leper marks the emergence of two primary mental health narratives, which have contributed to the social construction of mental illness and characterized its history. These narratives are "confinement" and "individual responsibility". Foucault (1967, p. 118) described the practice of confinement as having two important consequences. First, by locking away the debauched, the venereal, the alchemists, the libertines, witches, vagrants, the homeless, the idle, prostitutes, and the insane, the outcome was that all came to be considered as one "undifferentiated mass". Particularly for the mad, European society began to distinguish the mentally ill less clearly, with the "slightly deranged" and the "crazed lunatic" sharing the same label, and subsequently, the same stigma. This is not unlike twenty-first century western countries treating someone diagnosed with paranoid schizophrenia the same as someone diagnosed with an anxiety disorder. The second consequence was that in the depths of these European asylums, madness found its place in opposition to reason and progress. Foucault (1967, p. 28) describes the relationship that developed.

Madness becomes a form related to reason, or more precisely madness and reason enter into a perpetually reversible relationship which implies that all madness has its own reason by which it is judged and mastered, and all reason has its madness in which it finds its own derisory truth. Each is a measure of the other, and in this movement of reciprocal reference, each rejects the other but is logically dependent upon it.

Within the four walls of these institutions, society's so called abnormal became one undifferentiated mass, and this mass was portrayed as opposing reason and progress. Outside lay progress and inside, its threat. As late as 1815, Bethlem Hospital in London showed its insane every Sunday for one penny, with the institution accruing an annual revenue of almost 400 pounds from 96,000 visitors who came to see the mad each year (Foucault, 1967, p. 143). This figure is the equivalent today of a little more than US$44,000. The portrayal of madness as a social spectacle and public scandal emphasizes the place of the mad in the consciousness of European populations. They were the abnormal other, not unlike the lepers centuries before, and it is important to consider this history when evaluating present day attitudes towards the mentally ill.

The second narrative – individual responsibility – is one with firm historical roots cultivated and fostered throughout the seventeenth and eighteenth centuries. The earliest depictions of mental illness, dating back to 650BC, locate madness in the context of an inner devil (Porter, 2002). The seeds of modern Western medicine saw mental illness as originating from an imbalance in the body's basic fluids and juices; or "humours" as they were called (Porter, 2002, p. 37). For a long time, at least until the beginning of the seventeenth century, many behaviours considered mad "remained fixed within the tradition of these four humours", or more pointedly, within the individual (Foucault, 1967, p. 113). Early Greek attitudes towards madness found their place within the tragedy of literary figure *Oedipus*, while Shakespeare transposed his understanding into *King Lear*. In each of these works, madness is depicted as a self-created affliction, which, through introspection of the self, forms a potential road to self-discovery. In both cases, the disease is described as a problem for the individual. Society is an audience.

While the Christian view held reason and sanity were found walking in harmony with God, most early analyses of the origination of madness came from the Socratic belief that self-control held the key to one's living conditions. If one could summon free will and base one's actions on it, then madness could be abated. Western culture, according to Foucault (1967, p. 54), saw madness as "the weakening of discipline and the relaxation of morals", an overflowing measure of uncontrolled passion within the individual. Foucault (1967, p. 228) contends that this belief was pervasive among European populations during the seventeenth century.

The possibility of madness is offered in the very fact of passion. It is true that since long before the classical age, and for a series of centuries that has probably not yet come to an end, passion and madness have been kept in close proximity.

The belief that individuals were responsible for their own mental health continued throughout the nineteenth century. Edgar Sheppard (1872) was the Professor of Psychological Medicine at Kings College in London, and in 1872 he wrote that the majority of those he would describe as insane "have made themselves what they are by their own vice and wickedness". We can assume that the views of professionals during and before this time were reflected in the attitudes and perceptions of society as a whole. As Erica Bates (1977) explains, knowledge on the issue of mental health is a two-way process whereby "popular beliefs influence professional thinking, and professional thinking modifies popular beliefs". It is worth considering the extent to which these two narratives persist in the twenty-first century.

Critiques of Foucault's *History of Madness*

Five decades following the publication of Foucault's (1967) *History of Madness*, the French historian's central thesis regarding the confinement of the mentally ill is still subject to critique, revision, and interpretation. As this chapter draws heavily on Foucault's narrative history, it is important to offer a short analysis of his critics' primary appraisals.

The most common critique of Foucault's history is that it is too simplistic and that his account of the confinement of the mentally ill is grossly over-generalized. Yannick Ripa (1990) agrees that madness is a social construction, one that can be interpreted as a product of changing social norms, but believes that his history neglected a "more intimate and fastidious examination of particular [social] groups" that were confined, in particular, to women. According to Ripa (1990), institutionalisation was the ultimate form of feminine repression at a time when women were being held to an absurd expectation of morality, one to which men were immune. Indeed, in his summary of the confinement of the idle, the vagrants, the homeless, and the mentally ill, Foucault (1967) makes little mention of the female asylum experience. There is very little debate on whether the movement to confine the "abnormal" took place, with Lawrence Stone (1982) describing it as "undeniable". But Midelfort (1992) and Porter (2002) both contend that Foucault misread the motivation behind society's institutionalisation of the mad. Porter (2002, p. 95) argues that the rise of the asylum was not an act of state, but a "side effect of commercial and professional society". As the affluent accrued more medical services that had previously been offered in the home, madhouse keepers were in the business of persuading the public that services in the asylum were therapeutic. By 1800, the confined mad in England were largely housed in private asylums. Midelfort (1992, p. 36) extends this argument, stating that the great confinement was aimed "not at madness or even deviance, but at poverty", and instead of a deliberate attempt to segregate the mad, the poor of every kind were locked away.

These critiques suggest that Foucault generalized French confinement and overlooked the unique characteristics of the movement in France's neighbouring countries, yet Foucault's legacy is in his depiction of confinement as a retrogressive step by which the mentally ill became one solid mass, within which variation would go undetected. Andrew Scull's (2015) account of the segregation of the mad offers support for that presented by Michel Foucault in his own description of the history of madness. Scull's (2015, p. 190) account reinforces the importance of the asylum in the history of mental illness, stating that the "presumed need to segregate the mad … remained so notable a feature of the Western response to mental disorder until the last decades of the twentieth century". Scull described this movement to confine and segregate the mad as "a new geography of suffering", and the asylum became the "chosen solution" to the broad set of problems posed by this deviant group (p. 190). As was documented by Michel Foucault (1967), Roy Porter (2002), and Elaine Showalter (1985), conditions in these institutions were as horrendous as those experienced by animals housed in factory farms in the twenty-first century. The following account from French physician Jean-Etienne Dominique Esquirol, who lived from 1772 until 1840, documents the conditions "inmates" encountered inside these institutions.

I have seen them [the mad] naked, clad in rags, having but straw to shield them from the cold humidity of the pavement where they lie. I have seen them coarsely fed, lacking air to breathe, water to quench their thirst, wanting the basic necessities of life. I have seen them at the mercy of veritable jailers, victims of their brutal supervision. I have seen them in narrow, dirty, infested dungeons without air or light, chained in caverns, where one would fear to lock up the wild beasts that luxury-loving governments keep at great expense in their capitals.

Scull (2015) argues that across England, Europe, and North America, it was not uncommon to find in those institutions that specialised in the confinement of the mad, infestations of fleas and rats. Beating and whipping were commonly employed as means for enabling greater control of "inmates", and Scull notes that "female patients were frequently raped" (Scull, 2015, p. 191). The presence of naked women "chained haphazardly to the walls" in these institutions was common, and this treatment was the same for men. At the York Asylum in England, Scull (2015) reports that conditions were the very worst, as filth and neglect were combined with the frequent rape and murder of patients.

By 1860, the asylum revolution was essentially complete. Countries sought to replicate the Western institutional model which began in France, where in 1838 the National Assembly "passed a law directing every department in the country to build an asylum at public expense to house the insane" (Scull, 2015, p. 192). The same took place in England in 1845, while Tsarist Russia embraced the asylum once the Crimean War ended in 1856. Scull (2015) notes that Britain's settler colonies, notably Australia, built their own institutions rapidly and modeled them on those established in Britain. Australia's "inmates", by contrast with those in Europe and England, were mostly men, and many were violent. Even China and Japan would adopt the Western asylum model roughly one century after Europe and North America. An American missionary named John Kerr opened China's first asylum in 1898, in what is now known as Guangzhou. Japan passed the Mental Hospitals Act in 1919. Argentina eventually yielded to the status quo, as supporters of the asylum regime argued that these institutions were the mark of a "civilized society" (Scull, 2015, p. 200). It appears that when confronted with the problem of mental disorder, and the mad, countries looked instinctively to the asylum instead of old modes of family care, and it was a collective movement that fueled the "Great Confinement" Foucault described.

The institutions described by both Foucault (1967) and Scull (2015) developed from madhouses into asylums, where care and proper treatment became paramount. Scull (2015, p. 206) noted that "just as reformed asylums run on moral treatment principles were nothing like the madhouses … so too the new generation of superintendents were necessarily quite unlike their predecessors". He explains that at the

York Retreat, established by William Tuke in 1792, all forms of physical violence and coercion were forbidden, and chains were dispensed with. This new approach, replicated in all asylums scattered across Western nations, transformed the asylum system into a "moral machine", that Scull and Foucault both argue was no less confining and no more liberating than the conditions characteristic of the madhouse.

Whether or not the motivation of confinement was to round up the mad or the poor is largely irrelevant because too much evidence exists to support the locking away of the mad as part of a broader group that threatened progress and reason. Inheriting the stigma and abnormality that had long been associated with the lepers, even the slightly deranged became synonymous with the dangerous lunatic. The mad were considered as one. Foucault might not have, as Lawrence Stone (1982, p. 26) puts it, "got his history right" in accordance with a strict adherence to facts and moments, but his depiction of the movement of confinement and its transition in varying forms into the twentieth century has been replicated by others of that time and has been undeniably powerful.

What is certainly clear is that Foucault did fail to account for the large number of asylum "inmates" who were women. Elaine Showalter (1985) explains that while Foucault's description of the repressive ideologies of confinement was "brilliantly exposed", he did not explore the possibility that the irrationality and abnormality that the asylum sought to confine was also the feminine (p. 6). It is worth noting that this critique mirrors the views of Midelfort (1992) and Porter (2002). Where these scholars argued that Foucault misread the motivation behind the "great confinement", pinning it on madness instead of poverty, Showalter argues for a similar misinterpretation. Showalter's work, entitled *The Female Malady*, demonstrated how cultural ideas about "proper" feminine behaviour have shaped the definition of female insanity for nearly two centuries, giving mental disorder in women a gender-specific connotation, one which eludes the sick man. Women's madness has historically been tied to the female body, with sickness derived from any one of an unfettered female sexuality that disturbs and threatens the intelligent man (Ussher, 1991); the reproductive functions of menstruation, pregnancy, and menopause; or even a simple tendency towards strong emotion (Russell, 1995). This is significant because if women's madness comes to be associated with the female body, and this is replicated historically, this link presents female suffering as inevitable. On this topic, Showalter (1985) states: "[women] are typically situated on the side of irrationality, silence, nature, and body, while men are situated on the side of reason, discourse, culture, and mind".

As a consequence of this linking of insanity with femininity, society came to seek the same symptoms in the male (Showalter, 1985; Wright & Owen, 2001). Since the beginning of the twentieth century, scholars have sought to revise this association, citing male representations of madness through literature and art which are equally powerful in comparison with the feminine images of suicidal Ophelia, crazy Jane and violent Lucia. Elaine Showalter describes in *The Female Malady* the three major Romantic images of female insanity – suicidal Ophelia, crazy Jane, and violent Lucia. She argues that all three were constructed to establish female sexuality as the primary source of madness. Wright and Owen (2001) state that "images such as the mad genius and the criminal lunatic portray men's madness as a 'malfunction' of masculine rather than feminine traits", suggesting that there has been movement beyond madness as being linked entirely with the female body (p. 145).

That Foucault overlooked the oppression of women within the asylum regime is certainly a shortcoming of his narrative history. But the purpose of his work and its resulting legacy still has important implications. Whether or not the movement to confine those perceived as threatening European reason and progress was aimed at the poor, the feminine, the mad, or all three, is largely irrelevant. The legacy of Foucault's work is in confinement as a deliberate system of control, and that the mentally ill were one part of a large, undifferentiated mass that fell under this oppressive system. This was not a new form of control, as even the institutions used to confine this mass had once been saved for the lepers. And similarly, even after these asylums and the institutions known as madhouses had closed, our modern world has sought new ways to control and confine those who appear as abnormal, undesirable, or threatening. Sometimes this confinement is physical, sometimes more subtle, as is the case through the use of language.

Mad, Bad or Sick

Early asylums across Europe, Great Britain, and North America came in "all shapes and sizes", and according to Porter (2002), many were atrociously run given medical supervision was not a legal requirement until well into the nineteenth century (p. 97). Treatments were basic and mostly ineffective, as was the case with either hot drinks or ice-cold baths that Foucault (1967) describes were a means to return the human flesh to its "natural suppleness" (p. 316).

In the cold shower proper, "the lunatic was tied to a chair and placed under a reservoir filled with cold water, which poured down directly onto his head through a wide pipe". The variant was the surprise bath where "the patient was … tipped backwards into the water". This violence promised the rebirth of a baptism (Foucault, 1967, p. 317).

In the years preceding the seventeenth century, the mad who were placed on foreign-bound boats searched for their reason out on the high seas. Even throughout the eighteenth century, Foucault's quote illustrates how this image persisted, as water remained the dominant purifying method for the treatment of madness. Yet among this prolonged ill-treatment were periods of progress where compassionate ideals were adopted. These began most clearly in 1794 when Philippe Pinel liberated the mad in chains at Bicêtre, an asylum in the south of Paris. It was Pinel who would pioneer moral therapy in revolutionary France, promoting more compassionate ideals that were to be mirrored by physician William Tuke in England (Porter, 2002, p. 106).

Despite the rapid increase in the number and scale of mental hospitals throughout Europe in the nineteenth century, reforms were introduced that minimized restraint and delivered some freedom back to the insane. Roy Porter describes the rate at which non-restraint methods were adopted at the Lincoln Asylum in London. Between the years 1829 and 1838, the total number of patients restrained went from 39 to 0; the total number of instances of restraint went from 1727 to 0; and the total number of hours passed under restraint declined from 29424 to 0 (Porter, 2002, p. 115). This example serves to illustrate the power of human beings to construct the lived experience of mental illness. In the short span of nine years, the asylum experience had changed dramatically, transforming from a life characterised by restraint to one with the possibility of autonomy and freedom. Discarding methods of restraint, the mad were treated with greater levels of compassion throughout the nineteenth century, contributing to a process whereby madness would transition from "badness" to "sickness".

For present day understandings of attitudes towards mental illness, the asylums of Europe, Great Britain and North America would develop into locations and structures for the delivery of psychological treatments, largely on the back of the pioneering work of William Tuke and Philippe Pinel. It was these individuals who devised the first true methods of psychological treatment, ones that would form a platform for the work of Sigmund Freud. It is at this point in the history of unreason that the story of confinement takes a subtle turn. The following section depicts the psychiatric relationship as a modern means of confining the mad.

The Legacy of Sigmund Freud

The practice of confining the mad within asylums has formed one part of a broader narrative that has defined, and continues to define, the history of mental illness. As has been established in this chapter, western civilization has used this method for over three centuries, and has done so in both subtle and overt ways. In simplistic terms, the sixteenth century saw the mentally ill placed on boats, taken to foreign locations and dumped there. In the seventeenth and eighteenth centuries, western nations found convenience in segregating the mentally ill within workhouses, a system of confinement that would continue in varying forms until asylums were closed in the 1980s (Barham, 1992). In the nineteenth and twentieth centuries, following the pioneering treatments of William Tuke and Philippe Pinel, the expression and treatment of mental illness were confined within the institution of the psychiatric relationship. In proceeding with this chapter's account of the history of unreason, I argue that Sigmund Freud played a central role in connecting the physical confinement of the seventeenth century with the more subtle segregation of the twenty-first. In this section, I detail the legacy of Freud and place particular emphasis on his role in the birth of modern medicalization.

Born in 1856, Sigmund Freud came to prominence at a time when the legacy and effects of confinement had become two-fold. First, madness had become entwined with unreason. Both metaphorically and physically, the mad posed a threat to enlightened thought and progress, and so justified 'normal' society's sequestering of this group within asylums (Foucault, 1967). Second, within confinement the mad became one undifferentiated mass, with individual insanity distinguished less clearly. It is only with the value of hindsight that one is able to assess the relevance of these consequences for the development of Freud's work. Yet it is clear that these two effects formed a platform from which he could develop his psychoanalytic approach. The mad were guilty of unreason, and so required a treatment that could deliver them back to normality. And with the mad as one unbroken mass, theories and hypotheses could be freely developed for a group that was, during the eighteenth and nineteenth centuries, relatively static. If the mad were not this solid body of despair, threatening civilized society, they would have been too fragmented and fluid for the development of a large-scale therapeutic technique. Ironically, Sigmund Freud could thank confinement for ensuring the inception and ongoing relevance of his talking cure throughout the twentieth century.

Following the publication of his first major thesis, *The Interpretation of Dreams*, Freud began to develop and outline the fundamental tenets of his psychoanalytic approach, a set of theories that would become the dominant therapeutic method of the first half of the twentieth century (Porter, 2002). His work on the unconscious, the symbolic meaning of dreams, hysterical symptoms and infantile sexuality laid the foundations for the work of other prominent European psychologists, notably, Eugen Bleuler (1857-1939), Carl Jung (1875-1961), Pierre Janet (1859-1947), and Alfred Adler (1870-1937). Roy Porter argues that each would extend and reshape Freud's theories.

While asylums were still prominent well into the twentieth century, Freud's work allowed for the flourishing of a more subtle method of control, namely, "the doctor-patient relationship". As Michel Foucault explains, Freud's most powerful legacy was in opening up the possibility of a dialogue between madness and medical thought, and so bringing mental illness back in tandem with unreason (Foucault, 1967, p. 339). He argues that Darwinian-based positivism had reduced the experience of madness to silence because it locked it away inside the walls of the asylum and within the confines of incurability. The development of a therapeutic technique prefaced on conversation reopened the gateway between reason and madness, with the consequence that it concentrated the treatment of mental illness within the doctor-patient relationship, laying the foundations for twenty-first century medicalization.

This transformation was mostly subtle. Freud did not change the nature of the structures put in place by his predecessors, he simply moved them from the madhouses into the psychoanalytic situation. He did not change the nature of madness, but altered its location and so forced others to see it in a new light.

Freud made sure all the structures integrated by Pinel and Tuke into confinement were appropriated by the doctor. He freed the patient from that asylum experience ... but he failed to spare him the essential components of that existence. He concentrated its powers ... and placed them in the hands of the doctor. He created the psychoanalytic situation, where ... alienation became disalienating because, in the doctor, it became a subject (Foucault, 1967, p. 511).

The doctor came to be seen as the sole means by which a patient could be delivered from their suffering, as madness was now a subject for the doctor to decipher. This is a transition of power that remains to this day. Considering the development of this doctor-patient relationship with the growth of medicalization following the second World War (Conrad, 2007), and one would suggest that confinement did not end with the liberation of the mad in chains at Bicêtre, or the birth of psychoanalysis. Rather, the walls remained, but they became invisible.

Medicalization

Medicalization is the process of taking non-medical problems and reframing them as issues that require medical attention (Conrad & Schneider, 1992). It is not the direct work of Sigmund Freud, but there is little doubt that medicalization has benefited greatly from the platform of the doctor-patient relationship, without which its ability to expand in both breadth and scope would be greatly diminished. Medicalization is an important figure in the history of madness for two reasons. First, it represents a continuation of the confinement narrative, albeit in a more subtle form. Second, it is a social process that supports the constructionist view of health and illness, explored in the early stages of this chapter. Peter Conrad (2007) offers a suggestion for how mental health can be understood as socially constructed through a description of medicalization's bidirectional nature.

Medicalization is bidirectional, in the sense that there can be both medicalization and demedicalization ... For demedicalization to occur, the problem must no longer be defined in medical terms, and medical treatments can no longer be deemed appropriate interventions. A classic example is masturbation, which in the nineteenth century was considered a disease and worthy of medical intervention (Conrad, 2007, p. 7).

Conrad's thesis on the medicalization of society focuses on balding, erectile dysfunction and adult ADHD as more recent examples of non-medical problems that have been defined and treated under the umbrella of the medical model. This medical imperialism has been aided by major pharmaceutical companies and their development of medication designed to treat what Conrad (2007) argues are not illnesses, but "life problems" (p. 61). These developments became most evident in the second half of the twentieth century.

The introduction of penicillin in the 1940s and chlorpromazine in 1954 became precursors to the pharmacological revolution (Barham, 1992). Chlorpromazine was the first antipsychotic drug designed for the treatment of mental illness, and significantly changed the way the insane were treated in asylums during the twentieth century (Barham, 1992, p. 6). Elizabeth Bott (1976) explains that medication was useful in British institutions because it solidified the distance thought necessary between the insane and their carers. She states that "talking to patients is dangerous because it threatens to puncture the barrier that keeps sanity and madness in their proper places" (Bott, 1976, p. 133). The use of medication to confine and control, evident in Bott's description, represents an overlap in the confinement narrative. While the confinement of the psychiatric institution faced imminent closure towards the end of the twentieth century, the confining effects of medication and its inherent linking with the doctor-patient relationship were rapidly developing in its stead. Barham (1992) argues therefore that the legacy of the asylum is the "abolition of the *person* who suffers from mental illness", replaced by the mental patient, identity permanently spoiled, exiled on the margins of society (p. xi).

In 1987, Prozac was first introduced as a new type of medication to treat depression. Conrad and Schneider (1992) argue that the introduction of Prozac was important because while the 1980s saw the widespread closing of asylums and the end of physical confinement for those defined as needing treatment for mental illness across western countries, the mentally ill would find a new segregation within the doctor-patient relationship, the site at which they remain dependent for their antidepressant and antipsychotic medication. The uptake of prescription medication has been rapid and unrelenting. Between 1990 and 2007, there has been a 2.5-fold increase in the number of visits to a doctor in the United States that resulted in a prescription for a psychotropic medicine, suggesting that "problems that a decade or two ago would not have been deemed appropriate for medication are now managed with psychotropics" (Conrad, 2007, p. 129). Between 2011 and 2012, there were over 23 million prescriptions written for mental health medication alone (DoHA, 2012). According to Conrad, medicalization holds biological factors accountable, and it is here that prescription medication and the physician who prescribes them, present themselves as necessary for complete recovery. In describing the patterns of use for mental health medications in Australia, the Australian Bureau of Statistics (1995) reports:

Almost everyone who used ... anti-depressants did so on the advice of a health professional, mostly a General Practitioner or medical specialist ... Nearly all people who used medications in these groups obtained them either by prescription of from a doctor or a hospital. Patterns of use differed by the types of medications used ... of people who used antidepressants, 94% used them regularly and 91% used them daily. Of people who used antipsychotics, 90% used them regularly and 87% used them daily (ABS, 1995).

Peter Barham argues that this dependency on medication has been one of the major consequences of the closing of asylums in the 1980s. He also believes that it propelled the process of deinstitutionalization forward, arguing that multiple factors originating from the middle of the twentieth century combined to reinforce a focus on deinstitutionalization, namely, "the literature of protest against the indignities of the mental hospital regimes on the one hand, and the new-found psychiatric optimism about the major tranquilizers on the other" (Barham, 1992, p. 12). With inadequate community-based support set up to meet treatment and care needs, the mentally ill were discharged and expected to re-join the broader community outside the mental hospital seamlessly. Evidence suggests that doctors were the most vocal enthusiasts for community-care policies, based on their belief in the effectiveness of new drug treatments. Community care facilities were envisaged as a stepping-stone between a brief stay in a mental hospital and complete reintegration back into society (Barham, 1992, p. 12), and so it appears there was a discrepancy between the commitment to scale down mental institutions and the establishment of alternative forms of service. As a consequence, a vast majority of the mentally ill found new forms of confinement within prisons, on the streets as the homeless, and finally, through the confinement of the doctor-patient relationship, an institution that began with the work of Sigmund Freud at the beginning of the twentieth century. In the final section of this chapter, I shift the focus more locally, outlining how twenty-first century confinement is taking place in Australia.

AUSTRALIA

Australia's mental health history mirrors that which has been described throughout this chapter for seventeenth-century Europe, blended with some characteristics unique to Australia's rich Indigenous culture (Martyr, 2010). Brenda Happell (2007) reflects that in the 1800s, Australia's approach followed the British model, tending to "reflect the views of medical superintendents who migrated to the colonies to oversee the asylums" (p. 1440). By the year 1811, at the Castle Hill Lunatic Asylum in New South Wales, mental illness was still referred to as "madness", and its origins remained the product of "bad blood" or character flaws, as opposed to illness (Happell, 2007). This suggests that the "individual responsibility" narrative introduced in part two of this chapter was transposed from the British context into Australia. The mad were managed through methods of physical restraint and isolation, and there appears no evidence of mental treatment, with a far greater emphasis placed on the custodial role (Keane, 1987). The treatment of supposed mentally ill Indigenous Australians between 1870 and 1914 has emerged as a unique characteristic of Australia's mental health history also. Philippa Martyr found that between 1870 and 1914, a total of 30 Indigenous Australians, mostly from Western Australia, were charged and/or diagnosed with lunacy. The incarceration that followed forms part of White Australia's mistreatment of Aboriginal Australians following colonisation. Yet as the moral therapy pioneered by Tuke and Pinel signaled the transformation of European attitudes towards mental ill-health, Australia's approach began to consider mental illness less as a moral failing and more as an issue requiring behavioural treatment and change (Happell, 2007).

In line with broader changes occurring in most western countries at the time, mental illness was shifting from "badness" to "sickness". In 1867, an Act of Parliament ensured that the mentally ill were sent to asylums rather than prisons, and by the middle of the nineteenth century, mental patients were being transferred from jails to newly opened asylums in all major Australian cities (Happell, 2007). Responsibility for mental illness was becoming less individual and more societal. In 1955, the Stoller Report became the first document to outline the consequences of social indifference towards public mental health services, and the effect this lack of attention could have on the mentally ill (Bates, 1977). Erica Bates (1977) described the report as "the first public recognition that the problem of mental illness is a general problem, and not one to be blamed on the individual" (p. 20). The Stoller Report proved prophetic. Following deinstitutionalization, Australia's mental health approach accelerated towards community-based care, ensuring the responsibility for mental illness came to rest on society more broadly. How effective this process has been for the treatment of the mentally ill is debatable, yet community mental health organisations naturally increased in prominence as a result of this trend, with *Reach Out* founded in 1996, *beyondblue* in October 2000, and *Black Dog* in 2002.

Despite this increase in community-based care practices, western medicalization continues its rapid expansion, of what has been described in this chapter as a modern form of mental health confinement. This control, enabled through psychiatric diagnosis and psychotropic medication, has been no less pronounced in Australia. Following the publication of the DSM-V in 2013, the Australian Broadcasting Commission (2014) reported that current definitions of mental illness were so broad that "50% of western populations can be diagnosed with a mental disorder". To an extent, this is exactly what is taking place. The prevalence of mental illness in countries like Australia has become a problem taking on epidemic proportions. According to the World Health Organisation (2013), major depression is the most prevalent psychological disorder in the west, affecting approximately 350 million people, and surpassing heart disease as the world's leading cause of disability. This growth is symptomatic of a society seeking to solidify the boundaries between normality and abnormality, reason and unreason. In clarifying this divide, western civilizations have re-enacted an historically effective method of controlling the mentally ill. This method is confinement.

The process of identifying more and more behaviours as symptomatic of mental illness segregates the mentally ill because it concentrates the site at which mental health issues are treated: within the doctor-patient relationship. It also focuses the problem within the individual at the expense of a thorough exploration of broader social causes. From the leprosaria to *The Ship of Fools*, and from the madhouse to the therapeutic relationship, society has developed the "deep disposition to see madness as essentially Other" (Porter, 1987, p. 35). As a consequence, modern society seeks to segregate and control this deviance, and since the closing of asylums in the 1980s, medicalization has been an effective means of enabling this control. Peter Barham suggests that to some extent, the asylum provided a more certain system of care than the one offered today.

It is clear that people with long-term mental illness in the community may find themselves as structurally isolated as ever they were in the asylums, and in addition their health needs may now be ignored (Barham, 1992, p. 32).

Within the asylum, the mentally ill were neglected as patients. Released into the community, they are now neglected as both patients and citizens, in equal measure. In this way, Western society has developed a subtle continuation of seventeenth century European confinement, representative of a powerful arm in the social construction of mental illness.

CONCLUSION

This chapter charted the history of mental illness as a means for illustrating how it can be understood as socially constructed. Drawing on the work of Roy Porter (2002) and Michel Foucault (1967), we have shown that social norms, attitudes, beliefs, and institutions within which treatments are delivered define the lived experience of mental illness. These phenomena, particularly social institutions, are all dependent on social forces. The individual confined in a Parisian Hôpital-Général in 1656 experienced their illness differently from an American teenager diagnosed with depression in 2018. Their social worlds were different and so also were the understandings of mental illness – madness in the case of the Frenchman – and the treatments they received. The mark of stigma affects the way an individual understands their illness, and we have shown in this chapter that this stigma has distinct historical origins.

Roy Porter's (2002) description of the rate at which non-restraint methods were adopted at the Lincoln Asylum in London between 1829 and 1838 illustrates how quickly human beings can reshape and reconstruct the lived experience of mental illness. The central argument of this chapter is that while methods, treatments, and institutions have changed over time, the purpose of these changes has almost exclusively been to exercise a tighter form of social control. Institutions like the Lincoln Asylum eventually discarded their shackles in the mid-late nineteenth century, but Porter (2002) and Foucault (1967) argue that the institution then became a site for moral segregation, moving mental illness from "badness" to "sickness".

The dominant mental health narratives that characterised this history have been "confinement" and "individual responsibility". While the *Ship of Fools* no longer exists, nor the madhouses that were borne out of what Foucault called "The Great Confinement", we argue that this narrative persists in more subtle forms, namely, through the invisible walls of stigma and medicalization, which continue to frame the mentally ill as a distinct, abnormal "other". An appreciation of this history allows for an acknowledgment of our ability to construct and reconstruct the mental health lived experience.

REFERENCES

American Psychiatric Association. (1952). *Diagnostic and statistical manual of mental disorders* (1st ed.). Washington, DC: APA.

American Psychiatric Association. (1994). *Diagnostic and statistical manual of mental disorders* (4th ed.). Washington, DC: APA.

Aneshensel, C. S., Phelan, J. C., & Bierman, A. (2013). *Handbook of the sociology of mental health.* New York: Columbia University. doi:10.1007/978-94-007-4276-5

Australian Broadcasting Commission. (2014). Mental illness – a history. *Rear vision.* Available at http://www.abc.net.au/radionational/programs/rearvision/mental-illness---a-history/5611268

Australian Bureau of Statistics. (1995). *National health survey: use of medications, Australia, 1995. cat No. 4377.0.* Canberra: ABS.

Barham, P. (1992). *Closing the asylum: the mental patient in modern society.* London: Penguin.

Barnes, B. (1977). *Interests and growth of knowledge.* London: Routledge and Kegan Paul.

Bastien, J. (1992). *Drum & stethoscope.* Salt Lake City, UT: University of Utah Press.

Bates, E. M. (1977). *Models of madness.* St Lucia: University of Queensland Press.

Bott, E. (1976). Hospital and society. *The British Journal of Medical Psychology, 49*(2), 97–140. doi:10.1111/j.2044-8341.1976.tb02357.x PMID:821510

Bury, M. R. (1986). Social constructionism and the development of medical sociology. *Sociology of Health & Illness, 8*(2), 137–169. doi:10.1111/1467-9566.ep11340129

Conrad, P. (2007). *The medicalization of society: on the transformation of human conditions into treatable disorders.* Baltimore, MD: The John Hopkins University Press.

Conrad, P., & Schneider, J. W. (1992). *Deviance and medicalization: from badness to sickness.* Philadelphia: Temple University Press.

Cooper, N., Stevenson, C., & Hale, G. (1996). *Integrating perspectives on health*. Buckingham, UK: Open University Press.

Department of Health Australia. (2012). *Australian statistics on medicines 2010*. Canberra: Commonwealth of Australia.

Engel, G. L. (1977). The need for a new medical model: A challenge for biomedicine. *Science*, *8*(4286), 129–136. doi:10.1126cience.847460 PMID:847460

Foucault, M. (1967). *Madness and civilization*. London: Routledge.

Goffman, E. (1959). *The presentation of self in everyday life*. London: Penguin.

Goffman, E. (1963). *Stigma: notes on the management of spoiled identity*. New York: Touchstone.

Greene, S. (1998). The shaman's needle: Development, shamanic agency, and intermedicality in Aguarana Lands, Peru. *American Ethnologist*, *25*(4), 634–658. doi:10.1525/ae.1998.25.4.634

Greider, T., & Garkovich, L. (1994). Landscapes: The social construction of nature and the environment. *Rural Sociology*, *59*(2), 1–24.

Happell, B. (2007). Appreciating the importance of history: A brief historical overview of mental health, mental health nursing and education in Australia. *The International Journal of Psychiatric Nursing Research*, *12*(2), 1439–1445. PMID:17283958

Harris, K. M., & Edlund, M. J. (2005). Self-medication of mental health problems: New evidence from a national survey. *Health Services Research*, *40*(1), 117–134. doi:10.1111/j.1475-6773.2005.00345.x PMID:15663705

Hepworth, J. (1999). *The social construction of anorexia nervosa*. London: Sage Publications.

Kalanithi, P. (2017). *When breath becomes air*. London: Penguin Random House.

Keane, B. (1987). *Study of mental health nursing in Australia. Commonwealth department of Australia*. Canberra: Australian Government Printing Service.

Latour, B., & Woolgar, S. (1979). *Laboratory life: the social construction of scientific facts*. Princeton University Press.

Martyr, P. (2010). Behaving wildly: Diagnoses of lunacy among Indigenous persons in western Australia, 1870-1914. *Social History of Medicine*, *24*(2), 316–333. doi:10.1093hm/hkq046

Mehl, L. E. (1988). Modern shamanism: integration of biomedicine with traditional world views. In Shaman's path (pp. 127-138). Boston: Shambhala.

Midelfort, H. C. E. (1992). *Madness and civilization in early modern Europe: a reappraisal of Michel Foucault. In Critical thought series: 2, critical essays on Michel Foucault*. Scolar Press.

Porter, R. (1987). *A social history of madness: stories of the insane*. London: Phoenix Giants.

Porter, R. (2002). *Madness: a brief history*. New York: Oxford University Press.

Ripa, Y. (1990). *Women and madness: the incarceration of women in nineteenth century France*. Cambridge, UK: Polity Press.

Russell, D. (1995). *Women, madness & medicine*. Cambridge, UK: Polity Press.

Scull, A. (2015). *Madness in civilization: a cultural history of insanity, from the bible to Freud, from the madhouse to modern medicine*. Princeton University Press. doi:10.1515/9781400865710

Shapin, S. (1982). History of science and its sociological reconstructions. *History of Science*, *20*(3), 157–211. doi:10.1177/007327538202000301

Sheppard, E. (1872). On some of the teachings of insanity. *The Journal of Mental Science*, *17*(80), 499–514. doi:10.1192/bjp.17.80.499

Showalter, E. (1985). *The female malady: women, madness, and English culture, 1830-1980*. London: Virago.

Stone, L. (1982). *Madness. In Critical thought series: 2, critical essays on Michel Foucault*. Scolar Press.

Szasz, T. (2007). *The medicalization of everyday life: selected essays*. New York: Syracuse University Press.

Ussher, J. (1991). *Women's madness: misogyny or mental illness?* Boston: University of Massachusetts Press.

World Health Organisation. (2013). *Depression: factsheet no. 369*. Available at http://www.who.int/medicalcentre/factsheets/fs369/en/index.html

Wreford, J. (2005). Missing each other: Problems and potential for collaborative efforts between biomedicine and traditional healers in South Africa in the time of AIDS. *Social Dynamics*, *31*(2), 55–89. doi:10.1080/02533950508628708

Wright, N., & Owen, S. (2001). Feminist conceptualizations of women's madness: A review of the literature. *Journal of Advanced Nursing*, *36*(1), 143–150. doi:10.1046/j.1365-2648.2001.01951.x PMID:11555058

Chapter 2
Risk:
What Is It, Whom Does It Protect, and What Happened to Care?

Kellie Grant
Monash University, Australia

Jenny Martin
Swinburne University, Australia

Jenni White
Monash University, Australia

Terry Haines
Monash University, Australia

ABSTRACT

Risk assessment and management are considered core elements of healthcare practice. However, a brief examination of the theoretical literature on risk demonstrates that it is not a fixed concept. This chapter will critically analyze the impact that focusing on risk has on healthcare practice. The authors will join many others in pointing out the many potential negative impacts of viewing healthcare through the lens of risk. One risk type, suicide risk, will be examined closely. It will be shown that health professionals often fear liability when risk is a factor. In order to dissuade these fears, the legal elements of liability will be outlined, and relevant common law judgements will be discussed. Finally, future directions will be discussed.

INTRODUCTION

The assessment and management of risk are now considered to be crucial elements of health care practice, in Australia and internationally (Clancy & Happell, 2014; Hillman, Tadd, Calnan, Calnan, Bayer, & Read, 2013; Lane & Reiger, 2013). Across a variety of practice contexts, health professionals encounter

DOI: 10.4018/978-1-5225-7402-6.ch002

the notion of risk on a daily basis. Risk is embedded throughout all tiers of health organisations: Directors, managers, and clinicians alike all have risk management responsibilities.

Risk is so deeply embedded in health services that it can be difficult to imagine a system which is not, in some way, ordered around this concept. This has not always been the case. Danger and uncertainty have always been facts of life. The concept of "risk", on the other hand, has gained increasing prominence over the past several decades. Several authors (Clancy & Happell, 2014; Horlick-Jones, 2005a; Lane & Reiger, 2013) have documented this rise in the focus on risk, including Eagleton-Pierce (2016), who discussed "problems which are now called risks" (p.164). Similarly, Beck (1992) referred to "(r) isks, as opposed to older dangers" (p.21). The increasing focus on risk in health care does not reflect that patients are exposed to greater dangers compared with a prerisk era. To the contrary, advances in health care mean that it is constantly becoming safer for people to access treatment. Risk is simply a new way of relating to the age-old reality that many aspects of life (health care included) contain dangers, uncertainties, problems or contingencies.

This chapter will begin by exploring theoretical approaches to risk. It will show that risk is an ambiguous concept, as it takes on different meanings in different disciplines. Risk will then be examined linguistically by discussing the many different uses of this term in health care. This will further trouble the concept of risk, by demonstrating that risk is often morally loaded and contingent on an unspoken norm. Subsequently, the chapter will examine the impact of risk on health care practice. As a case study of a risk type, suicide risk will be explored in depth. This will illustrate the many potential negative impacts of ordering health care around the paradigm of risk. One such impact is that risk can lead clinicians to focus on liability. The chapter will examine the legal requirements of liability. Relevant common law judgements of negligence claims will be explored, to demonstrate that negligence claims often favour health services and practitioners (Popa, 2017). Having outlined the many potential issues of a risk focus in health care, the chapter will discuss future directions.

Risk Is Important, but What Is It?

Risk takes on different meanings, depending on the lens through which it is viewed. Although exceptions occur, approaches to theorising risk can be broadly grouped into three categories: Sociological, economic (/"objective" sciences), and psychological. These will be briefly examined, to demonstrate that risk is not a concept with a universally accepted meaning.

THEORETICAL APPROACHES TO RISK

Sociological

In sociology, risk may be understood as both a product and a condition of a collective cultural group. Beck's (1992) idea of "the risk society" is an example of a sociological risk theory. Beck (1992; 2009) theorised that Western societies have become preoccupied with risk in response to new threats produced by globalisation. He posited that the concept of risk has been reinvented through the process of modernisation, to reflect growing dangers in the modern world: Nuclear energy, climate change, the threat of environmental catastrophes (Beck, 1992), and, later, genetic technology, nanotechnology (Beck, 2002), terrorism, and economic collapse (Beck, 2008). Beck understood risk as a socially and culturally contingent phenomena. He asserted that globalisation and modernisation produced objective risks, while simultaneously producing social and cultural conditions which fostered the spread of fear and anxiety concerning these risks (Beck, 1992).

Douglas (1992) proffered another sociological risk theory. She claimed risk is a forensic resource: A conceptual tool produced by a social world that is preoccupied with assigning blame in the event of harm. As Beck, Douglas conceptualised risk as being socially and culturally contingent. Douglas (1990) suggested risk was a discourse that had evolved from prior concepts, such as danger, taboo, or sin. She asserted that being "at risk" has similarities with the earlier concept of being "in sin", the former reflecting a social world oriented towards an epistemology of science, the latter reflecting a religious era (Douglas, 1990). Douglas's (1990) key assertion was that risk is a forensic resource: It's primary purpose being the attribution of blame. Further, she asserted that the language of risk implies that danger is calculable and controllable, with the result being that any event of harm can be seen as a systemic failure. Douglas (1990) stated:

Risk is unequivocally used to mean danger from future damage, caused by the opponents. How much risk is a matter for the experts, but on both sides of the debate it has to be taken for granted that the matter is ascertainable. Anyone who insists that there is a high degree of uncertainty is taken to be opting out of accountability. (p. 9)

In sociology, risk can be understood as a discourse, a social construction, an epistemology, or the consequence of a particular political lens (Beck, 1992; Douglas, 1990). Sociologically, risk is often conceptualised as a complex cultural phenomena.

Economic

These sociological approaches contrast with risk as conceptualised in the "objective" sciences, which often draw on models of risk originally developed in economics. Economic risk theories tend to represent risk as the probability and severity of possible events (Douglas, 1990; Ryan, Nielssen, Paton, & Large, 2010). Utility theory is an example of an economic approach, which represents risk as a mathematical function (Moscati, 2016). In utility theory, risk is conceptualised as the possibility of an event, the likelihood that said event will occur (probability), and the degree of either loss or gain should it occur (severity) (Moscati, 2016).

In economic models, risk can be discussed using mathematical formulas. Utility theory is described by Moscati (2016, p.219) as follows:

(T)he utility of a lottery yielding either a trip to London with probability p or a payment of $2,000 with probability (1 − p) is given by (u(trip to London) × p) + (u($2,000) × (1 − p)). ...(T)he decision maker will choose among these risky prospects...and will choose the one with the highest expected utility.

The change in language that is used when describing risk between sociological and economic models is reflective of the divergent conceptualisations of risk. In economics, risk can be mathematically calculated, and, hence, it may be discussed using a mathematical formula. In sociology, risk is a cultural condition, and it is regarded as not amenable to quantification (Douglas, 1990).

Psychological

Psychological approaches provide yet another conceptualisation of risk. In psychological risk models, emphasis is often placed on the perceiver of risk (Lupton, 2013). Some psychological risk models assert that decision makers will perceive risk based on their emotional states. Therefore, risk is conceptualised as the interaction between an objective threat and an individual's perception of said threat (Chen, 2015). For instance, the affect heuristic model asserts that emotions (affect) provide mental shortcuts (heuristics) which influence decision makers in both their perceptions of risk and their decisions (Chen, 2015; Lupton, 2013). Thus, it suggests that risk is evaluated emotionally, either instead of or in addition to rationally. For example, a person who is experiencing a positive affect may pay more attention to the benefits of a risky decision, leading them towards a risk taking choice, whereas a person experiencing a negative affect may focus more on the risks of the same decision, leading to a decision of risk aversion (Chen, 2015).

Another psychological model, protection motivation theory, asserts that decision makers will act to mitigate a risk (achieve protection) under circumstances where particular motivational elements are satisfied (Rogers, 1975). These are: The presence of fear, a perceived likelihood that the threatening event will occur, and a pathway to mitigate the risk which is perceived as effective. Protection motivation theory is one of many theories on fear appeals, which seek to understand how fear can act as a motivating element to reduce actions that may have aversive results, such as smoking (Rogers, 1975). According to this theory, action to mitigate risk occurs due to the combination of fear, likelihood of harm, and an available option that will effectively achieve protection.

In psychological models, risk may relate to an objective danger, but it is also in the eye of the beholder. Psychological models provide yet another lens through which risk can be understood.

Which Risk Theories Shape Health Care Practice?

Economic conceptualisations of risk exert influence well beyond the field of economics (Horlick-Jones, 2005a). Risk management in health care often involves efforts to quantify danger (Hillman, Tadd, Calnan, Calnan, Bayer, & Read, 2013) or estimate the probability of harm (Clancy & Happell, 2014; De Bortoli, Ogloff, Coles, & Dolan, 2017). This most closely aligns with economic understandings of risk. As psychology is a health discipline, risk models from this field are directly relevant to health care. While psychological models provide their own distinct understanding of risk, the field of psychology has been heavily influenced by economic risk models (Horlick-Jones, 2005a). The psychological and economic models, despite being divergent in many ways, also have many points of alignment. The sociological models, however, understand risk in a way that is quite different to both the economic and psychological models (Lupton, 2013). Sociological models also exert considerable influence in health care. Research exploring risk in health care practice frequently draws on sociological risk models to make sense of the observed risk practices (Clancy & Happell, 2014; Hillman, Tadd, Calnan, Calnan, Bayer, & Read, 2013; Manuel & Crowe, 2014).

Risk: A Nebulous Concept

Risk is widely considered to be an important element of health care practice (Clancy & Happell, 2014; Hillman, Tadd, Calnan, Calnan, Bayer, & Read, 2013; Lane & Reiger, 2013). Despite this, the theoretical literature on risk demonstrates that many competing conceptualisations of risk are at play, all exerting influence in health care. It cannot be assumed that a shared understanding of the term risk exists. The divergent conceptualisations of risk across disciplines is problematic (Horlick-Jones, 2005a; Lupton, 2013). In Victoria, Australia, the management of risk is a requirement for all health services, set by the Victorian State Government (2017). This requirement could be interpreted in entirely different ways, depending on the theoretical lens through which risk is being viewed.

Therefore, what the term risk is used to mean in the context of health care warrants further examination. The following section will examine how the language of risk is used in the health care context. The authors will show that the composition of the risk varies across many of the common uses of the term.

LINGUISTICS OF RISK

Risk as a Status: High Risk, at Risk, Risky

Risk can be a status used to describe an individual or group. In health care, status words, such as "high risk" "at risk" or "risky" tend to be applied to people by their treating professionals (Szmukler & Rose, 2013). As a result, this use of the term (risk) has a static quality: As distinct from people displaying risky behaviours or being risky, in this case, people are risky. Labelling an individual as risky is "to constitute the subjectivity of the person....so that people themselves are characterized as 'high-risk' or 'risky'" (Pollack, 2010, p. 1271). When a risk status has been assigned, harm is a possibility. The harm may be to the holder of the risk status, as is the case with a person who is "at risk" of suicide (Chehil & Kutcher, 2012). Alternatively, harm may be to the community, if a "risky" individual is deemed to be a danger to others (Szmukler & Rose, 2013).

Risk statuses such as "high risk" depend upon the existence of less risky individuals or groups. In this scenario, the term risk is relative, and a risk status will apply to those who "present a risk above a certain threshold" (Szmukler & Rose, 2013, p.131). For an individual to be "high risk", they must be deviating from a less risky norm. The norm, however, is usually not explicitly stated.

As well as being implicitly deviant from the norm, risk as a status is also implicitly negative, resulting in risk status being a state to be fixed. Just as risk status is assigned by professionals, the task of regulating the risky individual and returning them to the norm is also delegated to professionals (Szmukler & Rose, 2013). Risk as a status is assumed to be manageable and the risky person is assumed to not have the capability of managing their own risk (Pollack, 2010). The focus of the at-risk status is largely regulatory. Relative to this, the lived experience of suffering of the risk holder is often not a focus (Lupton, 2013).

Risk as an Action, Taken by Patients: Risky Behaviours, Health Risk Behaviour, High Risk Behaviour, Risk Taking

Risk can also be an action: People can engage in "risky behaviours" and "high-risk behaviours", lead "high-risk lifestyles", or make "risky choices". Risky actions are usually characterised as negative. Self-harm is an example of how actions can be positioned as risky behaviour (Ghafoor, 2008). These actions may be undertaken by persons with a risk status (high risk), or, alternatively, the risk actions may lead a person to be labelled with a risk status. The risk is usually one of harm that may befall the person taking the risky action.

As is the case with risk status, risky actions are dependent on an implicit norm. For example, the norm of nonself-harm is usually not explicitly stated (Ghafoor, 2008), but is implicit in the framing of self-harm as a risky behaviour. Self-harm, in the form of scarification, is a norm in some cultures, where it has cultural significance as a rite of passage or to mark coming of age (Garve, Garve, Türp. Fobil, & Meyer, 2017). Within this context, self-harm would not be understood as a risky behaviour. It is not a potentially dangerous action which constitutes "risk taking", but a potentially dangerous action which deviates from the accepted norm.

The professional regulation of risky behaviours is similar to that of risk status: Risky behaviour is something to be regulated and returned to the norm. Said regulation is implicitly delegated to treating professionals [as seen in strategies for mitigation of self-harm risk discussed by Ghafoor (2008)].

Risk Professionals

"Risk professionals" are those whose role involves assessing and managing risk (Horlick Jones, 2005b). They include health professionals, police, and correctional workers. Their job is "to predict, control and manage the risk of marginalized people who come under their gaze" (Pollack, 2010, p. 1267). The form said harm may take, and to whom the harm may occur, can vary depending on the type of risk professional.

Determining Levels of Risk: Risk Analysis, Risk Calculation, Risk Assessment

Levels of risk may be determined by risk analysis, risk calculation, or risk assessment. In health care, the term risk assessment is typically used. Risk assessment is an action performed by professionals, who use "expert" knowledge to determine the risk status of an individual, based on their individual characteristics (Szmukler & Rose, 2013). Risk assessment is based in the future: It predicts the likelihood of occurrence of future harm (Lupton, 2013). Who may be harmed depends on the type of risk being assessed. It may relate to the risky person being harmed, often by their own actions (Ghafoor, 2008) or it may relate to the risky person harming another person. Risk assessment routinely excludes certain types of harm, such as the risk of coercive or discriminatory treatment of at-risk persons. Risk assessment relates to the possibility of harm, but only specific types of harm: Those which may cause moral outrage in the broader society (Szmukler & Rose, 2013). In risk assessment, risk is understood to be calculable uncertainty, the domain of experts (i.e., a professional action), uncertainty located in the future, and implicitly negative (Lupton, 2013; Szmukler & Rose, 2013) (perhaps due to its function as a way of assigning risk status). Risk assessment includes a regulatory element: Risk is knowable and known risk must be acted upon by professionals (Szmukler & Rose, 2013).

Risk assessment is also a professional risk action.

Professional Risk Actions: Risk Management, Risk Mitigation, Risk Assessment, Risk Aversion

Once risk in a person or population has been detected, risk professionals may employ a range of actions. The responsibility remains with professionals, whether they are engaging in risk aversion or risk management. However, what the risk is of and who the risk may affect varies depending on the action and context. In health care, risk management is a common risk action (Ghafoor, 2008). Risk in risk management has the same composition as risk in risk assessment.

Risk Factors

Risk factors, uncovered by risk assessments, are used to determine risk status. Risk factors are characteristics individual people hold. As they determine risk status, the risk is similar in composition to that of risk status [i.e., implicitly negative, relative to an unspoken norm, relating to risk of harm of a patient or another person (Szmukler & Rose, 2013)]. The risk in risk factors is morally constituted: Risk factors are the types of risk that may cause moral outrage, such as harm resulting from negligence, risks that are do not cause moral outrage, such as restrictive treatment of risky individuals, are not usually described as risk factors (Szmukler & Rose, 2013). Risk factors may be weighed against their positive counterpart: Protective factors.

Risk as a Collective Condition: Risk Culture, Risk Discourse, Risk Regime, Risk Thinking

Risk can also be a collective experience. Organisations may have "risk cultures". Health care, in Australia and internationally, has been termed a "risk regime" (Lane & Reiger, 2013). "Risk discourses" may negatively shape practices of professional groups. These terms tend to be used to critically analyse the perceived societal focus on risk. Risk remains negative in this representation. "Risk thinking" is often framed as a negative practice (Pollack, 2010; Szmukler & Rose, 2013): Risk cultures (example.g., organisations which collectively engage in risk thinking) may also be represented as problematic (KPMG, 2011). When risk is discussed as a collective experience, the danger appears to be the concept of risk itself. The point is not an individual norm to be restored; rather, the implicit danger is the potentially oppressive influence of collective groups that have an overfocus on returning deviant individuals to the norm.

SECTION SUMMARY

Many voices note that an attentiveness to risk is considered an important part of health care practice (Clancy & Happell, 2014; Hillman, Tadd, Calnan, Calnan, Bayer, & Read, 2013; Lane & Reiger, 2013; Victoria State Government, 2017). However, significant uncertainty occurs as to what this important concept of risk actually is. The theoretical literature on risk represents risk in divergent ways. In health care, the word risk comes up in several terms, with varying compositions of the risk. Risk is often negative, relative to an unspoken norm, located in the future, and something to be controlled by professionals. However, this can vary, depending on how the term is used.

Risk is not a fixed or stable concept. Relying on implicit understandings of risk is likely to be problematic. Having deconstructed risk as a concept, the following section will examine the impact a focus on risk may have on health care practice.

RISK IN HEALTH CARE PRACTICE

Key Themes

Risk has a significant influence on the delivery of health services. However, there are widespread concerns that ordering health services around the paradigm of risk is not effective (Clancy & Happell, 2014; Manuel & Crowe, 2014; Wand, 2011; Wand, Isobel, & Derrick, 2015). Amongst these concerns is that risk assessment and risk management suggest that danger is calculable, thus that the future can be predicted and harm prevented with diligent care. Therefore, any adverse event carries the assumption that it has arisen from an error in the administration of care (Szmukler & Rose, 2013).

When risk is a factor, health professionals tend to focus on potential blame (Andersson & Liff 2012; Hillman, Tadd, Calnan, Calnan, Bayer, & Read, 2013; Horlick-Jones, 2005b; Manuel & Crowe, 2014; Szmukler & Rose, 2013; Wand, 2011). When clinicians fear blame, defensive practices can result. Defensive practice occurs when clinicians become primarily concerned with their own protection or the protection of their organisation. This can displace concerns of the person's best interests (Anderson & Liff, 2012; Grotto, Gerace, O'Kane, Simpson, Oster, & Muir-Cochrane, 2015; Hillman, Tadd, Calnan, Calnan, Bayer, & Read, 2013; Manuel & Crowe, 2014).

In the mental health context, suicide risk is a type of risk that illustrates many of the concerns of the risk paradigm particularly poignantly. Using the example of suicide risk, the next section will more closely examine the impact of a risk focus in practice.

SUICIDE RISK

Suicide is a major public health issue. In Australia, approximately 2500 people die from suicide each year, which equates to 1.7% of all deaths (Ridani, Shand, Christensen, McKay,Tighe, Burns, & Hunter, 2015). The risk of suicide is a difficult issue for treating clinicians, and can provoke negative feelings, such as fear and anxiety (Chehil & Kutcher, 2012). In response to this risk type, clinicians search for order. Risk assessment is the first step. As the previous sections outlined, risk assessment involves looking to the future to predict the likelihood of an event of harm occurring. Suicide risk assessment may take the form of an unstructured interview, wherein the clinician's goal is to elicit information on risk factors and protective factors in order to make a determination of low, moderate, or high risk (Chehil & Kutcher, 2012; Ryan, Nielssen, Paton, & Large, 2010). Increasingly, structured, "actuarial" risk assessment tools are being used to aid the risk assessment process (Ryan, Nielssen, Paton, & Large, 2010). Examples of such tools include the suicidal intent scale, Beck hopelessness scale, tool for the assessment of suicide risk, Beck depression inventory, and clinician hopelessness scale (Chehil & Kutcher, 2012; Large, Kaneson, Myles, Myles, Gunaratne, & Ryan, 2016). Scales such as these use itemised questions to give a numerical score, intended to indicate the likelihood that an event of harm will occur (Stone, 2011). Whether an unstructured clinical interview is used to determine risk level, or a scale is used to assign a numerical risk score, the focus is on calculating the likelihood of harm (Ryan, Nielssen, Paton, & Large, 2010). This reflects economic conceptualisations of risk.

Once a risk categorisation has been determined, this can have significant implications for people accessing mental health care. Care can be determined by risk (Chehil & Kutcher, 2012). A high-risk individual may receive a higher allocation of a clinician's time (Mullen, Drinkwater, & Lewin, 2014;

Ryan, Nielssen, Paton, & Large, 2010). In the Australian public mental health system, which is crisis driven, a low-risk status may actually be a barrier to accessing care (National Mental Health Commission, 2014). However, a high-risk status can lead clinicians to employ coercive practices, or may be used as a rationale for involuntary treatment, which can have iatrogenic consequences (Maylea, 2016; Ryan, Nielssen, Paton, & Large, 2010; Wand, 2011).

What Risks Appear to Be the Focus?

In suicide risk, the most obvious focus is the potential death of the suicidal individual (Chehil & Kutcher, 2012).

Perhaps, as an offshoot of the focus on death, a significant focus may be on liability or blame, should harm occur (Mulder, 2011; Wand, 2011). Szmukler and Rose (2013) argue that in mental health care there is a tendency to focus on types of risk which can incite moral panic, and to neglect types of risk which are not morally reprehensible. They explain the focus on liability in these terms, arguing that negligence is considered by society to be morally reprehensible, whereas other risk types, such as coercive practices, are not (Szmukler & Rose, 2013).

What Risks May Be Backgrounded?

Relative to these risks on which attention is focused, some risk types may be neglected. These include the risk of ineffective practices, the risk of harmful practices, and iatrogenic consequences of care.

Firstly, there is the risk of practice that is disconnected from evidence. In suicide risk, this is reflected in the common practice of categorising people into risk groupings (Ryan, Nielssen, Paton, & Large, 2010). Despite the importance placed on suicide risk assessment (Chehil & Kutcher, 2012), there are significant concerns that risk assessment lacks validity (Ryan, Nielssen, Paton, & Large, 2010). Highlighting this, Large, Sharma, Cannon, Ryan, and Nielssen (2011) conducted a metaanalysis and found that risk categorisation has no significant clinical utility in predicting suicide within a year post discharge from a psychiatric hospital. Results demonstrated that death by suicide occurred in only 3% of people categorised as high-risk and that more than 60% of suicides occurred in low-risk groups (Large, Sharma, Cannon, Ryan, & Nielssen, 2011). A subsequent metaanalysis (Large, Kaneson, Myles, Myles, Gunaratne, & Ryan, 2016) explored the efficacy of risk categorisation based on suicide risk assessment and concluded that "the psychometric properties of optimal suicide risk categorization remains uncertain... this uncertainty is profound and our results are not reassuring" (p.13). While the goal of helping suicidal individuals to survive is undoubtedly an important one, evidence suggests that a focus on risk assessment (Large, Kaneson, Myles, Myles, Gunaratne, & Ryan, 2016), or on addressing suicide risk factors (Large, Sharma, Cannon, Ryan, & Nielssen, 2011), may not be the best means to achieve this goal.

Ryan et al. (2010) argued that risk assessment is an ineffective practice. Subsidiary to the risk of ineffective practices, is the risk of ineffective resource use. As Undrill (2011) stated, "every hour spent on extensive risk assessment procedures is an hour not spent with a patient doing useful psychotherapeutic work" (p. 70). On a micro level, risk assessment (which lacks predictive validity) consumes clinicians time and detracts time from care (Ryan, Nielssen, Paton, & Large, 2010). On a macro level, perceived risk influences the structure of the service system, to the extent that scarce and insufficient resources are available in public mental health care for those categorised as low-risk (National Mental Health Commission, 2014; Ryan, Nielssen, Paton, & Large, 2010). Risk assessment heavily shapes mental health care despite it's 'strong mathematical and ethical' (Ryan, Nielssen, Paton, & Large, 2010, p.398) flaws.

Such evidence against risk categorisation (Large, Sharma, Cannon, Ryan, & Nielssen, 2011; Large, Kaneson, Myles, Myles, Gunaratne, & Ryan, 2016) is of particular concern when considering that a risk status is often used as a rationale for the restriction of liberties (Ryan, Nielssen, Paton, & Large, 2010), or for coercive (Wand, 2011) or discriminatory (Maylea, 2016) practices. This highlights the second potentially backgrounded risk: The risk of providing care that is harmful to consumers. Inpatient risk management for suicidal individuals may involve forced medication, reduction or denial of free movement, seclusion, locked wards, and constant observation (Larsen & Terkelsen, 2014; Slemon, Jenkins, & Bungay, 2017). Some argue that tactics such as these are necessary to secure the safety of the high-risk individual (Chehil & Kutcher, 2012). However, these strategies, which involve either a loss of privacy or a loss of liberty, can be experienced as traumatising and dehumanising (Slemon, Jenkins, & Bungay, 2017). Others similarly acknowledge that perceived high risk can trigger unnecessary (Szmukler & Rose, 2013), ineffective (Wand, 2011), or unethical (Slemon, Jenkins, & Bungay, 2017) restrictive interventions. The decision to employ involuntary treatment is often made on the basis of risk (Maylea, 2016; Ryan, Nielssen, Paton, & Large, 2010). Maylea (2016) asserted that involuntary mental health treatment has strong potential iatrogenic consequences, can act as a deterrent to help-seeking, and contravenes international law by constituting discrimination on the basis of disability. It would be difficult to argue that involuntary treatment in mental health is not discriminatory, considering, as Maylea (2016) did, that people who have lung cancer and smoke are not involuntarily treated for their own protection, and likewise, that high-risk spouse abusers are not involuntarily treated for community protection (Szmukler & Rose, 2013).

The obvious counter to the above critiques is that a focus on risk is necessary to achieve safety. The argument that suicide can be prevented through focusing on risk is a seductive one, and one that is certainly still being mobilised (Chehil & Kutcher, 2012; Goldney, 2012). Coercive risk management practices can damage trust for consumers who may grow wary of care providers motives (Szmukler & Rose, 2013). Were these risk management approaches to be effective in saving lives, an argument might arise for their use. However, there are concerns coercive tactics are not underpinned by evidence of efficacy (Wand, 2011) nor is the high-risk status that on which they may be justified (Large, Sharma, Cannon, Ryan, & Nielssen, 2011). It is possible tactics such as these actually create access issues for those in need of treatment (Maylea, 2016; Wand, 2011). Treating people with disrespect has potential to actually increase the rate of incidents (Larsen & Terkelsen, 2014).

CASE STUDIES

The following are real case studies drawn from the authors' practice experience. Some details have been changed to ensure anonymity.

Case Study 1: "Sue"

Sue was a young Sudanese woman. She came to Australia four years ago as an asylum seeker, after spending some time in a refugee camp. On arrival, Sue had experienced mental health issues relating to the trauma she had experienced in Sudan and her cultural dislocation. At this time, she had thoughts of ending her life. She had sought help from her G.P, who had contacted a Crisis Assessment and Treatment Team (CATT). Sue was assessed as being at risk of suicide and was involuntarily hospitalised for three weeks. Sue experienced this as retraumatising. Hospital reminded her of her experience in the refugee camp and made her feel like a prisoner. She reported that, while in hospital, her belongings were searched regularly. She experienced this as stigmatising and dehumanising. Through this experience, she had become fearful of accessing mental health care. She recounted that she was discharged from hospital with the provision that she would engage in follow-up appointments. She stated these appointments were not helpful to her, and she requested no further contact with the care providers. She reported that she was not placed on a Community Treatment Order, but was coerced to continue follow-up care, with what she recounted as vague implications that she would otherwise be treated involuntarily. While she continued to experience mental health issues, including persistent low mood, occasional suicidal ideation, and traumatic symptoms, she no longer discussed these with health professionals.

Four years later, an endocrinologist who had examined Sue in a hospital outpatient clinic and who had noticed her flat affect referred her to a social worker. Sue met with the social worker, believing that she had to, but was quite guarded in her interactions. She recounted her experience of involuntary treatment to the social worker, stating openly that she had learned from this that it was not safe to be honest with health professionals. Relating to her current mental health status, she disclosed that she experienced depressive symptoms, such as persistent low mood, sleep difficulties, loss of motivation, and loss of interest in daily activities. When the social worker asked if she experienced suicidal ideation, she told she did not, stating quickly "I have plenty to live for", and "I want to live". The social worker was concerned Sue may be concealing suicidal ideation, so the social worker probed deeply around suicide. Sue continued to reiterate that she was not in any danger and denied any thoughts of suicide. This appeared defensive to the social worker. At this time, Sue did not meet the criteria for involuntary treatment. The social worker suggested a referral to the hospital psychiatrist on an outpatient basis. Sue declined this, stating "I don't want to go back to hospital." The social worker encouraged her to reconsider it and explained that it would be an outpatient referral, but Sue still declined, stating "I don't want to take the risk."

Sue continued to decline all professional mental health care referrals. She acknowledged her mental health issues and reported that she was suffering. She wanted to help alleviate her own suffering. Sue agreed to the following plan: She would use the online platform Moodgym, she would work through one of the consumer self-help books from the Centre for Clinical Interventions, and she would attend a peer support group in a local migrant resource centre. She did not want further appointments with the hospital social worker, stating "you seem nice, but I don't trust hospital people." When she was offered details of phone crisis counselling services, Sue queried whether these services could trace the call and locate her, asking "what if they could find me?" This prompted further questioning around suicidality from the social worker, but Sue continued to reiterate that she was safe and had many reasons to live. She accepted the details of these phone counselling services, but only after extensive discussion of how she could access these services safely, such as by calling from a pay phone, or asking at the start of the call that they clarify the circumstances which could trigger a risk management response.

Reflection: Risk Types

In the case study above, suicide risk was a rationale for the detainment and involuntary treatment of Sue. The risk of death was the focus. Sue's belongings were searched, likely to ensure she did not have any means to harm herself in her possession. Physical safety was the focus. This may also have been informed by the risk of liability in the event of harm. Research has shown clinicians employ many restrictive strategies during psychiatric admission, informed by fears of liability or blame (Slemon, Jenkins, & Bungay, 2017).

Due to the lack of predictive validity of suicide risk assessment (Large, Sharma, Cannon, Ryan, & Nielssen, 2011; Large, Kaneson, Myles, Myles, Gunaratne, & Ryan, 2016), it is not possible to know that Sue was at high risk of suicide, yet she was detained on this basis. The risk of poor adherence to evidence was deprioritised, relative to the prioritised risks. By association, the risk of ineffective resource use was also deprioritised.

Sue's experience of involuntary care as traumatic is reflected in research (Larsen & Terkelsen, 2014). There was a known risk of iatrogenic harm. This iatrogenic harm was likely exacerbated by strategies such as searching her belongings. This risk was also deprioritised. Sue's negative experience has shaped her beliefs about mental health care and created an access issue for her. Thus, when she met the social worker four years later, she refused all professional referrals. As Maylea (2016) argued would occur, involuntary treatment in this case acted to prevent future help seeking.

When offered a psychiatry referral as an outpatient, Sue's response was "I don't want to take the risk." Health practitioners can construct mental health patients as threats to be protected against, when viewing them through the lens of risk (Anderson & Liff, 2012; Wand, 2011). Following her negative experience, Sue has constructed mental health care as a threat to be protected against. The risk has been transferred from the health organisation to the patient.

This case study highlighted the potential for risk management to result in iatrogenic harm.

A perhaps less drastic, though still very meaningful concern, is that a focus on risk can impede health professionals' ability to see their patient holistically, as a person. Szmukler and Rose (2013) noted that a focus on risk factors "moves us away from an attempt to understand the individual patient as an agent, with intentions, feelings, desires, preferences, specific needs and so on" (p. 132). Instead, risk makes health professionals cognisant of their perceived duty to protect and control (Szmukler & Rose, 2013). This focus, coupled with the fear of blame should they "fail", may account for the finding that mental health patients can become "risk objects", resulting in a perceived need for health professionals to protect themselves against the risk their patients pose (Anderson & Liff, 2012, p.260). Others (Clancy & Happell, 2014; Mulder, 2011; Wand, 2011) similarly note that a focus on risk can equate to a focus on protection of the organisation against blame, with the patient being constructed as a threat to be protected against (Mulder, 2011). The fear of blame can result in negative feelings, such as fear and anxiety, amongst treating professionals. Mulder (2011) suggests it may be this that underpins restrictive care pathways: "(P)atients may therefore be detained not for treatment needs but because not detaining them produces intolerable anxiety in the staff involved in the assessment" (p. 606). Overall, a focus on risk can lead to a focus on liability or blame, and a loss of focus on the patient as a person.

Case Study 2: "Mary"

Mary was assessed by a hospital social worker for suicidality. She had many risk factors commonly understood to be linked to suicide (i.e., suicidal thoughts, planning, persistent low mood, recent psychosocial stress, and hopelessness). While she had disclosed suicidal planning, she had denied the intention to act on this plan and did not have access to means to carry out the plan. The social worker, who was not a mental health social worker, regarded Mary as high-risk and encouraged her to remain in hospital to be assessed by a CATT clinician. Mary could not be persuaded to stay to wait for the CATT clinician. However, Mary agreed that the social worker could refer her to the CATT, and that she would be happy to have a CATT clinician visit her at home to assess her later that day. CATTs are responsible for assessing whether a psychiatric hospital admission is required and, when appropriate, providing support in the community as an alternative to inpatient care. Mary expressed relief on learning of the CATT service, stating that she was not aware there were people who could visit her at home, and that she found the knowledge of this support comforting. Mary also expressed the support the social worker had provided in their session, and the future support promised by the social worker, were comforting and helped Mary to feel less hopeless. The social worker referred Mary to the CATT, requesting Mary be followed up urgently.

On receipt of the referral, the CATT clinician expressed anger, stating that the social worker should not have allowed Mary to leave and should have informed Mary the police would be called if she would not stay. The CATT clinician stated that the referral was inappropriate, as CATTs do not have capacity to provide an urgent response, stating (incorrectly): "We are not a crisis service.". The CATT clinician told the social worker that they should phone the police and request a welfare check, as it was not possible to know when the CATT would be able to follow up on the assessment. The social worker expressed concern that a police welfare check would likely not be helpful, and, as a breach of trust, it may increase the risk, especially given Mary had expressed relief at the prospect of the CATT visiting. The CATT clinician reiterated that the social worker should phone the police, stating "this isn't my responsibility" and "you have dumped this on me."

The social worker relayed this exchange to their supervisor. The supervisor advised it was a liability issue and that, as CATTs has psychiatric expertise, their advice must be followed, even if it is not likely to be helpful. After some debate, the social worker phoned the police and requested they perform a welfare check (a home visit to ascertain if an individual is safe). The police attended Mary's home, confirmed Mary was safe, and left. Mary phoned the social worker expressing anger at the police visit and stating she did not want further contact with the social worker. The CATT clinician attended Mary's home 45 minutes after the police had left. The CATT reported that Mary had been "guarded" during their assessment. Mary had told the CATT clinician she was safe and did not need their help. The CATT assessed that Mary was not in imminent danger. The CATT followed up over the next two days, continuing to assess that Mary was not in imminent danger, then discharged Mary.

Reflection: Risk Types

This case study highlighted the focus on the risk of liability. Mary's risk was transferred into personal risk for the CATT clinician. The CATT clinician responded with anger, and acted to transfer the risk to the social worker. The social worker liaised with their supervisor, which may have been perceived as transferring the risk to the supervisor. The police were phoned, despite agreement that this had no therapeutic value. Concerns of liability displaced concerns of Mary's best interests. Mary has ultimately ended up with less support, as she has withdrawn consent for social work follow up, and will not be followed up by the CATT. Mary reported feeling that her trust had been breached. This may act as a deterrent for future help seeking. Mary's current fate is unknown.

Risk and Blame: Culpability and Liability

The above case study explored how fears of blame can shape practice. This was anecdotal, drawing on the authors' practice experience.

Research has also shown that both culpability and liability are common concerns health professionals hold when they make decisions concerning risk. Health research (Anderson & Liff, 2012; Grotto, Gerace, O'Kane, Simpson, Oster, & Muir-Cochrane, 2015; Hillman, Tadd, Calnan, Calnan, Bayer, & Read, 2013) often does not carefully distinguish between liability and culpability; rather, the two concepts can be either conflated, or addressed together. While they are interconnected concepts, as both relate to blame, it is useful to distinguish between them.

Culpability is a broad construct. Individuals may be held culpable through media, internal disciplinary action, judgement, or perceived judgement from colleagues, patients, community members, or other stakeholders. It is difficult to set parameters around what exactly culpability is and what circumstances lead to health professionals being held culpable. Unlike culpability, liability is a legal concept. It is much easier to set parameters around liability, as these are set in legislation and by the judgements enacted by courts. Given the importance of liability for decision making concerning risk, it is worthwhile for clinicians to understand exactly what liability is. An informed understanding of this legal concept could help to dissuade fears that are commonly attached to liability and risk. This is important, as such fears can lead to practices which are not in the best interests of the people accessing care (Anderson & Liff, 2012; Grotto, Gerace, O'Kane, Simpson, Oster, & Muir-Cochrane, 2015; Hillman, Tadd, Calnan, Calnan, Bayer, & Read, 2013).

The next section will begin by outlining the legal elements of liability. It will then provide examples, drawing on negligence case law relevant to suicide risk, of how this has been interpreted by the courts.

Liability and Negligence

Liability is a condition which must be proven for a negligence claim to succeed. In Victoria, Australia, while negligence can be a criminal matter under the Crimes Act 1958 (Austl.), medical negligence is normally a civil matter under the Wrongs Act 1958 (Austl.). This means it relies on an injured party initiating court action against a treating practitioner or health organisation. Several elements must be met for a negligence claim to succeed. A duty of care must be shown to exist and to have been breached. It must also be proven that harm occurred (Ryan, Callaghan, & Large, 2015). The harm must have resulted from a risk which was both "foreseeable" and "not insignificant", according to Section 48 of the Wrongs Act 1958 (Austl.). Further, a causal link must be established: A lack of proper care must be demonstrated to have caused the resulting harm (Popa, 2017).

This criteria that harm is foreseeable is interesting in light of the evidence of the metaanalysis that was outlined earlier on suicide risk. In brief, this evidence highlights that "(a) statistically strong and reliable method to usefully distinguish patients with a high risk of suicide remains elusive" (Large, Kaneson, Myles, Myles, Gunaratne, & Ryan, 2016, p.2). In light of this, the authors set out to explore common law judgements of negligence cases involving suicide. While this exploration did not find that the argument that risk was not "foreseeable" is being applied in court, it found that negligence is remarkably difficult to prove. Popa (2017) stated that the current Victorian system "has not yet achieved the balance" (p. 88), arguing that, on the whole, defendants in meritorious medical negligence claims are overly protected in a way which is "arguably unfair" (p.69) for injured claimants. Even some fairly extreme circumstances have been interpreted by the courts to not constitute negligence.

A striking illustration of this is seen in Stuart v. Kirkland-Veenstra (2009). In this case, police attended a scene to find an individual sitting in his vehicle with a hose connected to the exhaust pipe running into the car window (Victorian Government Solicitor's Office, 2015). The police assessed that the man was neither at risk of self-harm, nor suffering from a mental illness, and chose not to detain him under the (then) Mental Health Act 1986. The man committed suicide later that day. His partner sued the State of Victoria and the attending police officers for negligence. The claim for negligence was ultimately determined by the High Court to be unsuccessful (it was initially dismissed by the County Court, then taken to Court of Appeal and upheld, then appealed to the High Court where it was again dismissed). The High Court found that a duty of care was not owed, and the police officers did not have control over the source of the risk; rather, it was the deceased who controlled the risk (Victorian Government Solicitor's Office, 2015).

This case certainly supports Popa's (2017) suggestion that negligence is quite difficult to prove. This assertion is further supported by court judgements of negligence claims in the health sector. For instance, in Hunter and New England Local Health District v. McKenna (2014), a health service had detained a man under mental health legislation, having assessed and documented that he was at risk of suicide and posed a risk to others. The following day, the health service discharged the man into the care of his friend, despite very minimal change in his presentation. The man killed his friend shortly after discharge and then, later, committed suicide. Friends of the murdered man sued the health service for negligence. The claim was ultimately unsuccessful. The High Court found that, while a duty of care existed, it had not been breached. The High Court found that the duty of care required the treating psychiatrist to discharge the man into the care of his friend as had been done, as mental health legislation prohibited detainment unless the treating psychiatrist had formed the opinion that no less restrictive means of care existed.

A key point that can be drawn from examining how the courts are interpreting negligence claims, is that harm does not guarantee liability. Judges are not permitted to use hindsight when evaluating the circumstances that lead to harm (Australian Government Solicitor, 2012). Even the occurrence of avoidable harm does not equate to liability. In fact, this is specifically addressed in the Victorian legislation governing civil negligence, the Wrongs Act 1958 (Austl.), which states: "The fact that a risk of harm could have been avoided by doing something in a different way does not of itself give rise to or affect liability" [S.49(b)]. Further, there are examples of judgements which specifically give regard to the detrimental impact on public good of promoting defensive practices. In Hunter Area Health Service v. Presland (2003) (cited in Scott, 2006), a health service was sued for negligence by a claimant who asserted that the treating psychiatrist acted negligently by not detaining a person under mental health legislation. The presiding judge did not award damages despite accepting that the psychiatrist acted negligently. In his judgement, NSW Court of Appeal Judge Santow J. A. considered that the mental health system may be negatively impacted should the claim succeed, as it may introduce a "detrimentally defensive frame of mind and promote a bias toward detention" (Santow, cited in Scott, 2006, p.55). In this case, the judge gave specific regard to the potential negative impact of a judgement which could promote defensive practices in health care.

The argument being made here is not that health practitioners have a free license to be negligent without fear of repercussions. Rather, it is that no evidence is available to suggest that there is a legal expectation that health practitioners eliminate all risks and dangers, nor that the occurrence of harm automatically means someone is liable. Risk research repeatedly finds that practitioners fear liability (Anderson & Liff, 2012; Grotto, Gerace, O'Kane, Simpson, Oster, & Muir-Cochrane, 2015; Hillman, Tadd, Calnan, Calnan, Bayer, & Read, 2013) and then engage in defensive practice (Anderson & Liff, 2012; Grotto, Gerace, O'Kane, Simpson, Oster, & Muir-Cochrane, 2015), when risk is a factor. Grotto et al. (2015) found that mental health nurses feared being held liable should patients abscond after a nurse's assessment found they are not in need of restrictive measures to prevent absconding. Hillman et al. (2013) found that a manager believed staff feared being "neglectful" should they choose not to raise bed railings, even in circumstances when it is in the patient's best interests to leave bed railings down. Contrasting starkly with these fears, is the reality that police can attend a scene to find a person with a hose connected from their exhaust to their car window, and not be found negligent when they suicide hours later. While these studies (Grotto, Gerace, O'Kane, Simpson, Oster, & Muir-Cochrane, 2015; Hillman, Tadd, Calnan, Calnan, Bayer, & Read, 2013) were not in the Australian context, Manuel and Crowe (2014) noted that the connection between risk and liability is made by health practitioners in multiple countries, including countries with health systems underpinned by no-fault legislation. The central message is that while practitioners may fear liability when risk is a factor, it cannot be inferred that these fears are reflective of an actual legal threat.

SOLUTIONS AND RECOMMENDATIONS

This chapter has demonstrated that the concept of risk, despite being of central importance in health, is a nebulous notion. Risk heavily influences the delivery of health services (Clancy & Happell, 2014; Hillman, Tadd, Calnan, Calnan, Bayer, & Read, 2013; Lane & Reiger, 2013), despite a lack of agreement on what exactly risk is.

Clinicians are concerned about liability, when risk is a factor (Szmukler & Rose, 2013). There appears to be a perception that blame will automatically be attributable in the event of harm. In this chapter, the concepts of liability and culpability have been separated carefully. Culpability is less chartable than liability, so it is not as easy to dissuade these fears. Having highlighted the legal requirements of liability, and having examined how this is being interpreted by the courts, the authors assert that this fear of liability is largely unfounded. While liability is a possibility if negligence can be proven, it has been shown that this is quite difficult to achieve (Popa, 2017). The health sector, and indeed patient care, would benefit from educating clinicians about liability. Education on liability could help to dissuade fears that appear to be disproportionately held, relative to the legal threat. This could take place in both the health sector and in the tertiary education context. Mulder (2011) stated that "the best way to manage organizational risks is to improve core tasks of patient care" (p. 606). Reducing unfounded fears of liability may reduce defensive practices, and, ultimately, this could make mental health services more accessible. Decreasing defensive practice would improve patient care, and, following Mulder's (2011) argument, this would actually decrease organisational risk.

Suicide is a major public health issue, and one which certainly warrants attention and careful provision of care. However, in light of evidence suggesting that there is profound uncertainty regarding the prediction of individuals at high risk of suicide (Large, Sharma, Cannon, Ryan, & Nielssen, 2011; Large, Kaneson, Myles, Myles, Gunaratne, & Ryan, 2016), it is worth reflecting on whether risk is a useful frame. The authors assert that it is not. Noting the many issues with risk, some voices in mental healthcare have suggested shifting from risk to safety (Undrill, 2011) or to capacity (Ryan, Nielssen, Paton, & Large, 2010). The concerns with risk extend well beyond mental health care and into areas such as corrections (Pollack, 2010) and general health care (Hillman, Tadd, Calnan, Calnan, Bayer, & Read, 2013). Hence, a shift away from risk ideally needs to be applicable to these other areas also. Capacity may be applicable to mental health care, but would not resolve some of the issues observed in general health care (Hillman, Tadd, Calnan, Calnan, Bayer, & Read, 2013), which can occur in the absence of questioned capacity. Clinicians could consider shifting their focus from risk to well-being. A clinician who is motivated to protect a person's well-being will of course be motivated to ensure the person's survival. Returning to the case study of suicide risk, should a reliable tool that can predict suicide be developed in the future, this would surely be adopted by the clinician who has a well-being agenda. The lens of risk is not necessary to achieve the goal of safety. However, the lens of risk is firmly entrenched in the discourse of blame. It incites fear, can lead to defensive practices which disregard the patient's interests (Anderson & Liff, 2012), can create a false sense of security amongst clinicians (Wand, 2011), and a "them and us" dynamic between care providers and recipients (Hillman, Tadd, Calnan, Calnan, Bayer, & Read, 2013, p.950). Risk is a negative discourse and it needs to be removed. This may seem radical or unachievable, given the importance placed on risk (Clancy & Happell, 2014; Hillman, Tadd, Calnan, Calnan, Bayer, & Read, 2013; Lane & Reiger, 2013). However, it is worth reiterating that health has not always been ordered around the concept of risk; rather, it has risen over the past several decades (Eagleton-Pierce, 2016; Lane & Reiger, 2013). Any concept that can be introduced can also be removed.

In considering that a new lens, well-being, could replace risk, it is worth asking whether the same issues would arise with any frame used to provide care. Risk is strongly connected with blame and liability. It would be ideal to understand how this came to be in order to know how to prevent it happening again with a new conceptual frame. It is noteworthy that the language of risk can be seen often in legislation. For example, in Victoria, "foreseeable risk" is specifically named as a requirement for liability to be met under the Wrongs Act 1958 (Austl.) [S.48(1)(a)]. It also is a condition in other legislation, such as the Occupational Health and Safety Act 2004, [Austl.S.20(1)(a)], which asks employers to aim to "eliminate risks," the Bail Act 1977, [Austl.S.4(2)(d)(i)], which stipulates responses when "unacceptable risk" is assessed, and it appears in mental health legislation nationally (Ryan, Nielssen, Paton, & Large, 2010). It may be that risk is a concept with a legal history, hence in being employed in health care it has become intertwined with liability and blame. Well-being does not appear to have this same legal history.

Caring for suicidal and other "at risk" individuals can be a difficult experience for clinicians, as it can incite fear and anxiety (Chehil & Kutcher, 2012). Current practice appears to be to respond to this fear and anxiety with risk assessment and risk management (Mulder, 2011), which can be defensive, restrictive, or coercive (Ryan, Nielssen, Paton, & Large, 2010; Wand, 2011). Education on liability can help to reduce fear and anxiety relating to blame. However, there may still be fear and anxiety relating to the uncertainty or the chance of harm befalling the recipient of care. Regardless of the source of the fear and anxiety, it is important that it is separated from the task of care. The emotional experience of clinicians is not a patient care issue; it should not determine or unduly influence patient care. Clinicians could consider employing emotion regulation strategies to address their own fear and anxiety, before returning focus to the well-being of the person with whom they are working.

CONCLUSION

The concept of risk significantly influences the delivery of health services. Despite the importance placed on risk, there is not a universally accepted understanding of what risk is. Seen through one lens, it refers to the probability and severity of harm (Moscati, 2016). Through another, it is a discourse of accountability and blame (Douglas, 1990). The lack of agreement on the definition of risk is problematic (Lupton, 2013). This chapter has examined how the language of risk is used in health care. It has been shown that risk is often negative, relative to an unspoken norm, and morally loaded. It is something to be held by patients, yet controlled by professionals.

This chapter has demonstrated health professionals' tendency to focus on liability and blame when they make decisions concerning risk. Further research is needed on the blame elements of risk and how this effects risk taking amongst health professionals. In this chapter, the authors have suggested that fears of liability are likely disproportionate to the actual legal threat. Future research could explore the frequency at which blame events (relating to both liability and culpability) are actually occurring. This knowledge may be of use in helping to reduce the fear that is associated with risk.

ACKNOWLEDGMENT

This first author of this chapter is supported by an Australian Government Research Training Program (RTP) Scholarship and a Monash Research Scholarship.

REFERENCES

Andersson, T., & Liff, R. (2012). Does patient-centred care mean risk aversion and risk ignoring? Unintended consequences of NPM reforms. *International Journal of Public Sector Management*, *25*(4), 260–271. doi:10.1108/09513551211244098

Australian Government Solicitor. (2012). *Express Law*. Retrieved October 2, 2017, from http://www.ags.gov.au/publications/express-law/el178.pdf

Beck, U. (1992). *Risk society: Towards a new modernity*. London: Sage.

Beck, U. (2002). The terrorist threat: World risk society revisited.(State of Emergency). *Theory, Culture & Society*, *19*(4), 39–55. doi:10.1177/0263276402019004003

Beck, U. (2008). Global generations in world risk society. *Revista CIDOB d'Afers Internacionals*, (82/83), 203-216.

Beck, U. (2009). *World at risk*. Cambridge, UK: Polity.

Chehil, S., & Kutcher, S. (2012). *Suicide risk management a manual for health professionals*. Chichester, UK: Wiley.

Chen, N. (2015). Predicting vaccination intention and benefit and risk perceptions: The incorporation of affect, trust, and television influence in a dual-mode model. *Risk Analysis*, *35*(7), 1268–1280. doi:10.1111/risa.12348 PMID:25808562

Clancy, L., & Happell, B. (2014). Tensions of difference: Reconciling organisational imperatives for risk management with consumer-focused care from the perspectives of clinicians and managers. *Journal of Clinical Nursing*, *23*(21-22), 3177–3187. doi:10.1111/jocn.12564 PMID:25453122

Crimes Act. 1958. (Vic) (Austl.)

De Bortoli, L., Ogloff, J., Coles, J., & Dolan, M. (2017). Towards best practice: Combining evidence-based research, structured assessment and professional judgement. *Child & Family Social Work*, *22*(2), 660–669. doi:10.1111/cfs.12280

Douglas, M. (1990). Risk as a forensic resource. *Daedalus*, *119*(4), 1–16.

Douglas, M. (1992). *Risk and blame: Essays in cultural theory*. London: Routledge. doi:10.4324/9780203430866

Eagleton-Pierce, M. (2016). *Neoliberalism: The key concepts*. New York: Routledge.

Garve, R., Garve, M., Türp, J. C., Fobil, J. N., & Meyer, C. G. (2017). Scarification in sub-Saharan Africa: Social skin, remedy and medical import. *Tropical Medicine & International Health*, *22*(6), 708–715. doi:10.1111/tmi.12878 PMID:28380287

Ghafoor, S. (2008). Out of harms way. *Nursing Standard (through 2013)*, *22*(43), 61-61.

Goldney, R. D. (2012). Problems with suicide risk assessment. *The Australian and New Zealand Journal of Psychiatry*, *46*(2), 172–173. doi:10.1177/0004867411433223 PMID:22311534

Grotto, J., Gerace, A., O'Kane, D., Simpson, A., Oster, C., & Muir-Cochrane, E. (2015). Risk assessment and absconding: Perceptions, understandings and responses of mental health nurses. *Journal of Clinical Nursing*, *24*(5-6), 855–865. doi:10.1111/jocn.12671 PMID:25209549

Hillman, A., Tadd, W., Calnan, S., Calnan, M., Bayer, A., & Read, S. (2013). Risk, governance and the experience of care. *Sociology of Health & Illness*, *35*(6), 939–955. doi:10.1111/1467-9566.12017 PMID:23356787

Horlick-Jones, T. (2005a). Informal logics of risk: Contingency and modes of practical reasoning. *Journal of Risk Research*, *8*(3), 253–272. doi:10.1080/1366987042000270735

Horlick-Jones, T. (2005b). On 'risk work': Professional discourse, accountability, and everyday action. *Health Risk & Society*, *7*(3), 293–307. doi:10.1080/13698570500229820

Hunter and New England Local Health District v. McKenna (2014) (HCA) (Austl.).

KPMG. (2011). *Child FIRST and integrated family services final report: Prepared for the Department of Human Services*. Retrieved September 2016, from http://www.dhs.vic.gov.au/_data/assets/pdf_file/0008/646820/childFIRSTandintfamservicesfullreport_09082011.pdf

Lane, K., & Reiger, K. (2013). Regime change in Australian maternity hospitals. *Social Theory & Health, 11*(4), 407–427. doi:10.1057th.2013.7

Large, M., Kaneson, M., Myles, N., Myles, H., Gunaratne, P., & Ryan, C. (2016). Meta-analysis of longitudinal cohort studies of suicide risk assessment among psychiatric patients: Heterogeneity in results and lack of improvement over time. *PLoS One, 11*(6), 1–17. doi:10.1371/journal.pone.0156322 PMID:27285387

Large, M., Sharma, S., Cannon, E., Ryan, C., & Nielssen, O. (2011). Risk factors for suicide within a year of discharge from psychiatric hospital: A systematic meta-analysis. *The Australian and New Zealand Journal of Psychiatry, 45*(8), 619–628. doi:10.3109/00048674.2011.590465 PMID:21740345

Larsen, I. B., & Terkelsen, T. B. (2014). Coercion in a locked psychiatric ward: Perspectives of patients and staff. *Nursing Ethics, 21*(4), 426–436. doi:10.1177/0969733013503601 PMID:24106262

Lupton, D. (2013). Risk and emotion: Towards an alternative theoretical perspective. *Health Risk & Society, 15*(8), 634–647. doi:10.1080/13698575.2013.848847

Manuel, J., & Crowe, M. (2014). Clinical responsibility, accountability, and risk aversion in mental health nursing: A descriptive, qualitative study. *International Journal of Mental Health Nursing, 23*(4), 336–343. doi:10.1111/inm.12063 PMID:24548741

Maylea, C. (2016). A rejection of involuntary treatment in mental health social work. *Ethics & Social Welfare, 1*(1), 1–17.

Moscati, I. (2016). Retrospectives: How economists came to accept expected utility theory: The case of Samuelson and Savage. *The Journal of Economic Perspectives, 30*(2), 219–236. doi:10.1257/jep.30.2.219

Mulder, R. (2011). Problems with suicide risk assessment. *The Australian and New Zealand Journal of Psychiatry, 45*(8), 605–607. doi:10.3109/00048674.2011.594786 PMID:21870919

Mullen, A., Drinkwater, V., & Lewin, T. J. (2014). Care zoning in a psychiatric intensive care unit: Strengthening ongoing clinical risk assessment. *Journal of Clinical Nursing, 23*(5-6), 731–743. doi:10.1111/jocn.12493 PMID:24329872

National Mental Health Commission. (2014). *The national review of mental health programmes and services*. Sydney: National Mental Health Commission.

Pollack, S. (2010). Labelling clients 'risky': Social Work and the neo-liberal welfare state. *British Journal of Social Work, 40*(4), 1263–1278. doi:10.1093/bjsw/bcn079

Popa, T. (2017). Righting Wrongs: Lawyers' reflections on the amendments to the Wrongs Act 1958 (Vic) on medical negligence and mental harm claims.(Australia). *Torts Law Journal, 24*(1), 64–82.

Ridani, R., Shand, F. L., Christensen, H., McKay, K., Tighe, J., Burns, J., & Hunter, E. (2015). Suicide prevention in Australian Aboriginal communities: A review of past and present programs. *Suicide & Life-Threatening Behavior, 45*(1), 111–140. doi:10.1111ltb.12121 PMID:25227155

Rogers, R. W. (1975). A protection motivation theory of fear appeals and attitude change. *The Journal of Psychology, 91*(1), 93–114. doi:10.1080/00223980.1975.9915803 PMID:28136248

Ryan, C., Nielssen, O., Paton, M., & Large, M. (2010). Clinical decisions in psychiatry should not be based on risk assessment. *Australasian Psychiatry, 18*(5), 398–403. doi:10.3109/10398562.2010.507816 PMID:20863176

Ryan, C. J., Callaghan, S., & Large, M. (2015). The importance of least restrictive care: The clinical implications of a recent High Court decision on negligence. *Australasian Psychiatry*, *23*(4), 415–417. doi:10.1177/1039856215590025 PMID:26104773

Scott, R. (2006). Hunter Area Health Services v Presland: Liability of Mental Health Services for Failing to Admit or Detain a Patient With Mental Illness. *Psychiatry, Psychology and Law*, *13*(1), 49–59. doi:10.1375/pplt.13.1.49

Slemon, A., Jenkins, E., & Bungay, V. (2017). Safety in psychiatric inpatient care: The impact of risk management culture on mental health nursing practice. *Nursing Inquiry, 24*(4).

Stone, G. (2011). *Self-orientation and relational-orientation in suicidal risk: Possible facilitative and protective aspects*. ProQuest Dissertations Publishing.

Szmukler, G., & Rose, N. (2013). Risk assessment in mental health care: Values and costs. *Behavioral Sciences & the Law*, *31*(1), 125–140. doi:10.1002/bsl.2046 PMID:23296543

Undrill, G. (2011). Calling time on risk assessments. *Journal of Psychiatric Intensive Care*, *7*(2), 67–72. doi:10.1017/S1742646411000045

Victoria State Government. (2017). *Clinical risk management.* Retrieved October 3, from https://www2.health.vic.gov.au/hospitals-and-health-services/quality-safety-service/clinical-risk-management

Victorian Government Solicitor's Office. (2015). *High Court decision- Stuart v Kirkland-Veenstra [2009] HCA 15.* Retrieved October 2, 2017, from http://vgso.vic.gov.au/content/high-court-decision-stuart-v-kirkland-veenstra-2009-hca-15

Wand, T. (2011). Investigating the Evidence for the Effectiveness of risk assessment in mental health care. *Issues in Mental Health Nursing*, *33*(1), 2–7. doi:10.3109/01612840.2011.616984 PMID:22224960

Wand, T., Isobel, S., & Derrick, K. (2015). Surveying clinician perceptions of risk assessment and management practices in mental health service provision. *Australasian Psychiatry*, *23*(2), 147–153. doi:10.1177/1039856214568227 PMID:25688130

Wrongs Act. 1958. (Vic) (Austl.)

Chapter 3
Healthcare Decision Making:
Allied Health and Equity

Haylee Lane
Monash University, Australia

Jennifer Martin
Swinburne University, Australia

Terry Haines
Monash University, Australia

ABSTRACT

The aim of this chapter is to explore the factors that health managers adopt when making decisions on how to allocate limited healthcare resources. The objective is to increase knowledge and understanding of decision making processes at the macro, meso, and micro levels and priority setting. An examination of current healthcare decision-making processes used for resource allocation around the world highlights the disparities in models and approaches and the often ad hoc nature of decisions made. A description of the allied health workforce highlights the size and significance of this workforce and why understanding decisions made in regards to allied health resources is of importance. Issues of access and equity are also considered in relation to notions of fairness and efficacy in relation to health outcomes.

INTRODUCTION

Health care and the needs of consumers and communities are changing, with increasing demand rapidly outgrowing service capability in the health care system. When health care resources are limited, questions of fairness, efficiency and effectiveness are raised: How should resources be allocated? Which services should be publicly funded? Who determines who has access to a particular service or if a service is needed? (Emanuel, 2000; Fleck, 2001; Rawls, 2009) Explicitly addressing and understanding the process of decision making (also known as priority setting or rationing) in health care resource allocation is needed to improve legitimacy and fairness of these decisions (Angelis, Kanavos, & Montibeller, 2017; Fleck, 2001).

DOI: 10.4018/978-1-5225-7402-6.ch003

Distribution of resources within the healthcare sector may follow many different paths depending on the stated aims or goals of that health system. These and other related principles of healthcare resource allocation have had a dramatic effect on health system structures and health outcomes when operationalised through a range of different healthcare policies and resource allocation decision making mechanisms worldwide (Jones, Bradley, & Oberlander, 2014; Marmot, Friel, Bell, Houweling, Taylor, & Health, 2008; Thomas, 1993).

The general aim of this chapter is to describe the factors taken into account by allied health managers and clinicians when making resource allocation decisions. This includes consideration of the different levels of decision making and factors influencing priority setting. A description of the main features of the Australian allied health workforce is followed by consideration of decision making processes, theories and frameworks. Key factors influencing equitable healthcare are discussed in relation to accountability for reasonableness.

RESOURCE ALLOCATION DECISIONS IN HEALTHCARE

Resource allocation decisions are made at all levels within the healthcare system (Klein, 1993). Macro level decisions include decisions that affect structures and processes at the policy level to fit with the health needs of populations across the continuum of care, e.g. the central government setting the overall budget for the health system. Meso level decisions include organisational decisions such as determining the services provided, coordination of care for particular groups of patients or the purchase of appropriate equipment to support a specific service (Adams, Jones, Lefmann, & Sheppard, 2016). Micro level decisions include the management of individuals at the service level including both clinical decision making (Klein & Maybin, 2012) and service level decision making (Adams, Jones, Lefmann, & Sheppard, 2016; Bærøe, 2008). The effects of macro level decisions filter down the decision-making chain, shaping the organizational level and service/clinical level decisions being made as seen in Figure 1.

Figure 1. Levels of healthcare decision-making

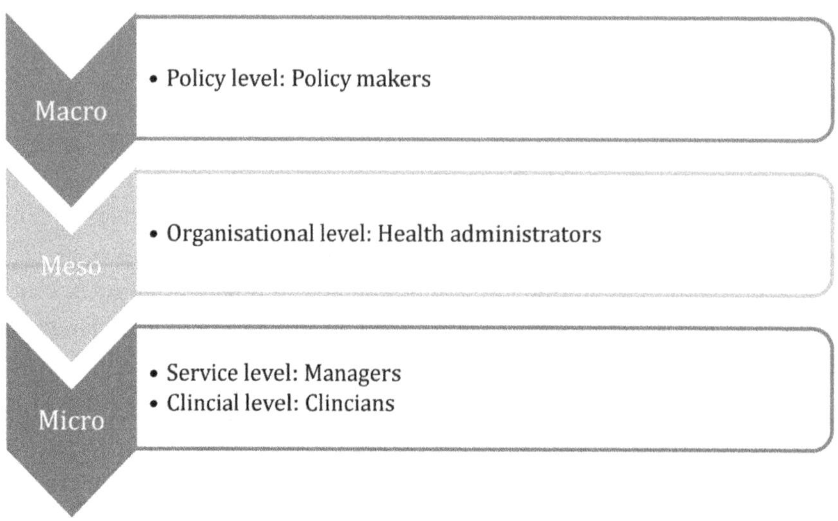

Decisions made at the macro level can often be from politically charged topics (Sabik & Lie, 2008). At the meso level, there is little evidence to guide decision-making in regards to service priorities of a health care system as a whole (Imison, Sonola, Honeyman, & Ross, 2014), with most approaches focusing on a single intervention or condition (Angelis, Kanavos, & Montibeller, 2017). Previous authors have labeled this kind of decision-making as an ad hoc process with intuitive or heuristic elements and has been more about "muddling through" (Figure 2) rather than explicitly following an operational procedure (Angelis, Kanavos, & Montibeller, 2017; Baltussen & Niessen, 2006; Parsons, 2002; Yancey, Cole, & McCarthy, 2010).

At the micro level, there are many decision-making algorithms and frameworks, such as evidence-based medicine and person-centered care, that have been constructed for use amongst health professionals (Graham, Logan, Harrison, Straus, Tetroe, Caswell, & Robinson, 2006; Offredy, 1998; Sackett & Richardson, 2006; Stacey, Murray, Legare, Sandy, Menard, & O'connor, 2008; Towle & Godolphin, 1999). These algorithms and frameworks usually concentrate on specific areas of decision making or specific conditions/disciplines commonly centered around a "bottom-up" decision-making approach as opposed to taking a "top down" approach and considering the holistic picture. Others have emerged from the quality improvement literature and incorporate both decision-making and subsequent practice change within the one framework (Graham, Logan, Harrison, Straus, Tetroe, Caswell, & Robinson, 2006). It is

Figure 2. Ad hoc priority setting (adapted from Baltussen & Niessen, 2006)

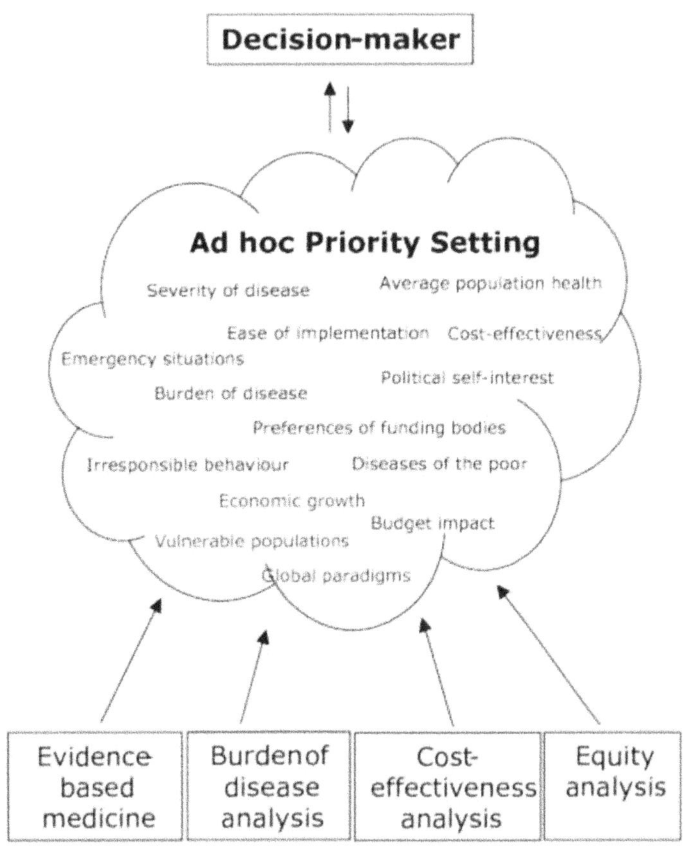

extremely difficult to identify a single best solution of allocating scarce resources regardless of whether there is common agreement of the causes of particular health problem due to the ambiguity in research outcomes, validity of generalising results to different populations, cost effectiveness judgments and politics (Robert, Harlock, & Williams, 2014; Yancey, Cole, & McCarthy, 2010).

HISTORICAL DECISION-MAKING PROCESSES

Around the world, many countries have implemented explicit decision-making processes. Sabik and Lie (2008) have completed an informative review on the historical decision-making efforts adopted by eight countries when setting health care priorities. Their paper summarises the details of the frameworks adopted (Table 1) in each of the countries efforts to adopt an explicit and transparent decision-making process (Sabik & Lie, 2008). The most common principle between the countries was "effectiveness" and/or "efficiency" with all eight countries referring to these terms to some degree. Several other principles overlapped between the frameworks adopted these countries including principles like solidarity and human dignity, however no two of the frameworks are consistent nor were the approaches adopted. The processes and those involved in the priority setting discussions was also explored. Some counties included government officials and/or involved public/lay representatives or government commission, with the only consistent factor in the priority setting efforts by all eight countries being the inclusion of health professionals in the decision making process (Sabik & Lie, 2008).

An operational approach in healthcare resource allocation decision making is needed to ensure resources are used in an efficient and fair way and to validate the decisions being made (Angelis, Kanavos, & Montibeller, 2017). The range of stakeholders involved and the competing principles to consider highlights the importance of having a clear and coherent approach for resource allocation decision-making in healthcare (Baltussen & Niessen, 2006).

ALLIED HEALTH

Allied health in conjunction with medicine and nursing, comprise the three major divisions of the health care workforce. Allied health encompasses a diverse range of professions with different knowledge, skill sets and practices, who work collaboratively with many other professionals throughout the care pathway (Allied Health Professionals Federation [AHPF], 2013). Professions are both nationally registered professions and self-regulated allied health professions including both professionals and assistants (Department of Health [DoH], 2014). Their duties cover many areas of care including prevention, health promotion, diagnosis, treatment, support and enabling independence. Allied health can work in a range of settings (including acute, sub-acute, specialist services, community health, primary care, aged care and non-health settings including schools and child welfare) and across different sectors (including public and private health services, not for profit organisations, government departments and higher education and research) (DoH, 2014).

Table 1. Overview of centralized priority setting efforts (reproduced from Sabik & Lie, 2008)

Country, Year, Process	Principles, Guidelines, Recommendations
Norway, 1987/1997, Lønning Committee I and II	Priority principles:
	• Severity
	• Potential effect
	• Cost-effectiveness
	Priority groups based on severity (and later funding):
	• Fundamental
	• Supplementary
	• Low priority
	• No public funding
The Netherlands, 1992/1995, Dutch Committee on Choices in Health Care (Dunning Committee)	Sieves/filters to determine basic package of services:
	• Is care necessary?
	• Is care efficient?
	• Is care effective?
	• Can care be left up to individual responsibility?
Sweden, 1993/1995, Commission of Parliament members and experts	Ethical platform principles:
	• Human dignity
	• Need and solidarity
	• Cost-efficiency
	Political/administrative and clinical priority groups:
	• Life-threatening acute diseases, severe chronic diseases and palliative terminal care
	• Prevention and habilitation/rehabilitation
	• Less severe acute disease
	• Borderline cases
	• Care for reasons other than disease
Denmark, 1997, Danish Council of Ethics	Core values:
	• Equal human worth
	• Solidarity
	• Security and safety
	• Freedom and self-determination
	General goal, framed in terms of "opportunity for self-expression...irrespective of social background and economic ability"
	Partial goals:
	• Social and geographical equity
	• Quality
	• Cost-effectiveness
	• Democracy and consumer influence

continued on following page

Table 1. Continued

Country, Year, Process	Principles, Guidelines, Recommendations
Israel, 1995, Medical Technology Forum and National Advisory Committee, In response to new National Health Insurance Law	Criteria for prioritization of recommended technologies:
	• Life-saving technology with full recovery
	• Potential to prevent mortality or morbidity
	• Number of patients to benefit
	• Financial burden on society and the patient
	• New technology for diseases with no alternative treatments available
	• Brings increase in longevity and quality of life
	• Benefits of reducing morbidity vs. improving quality of life
	• Net gain is higher than short- or long-term cost
	• Funding of efficacious treatment than is expensive to the individual, but of reasonable cost to society
New Zealand, Yearly, beginning in 1993, Core Services Committee/ National Health Committee	Set out principles to guide priority setting decisions:
	• Effectiveness
	• Efficiency
	• Equity
	• Acceptability
	'Consensus conferences' for specialized services;
	Recommend core services for given year
Oregon (US), Beginning in 1989, Health Services Commission	Developed Quality of Well-Being Scale;
	Used scale to establish cost-effectiveness rankings;
	Revised rankings after public backlash;
	Continued to use ranked list of condition-treatment pairs
	Recently more emphasis on evidence base for recommendations
UK, Ongoing, beginning in 1999, National Institute for Clinical Excellence (NICE)	Appraisal of new health technologies;
	Development of clinical guidelines;
	Explicit use of cost-effectiveness evaluations
	Appeal possible on narrow grounds

Defining Allied Health

There is currently no national or international consensus on the specific professions that fall under the umbrella term of Allied Health (Choon, Teo, Choo, Mun, Beng, Chua, . . . Wong, 2015; Turnbull, Grimmer-Somers, Kumar, May, Law, & Ashworth, 2009). It is generally accepted that allied health refers to the health professionals that work alongside the medical and nursing professions within the health care system (Choon, Teo, Choo, Mun, Beng, Chua, . . . Wong, 2015).

The national peak body representing the role of allied health professionals in Australia is the Allied Health Professions Australia (AHPA). AHPA define an allied health profession as a profession that has;

- A direct patient care role and may have application to broader public health outcomes;

- A national professional organisation with a code of ethics/conduct and clearly defined membership requirements;
- A university health sciences courses (not medical, dental or nursing) at Australian Qualifications Framework Level 7 or higher, accredited by their relevant national accreditation body;
- Clearly articulated national entry level competency standards and assessment procedures;
- A defined core scope of practice and;
- Robust and enforceable regulatory mechanisms.

With allied health professions working within the profession who;

- Are autonomous practitioners;
- Practice in an evidence-based paradigm using an internationally recognised body of knowledge to protect, restore and maintain optimal physical, sensory, psychological, cognitive, social and cultural function;
- May utilise or supervise assistants, technicians and support workers (AHPA).

In Australia, allied health account for 18% of the overall health workforce, greater than GPs and medical specialists (10%), but less than nursing (35%), and provide over 200 million services annually to improve the quality of life and/or life expectancy of consumers (Allied Health Professionals Australia, 2013). In Victoria, Australia, Allied Health includes 27 different professions with over 42,500 practitioners (Victorian State Government, n. d.) that are broken into two categories of Therapy and Science disciplines.

The therapy disciplines include; Allied Health Assistant, Art therapy, Chiropractry, Dietetics, Exercise Physiology, Music Therapy, Occupational Therapy, Oral Health (not dentistry), Osteopathy, Orthotics and Prosthetics, Physiotherapy, Podiatry, Psychology, Social Work and Speech Therapy. The Science disciplines include; Audiology, Biomedical Science, Diagnostic Imaging Medical Physics, Medical Laboratory Science, Nuclear Medicine, Optometry, Orthoptics, Pharmacy, Radiation Oncology Medical Physics, Radiation Therapy, Radiography and Sonography.

Whilst there are many professions that can fall under the allied health umbrella, it is important to note that each of these are distinct professions with diverse roles (AHPF, 2013). The assortment of professions within allied health each have different training requirements, practical experience, settings and sectors of practice and varying professional governance structures, making this group of professionals highly complex. This can be problematic when viewing allied health as a single entity group.

Allied health intervention is essential for improved health, quality of life and community participation, particularly for people who experience difficulty performing activities of daily living due to cognitive, neurological and physical impairments (Wilson, Lewis, & Murray, 2009). There is now a greater need and demand for allied health intervention due to the increased importance of allied health input into the health workforce and the increase in the proportion of older people in developed countries (Dew, Veitch, Lincoln, Brentnall, Bulkeley, Gallego, . . . Griffiths, 2012; Ortman, Velkoff, & Hogan, 2014). To meet these changes, the allied health services provided and the structure of these services will need to adapt. As well as implementing new interventions and services, organisations must recognise the need to cease performing activities that are no longer deemed essential or effective (Robert, Harlock, & Williams, 2014). Health outcomes may not necessarily improve with increased intensity and volume of a health care service, instead delivery of effective services at the right time, in the right place, responsive to individual need, within available resources is required (Allied Health Professionals Australia, 2013; Posnett, 2002).

Decision Making in Allied Health

Ultimately the goal for decision makers in allied health is to ensure that allied health services are being provided in a way that is most efficient and effective in order to maximise the health and wellbeing of the communities they serve. Little has been done focusing on resource allocation decision-making by allied health managers (Department of Health Hume Region, 2011). The problem that is faced when allocating resources within allied health is that there are many different potential ways of allocating these resources. There are many different services that can be provided, by many different disciplines, in many different settings, to many different populations. All of these choices require consideration of where that resource would be best allocated. There is also a large amount of inconsistency in how the allied health workforce is structured, and in the design and delivery of services across health settings and sectors. Thus, it makes it hard for a one size fits all approach to be adopted. The varied disciplines can put forward their own perspectives of how resource decisions should be decided, however there are often discrepancies between disciplines regarding the prioritisation of the key principles (Sibbald, Singer, Upshur, & Martin, 2009).

The need has arisen for a rational methodological approach that can aid decision-makers to understand, elicit and construct their preferences across a multitude of concerns in a transparent way. It is essential allied health managers are equipped and can follow a consistent approach to manage the increasing demands placed on the service being provided and their staff members (Scottish Executive National Health System, 2006). The decision-making process should be strongly embedded in the organisational context by using transparent and systematic processes that take into account all relevant criteria and involve all relevant stakeholders, rather than focusing on discipline specific areas (Baltussen & Niessen, 2006). Such an approach could help to improve the efficiency of resource allocation decisions across the field of health care with the ultimate goal of maximising societal health and well-being.

THEORIES AND FRAMEWORKS

Distributive justice theories have typically focused on justifying health care as a special social good (Ruger, 2004). Egalitarian theories advocate that all be provided with an equal distribution of certain goods such as health care (Ruger, 2004), placing focus on what each individual receives regardless of their current health state. In an egalitarian society, there would be no advantages to anybody. Hence if a health service is offered to a certain group of individuals then, in order to be equal, the service must be offered to all individuals. To the contrary, utilitarian theories propose choosing options that maximizes the goods for the population (Daniels, 1985), thus placing focus on maximising the overall health of a population rather than focusing individuals. The concept of equality on its own does not attract much attention until focusing in on what exactly is to be equalised (Sen, 2002), or what is considered to be equitable (Lane, Sarkis, Martin & Haines, 2017).

Equity is an ethical concept grounded in principles of distributive justice (Braveman & Gruskin, 2003; Soares, 2012). Equity is based on values and has vast implications on resource allocation decisions. Conflict can arise when there are decisions to be made regarding the competition for limited resources, generally evoking strong emotions that need to be addressed and managed appropriately for the conflict to be resolved (Martin, 2015). What may seem to be equitable for an individual or group may not be equitable for another individual or group of individuals. Human rights denote internationally recognized norms applying equally to all people everywhere in the world (Braveman, 2006; Braveman & Gruskin, 2003). International human rights law has been agreed upon by governments as a set of legal standards with the purpose of upholding and protecting these rights (Braveman & Gruskin, 2003). Human rights or distributive justice principles dictate striving for equal opportunity for health for all groups, despite socioeconomic, racial, ethnic or religious differences (Braveman, 2006; Braveman & Gruskin, 2003). These principles are often summoned by decision makers to endorse choices that create winners and losers and highlight the magnitude of the broad nexus that health rests on, due to the numerous factors including economic, social, cultural and political factors that can affect a person's overall health (Gruskin & Daniels, 2008; Gruskin, Mills, & Tarantola, 2007). Principles of distributive justice or human rights instruments provide a framework and legal obligation for international policies to work towards achieving equal opportunity to be healthy (Braveman & Gruskin, 2003). Governments therefore have a responsibility to assist the populations they serve to achieve better health by creating policies and services that promote and enforce these rights (Gruskin, Mills, & Tarantola, 2007). Advances in health and human rights can be achieved by advocacy, application of legal standards, and programming (Gruskin, Mills, & Tarantola, 2007).

EQUITY AND DECISION MAKING IN HEALTHCARE

Ensuring equity in healthcare decisions is an unarguable challenge as there is no consensus on how to define and measure the concept (Boeckxstaens, De Smedt, De Maeseneer, Annemans, & Willems, 2011). Health equity as a basic principle is described as all people despite race/ethnicity, gender, age, religion, geographic location, or sexual orientation have equal opportunity to lead healthy lives (Braveman, Kumanyika, Fielding, LaVeist, Borrell, Manderscheid, & Troutman, 2011). However, pursing health equity and equity in health care can be seen as multidimensional, involving several considerations (Culyer & Wagstaff, 1993; Sen, 2002; Tsuchiya & Dolan, 2009; Whitehead, 1991). It has been defined in a number of ways with several different definitions of equity endorsed in the published literature (See Figure 3), including equity of access (Asthana, Gibson, & Halliday, 2013; Ong, Kelaher, Anderson, & Carter, 2009; Richardson, Sinha, Iezzi, & Maxwell, 2012), equity of use (Dixon, Le Grand, Henderson, Murray, & Poteliakhoff, 2007) and equity in health outcomes (Bambra, Garthwaite, & Hunter, 2014).

It is important to understand how healthcare managers and professionals use considerations of equity to guide their resource allocation decisions and ensure there are not inconsistencies in service delivery between different stakeholders resulting in different services being provided to different groups of individuals (Figure 4). For example, a program was employed in Australia to publicly subsidise some allied health services for people with chronic disease. There was no clear direction as to the principles of equitable service delivery to be applied (Foster, Mitchell, Haines, Tweedy, Cornwell & Fleming, 2008), resulting in uncertainty among allied health practitioners as to who these services should be offered to. These uncertainties lead to inconsistencies in service delivery (Haines, Foster, Cornwell, Fleming, Tweedy, Hart, & Mitchell, 2010).

Figure 3. Different definitions of equitable healthcare

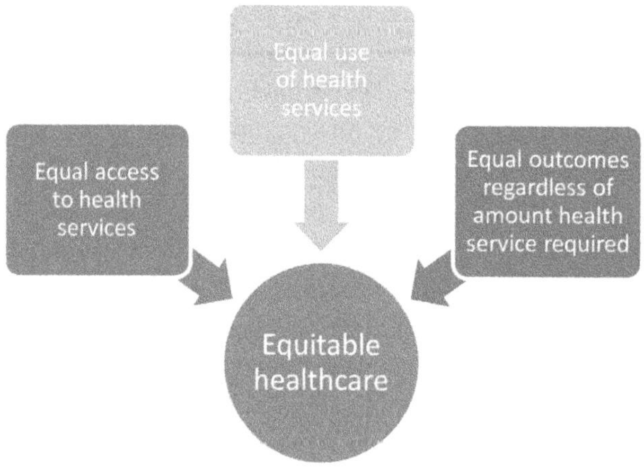

Figure 4. How the definition of equity can affect services provided

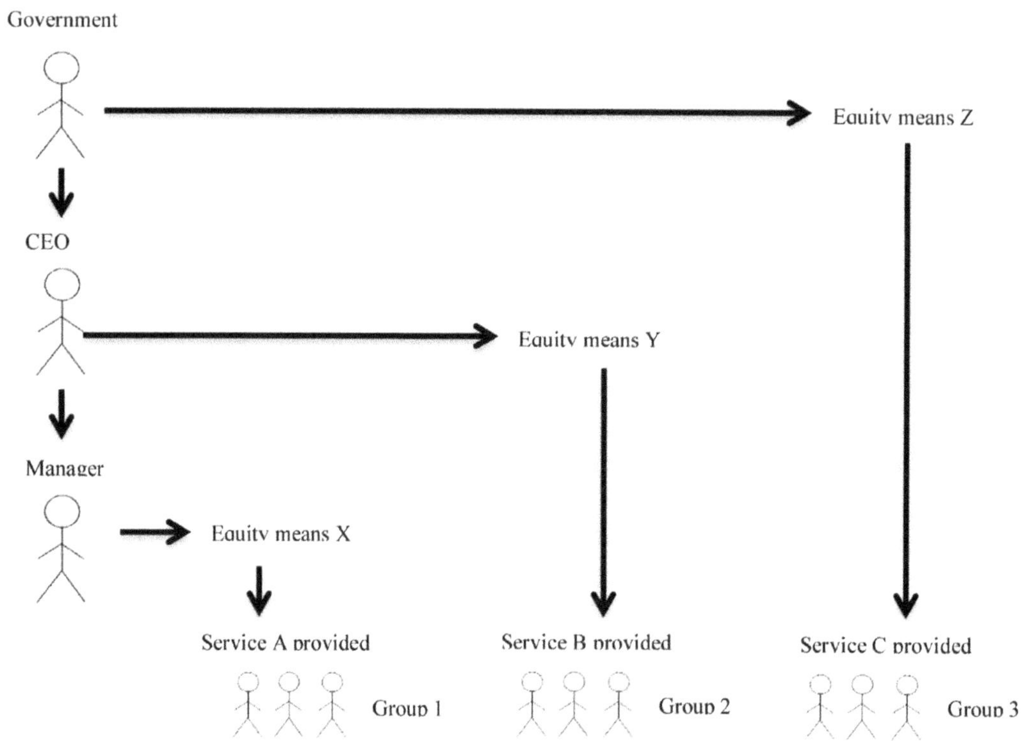

Table 2. Accountability for reasonableness (reporduced from: Daniels & Sabin, 2008)

Publicity condition	Decisions and their justifications should be transparent and made publicly accessible.
Relevance condition	The justifications of the decisions made should provide a reasonable explanation (i.e., evidence, principles, arguments) that can be agreed on and are relevant under the circumstances.
Revision condition	There should be process to revisit, revise and appeal decisions in light of further evidence or arguments.
Enforcement condition	There procedure must be either voluntary or public regulation of the process to ensure that the other three conditions are met.

ACCOUNTABILITY FOR REASONABLENESS (A4R)

Importance should be placed on the decision making process in order to assess the efficiency and fairness of the outcomes that follow (Angelis, Kanavos, & Montibeller, 2017). The Accountability for Reasonableness (A4R) (Daniels & Sabin, 2008) ethical framework has been cited to assist with this assessment (Daniels, 1999). The A4R was developed as a form of procedural justice for decision-making under resource constraints to be used as a fair and deliberative approach to decision-making (Gruskin & Daniels, 2008). This approach provides a coherent rationale highlighting key distributive justice principles (Gruskin & Daniels, 2008). It identifies four conditions of fair priority setting when making decisions within healthcare organisations, including conditions of publicity, relevance, revision and enforcement (Figure 5).

These four conditions are based on the concept that fair-minded people who are willing to cooperate should be able to agree on and justify, even when resources are constrained, the reasons for the priorities they determine necessary to meet health needs fairly (Gruskin & Daniels, 2008). As the allocation of health resources is also a political process, the application of such an ethical framework is very much needed (Angelis, Kanavos, & Montibeller, 2017). However, it is evident in areas of complex decision-making where resources are limited, that greater commitment from all parties and mechanisms to enforce decision-making are required.

SOLUTIONS, RECOMMENDATIONS AND FURTHER RESEARCH

The discussion in this chapter gives rise to a number of questions and identifies areas for further research including:

- How do allied health professionals define and apply equity when making resource allocation decisions?
- What are the published definitions and domains of equity in health care in regards to resource allocation decisions?
- How do allied health professionals conceptualize an equitable public health care system in regards to publically funded allied health resources?
- What domains of equity do allied health clinicians and managers think are more important than others in regards to publically funded allied health resources?

The responses to these questions will assist in developing solutions and recommendations for fair and equitable decision-making by allied health workers when deciding how to allocate limited resources.

CONCLUSION

Equitable decision-making is a key consideration in allied health resource allocation decision-making. The discussion in this chapter has highlighted the complexity of such decisions and the changing context within which these decisions are made. In Australia, a key consideration is the aging population and an increased demand for healthcare services that exceeds supply. Allied health managers are increasingly needing to make decisions on how to allocate limited resources fairly, efficiently and effectively. This includes decisions on whether or not a particular service continues or is no longer necessary and the introduction of new services. Decision-making occurs within government (setting the overall budget for the health system), healthcare organisations (deciding what services are provided) and by clinicians (making service delivery decisions). This chapter has highlighted the potentially ad hoc nature of allied health decision making and the lack of consistency between decision making frameworks and approaches currently available. Allied health workers are a sizeable workforce in healthcare and allied health managers need to be well-equipped to make equitable healthcare resource allocation decisions to improve the health and wellbeing outcomes of the members of the communities they serve. Effective decision-making processes are required that assist in assessing the efficacy and fairness of these health outcomes.

REFERENCES

Adams, R., Jones, A., Lefmann, S., & Sheppard, L. (2016). Service Level Decision-making in Rural Physiotherapy: Development of Conceptual Models. *Physiotherapy Research International, 21*(2), 116–126. doi:10.1002/pri.1627 PMID:25899820

Allied Health Professionals Federation. (2013). *Details of AHP Professions, their roles and Numbers.* Author.

Angelis, A., Kanavos, P., & Montibeller, G. (2017). Resource Allocation and Priority Setting in Health Care: A Multi-criteria Decision Analysis Problem of Value? *Global Policy, 8*(S2), 76–83. doi:10.1111/1758-5899.12387

Asthana, S., Gibson, A., & Halliday, J. (2013). The medicalisation of health inequalities and the English NHS: The role of resource allocation. *Health Economics, Policy, and Law, 8*(2), 167–183. doi:10.1017/S1744133112000126 PMID:22947257

Bærøe, K. (2008). Priority setting in health care: On the relation between reasonable choices on the micro-level and the macro-level. *Theoretical Medicine and Bioethics, 29*(2), 87–102. doi:10.100711017-008-9063-3 PMID:18528781

Baltussen, R., & Niessen, L. (2006). Priority setting of health interventions: The need for multi-criteria decision analysis. *Cost Effectiveness and Resource Allocation, 4*(1), 14. doi:10.1186/1478-7547-4-14 PMID:16923181

Bambra, C., Garthwaite, K., & Hunter, D. (2014). All Things Being Equal: Does it Matter for Equity How You Organize and Pay for Health Care? A Review of the International Evidence. *International Journal of Health Services, 44*(3), 457–477. doi:10.2190/HS.44.3.c PMID:25618985

Boeckxstaens, P., De Smedt, D., De Maeseneer, J., Annemans, L., & Willems, S. (2011). The equity dimension in evaluations of the quality and outcomes framework: A systematic review. *BMC Health Services Research, 11*(1), 209. doi:10.1186/1472-6963-11-209 PMID:21880136

Braveman, P. (2006). Health disparities and health equity: Concepts and measurement. *Annual Review of Public Health, 27*(1), 167–194. doi:10.1146/annurev.publhealth.27.021405.102103 PMID:16533114

Braveman, P., & Gruskin, S. (2003). Poverty, equity, human rights and health. *Bulletin of the World Health Organization*, *81*(7), 539–545. PMID:12973647

Braveman, P. A., Kumanyika, S., Fielding, J., LaVeist, T., Borrell, L. N., Manderscheid, R., & Troutman, A. (2011). Health disparities and health equity: The issue is justice. *American Journal of Public Health*, *101*(S1), S149–S155. doi:10.2105/AJPH.2010.300062 PMID:21551385

Choon, L. H., Teo, E., Choo, C. T. I., Mun, L. C., Beng, L. H., Chua, M., . . . Wong, G. (2015). Allied Health Professionals. *'Singapore's Health Care System': What 50 Years Have Achieved*, 155.

Culyer, A. J., & Wagstaff, A. (1993). Equity and equality in health and health care. *Journal of Health Economics*, *12*(4), 431–457. doi:10.1016/0167-6296(93)90004-X PMID:10131755

Daniels, N. (1985). *Just health care*. Cambridge University Press. doi:10.1017/CBO9780511624971

Daniels, N. (1999). Decisions about access to health care and accountability for reasonableness. *Journal of Urban Health*, *76*(2), 176–191. doi:10.1007/BF02344674 PMID:10924028

Daniels, N., & Sabin, J. E. (2008). *Setting limits fairly: learning to share resources for health*. Oxford University Press.

Department of Health Hume Region. (2011). *Review of HACC Allied Health Services*. Melbourne: Author. Retrieved from: http://www.health.vic.gov.au/hacc/publications/downloads/hume/allied_healthreport2011.pdf

Dew, A., Veitch, C., Lincoln, M., Brentnall, J., Bulkeley, K., Gallego, G., ... Griffiths, S. (2012). The need for new models for delivery of therapy intervention to people with a disability in rural and remote areas of Australia. *Journal of Intellectual & Developmental Disability*, *37*(1), 50–53. doi:10.3109/13668250.2011.644269 PMID:22211532

Dixon, A., Le Grand, J., Henderson, J., Murray, R., & Poteliakhoff, E. (2007). Is the British National Health Service equitable? The evidence on socioeconomic differences in utilization. *Journal of Health Services Research & Policy*, *12*(2), 104–109. doi:10.1258/135581907780279549 PMID:17407661

Emanuel, E. J. (2000). Justice and managed care: Four principles for the just allocation of health care resources. *The Hastings Center Report*, *30*(3), 8–16. doi:10.2307/3528040 PMID:10862365

Fleck, L. (2001). Healthcare justice and rational democratic deliberation. *The American Journal of Bioethics*, *1*(2), 20–21. doi:10.1162/152651601300168852 PMID:11951873

Foster, M. M., Mitchell, G., Haines, T., Tweedy, S., Cornwell, P., & Fleming, J. (2008). Does Enhanced Primary Care enhance primary care? Policy-induced dilemmas for allied health professionals. *The Medical Journal of Australia*, *188*(1), 29. PMID:18205560

Graham, I. D., Logan, J., Harrison, M. B., Straus, S. E., Tetroe, J., Caswell, W., & Robinson, N. (2006). Lost in knowledge translation: Time for a map? *The Journal of Continuing Education in the Health Professions*, *26*(1), 13–24. doi:10.1002/chp.47 PMID:16557505

Gruskin, S., & Daniels, N. (2008). Process is the point: justice and human rights: priority setting and fair deliberative process. *American Journal of Public Health*, *98*(9), 1573–1577. doi:10.2105/AJPH.2007.123182 PMID:18633088

Gruskin, S., Mills, E. J., & Tarantola, D. (2007). History, principles, and practice of health and human rights. *Lancet*, *370*(9585), 449–455. doi:10.1016/S0140-6736(07)61200-8 PMID:17679022

Haines, T. P., Foster, M. M., Cornwell, P., Fleming, J., Tweedy, S., Hart, A., & Mitchell, G. (2010). Impact of Enhanced Primary Care on equitable access to and economic efficiency of allied health services: A qualitative investigation. *Australian Health Review*, *34*(1), 30–35. doi:10.1071/AH09732 PMID:20334753

Imison, C., Sonola, L., Honeyman, M., & Ross, S. (2014). The reconfiguration of clinical services. *What is the evidence*.

Jones, D. K., Bradley, K. W., & Oberlander, J. (2014). Pascal's Wager: Health insurance exchanges, Obamacare, and the Republican dilemma. *Journal of Health Politics, Policy and Law*, *39*(1), 97–137. doi:10.1215/03616878-2395190 PMID:24193607

Klein, R. (1993). Dimensions of rationing: Who should do what? *BMJ (Clinical Research Ed.)*, *307*(6899), 309–311. doi:10.1136/bmj.307.6899.309 PMID:8374382

Klein, R., & Maybin, J. (2012). *Thinking about rationing*. King's Fund.

Lane, H., Sarkis, M., Martin, J., & Haines, T. (2017). Equity in healthcare resource allocation decision-making: A systematic review. *Social Science & Medicine*, *175*, 11–27. doi:10.1016/j.socscimed.2016.12.012 PMID:28043036

Marmot, M., Friel, S., Bell, R., Houweling, T. A., Taylor, S., & Health, C. (2008). Closing the gap in a generation: Health equity through action on the social determinants of health. *Lancet*, *372*(9650), 1661–1669. doi:10.1016/S0140-6736(08)61690-6 PMID:18994664

Martin, J. (2015). *Conflict Management*. Ginninderra Press.

Offredy, M. (1998). The application of decision making concepts by nurse practitioners in general practice. *Journal of Advanced Nursing*, *28*(5), 988–1000. doi:10.1046/j.1365-2648.1998.00823.x PMID:9840870

Ong, K. S., Kelaher, M., Anderson, I., & Carter, R. (2009). A cost-based equity weight for use in the economic evaluation of primary health care interventions: Case study of the Australian Indigenous population. *International Journal for Equity in Health*, *8*(1), 34. doi:10.1186/1475-9276-8-34 PMID:19807930

Ortman, J. M., Velkoff, V. A., & Hogan, H. (2014). *An aging nation: the older population in the United States*. United States Census Bureau, Economics and Statistics Administration, US Department of Commerce.

Parsons, W. (2002). From muddling through to muddling up-evidence based policy making and the modernisation of British Government. *Public Policy and Administration, 17*(3), 43-60.

Posnett, J. (2002). Are bigger hospitals better. *Hospitals in a changing. Europe*, 100–118.

Rawls, J. (2009). *A theory of justice*. Harvard University Press.

Richardson, J., Sinha, K., Iezzi, A., & Maxwell, A. (2012). Maximising health versus sharing: Measuring preferences for the allocation of the health budget. *Social Science & Medicine*, *75*(8), 1351–1361. doi:10.1016/j.socscimed.2012.05.036 PMID:22795915

Robert, G., Harlock, J., & Williams, I. (2014). Disentangling rhetoric and reality: An international Delphi study of factors and processes that facilitate the successful implementation of decisions to decommission healthcare services. *Implementation Science; IS*, *9*(1), 123. doi:10.118613012-014-0123-y PMID:25204900

Ruger, J. P. (2004). Health and social justice. *Lancet*, *364*(9439), 1075–1080. doi:10.1016/S0140-6736(04)17064-5 PMID:15380968

Sabik, L. M., & Lie, R. K. (2008). Priority setting in health care: Lessons from the experiences of eight countries. *International Journal for Equity in Health*, *7*(1), 4. doi:10.1186/1475-9276-7-4 PMID:18208617

Sackett, S., & Richardson, R. (2006). Evidence-based practice. *Found Evidence-Based Social Work Pract, 35*.

Scottish Executive National Health System. (2006). *Allied Health Professions: Workload Measurement and Management*. Retrieved from http://www.sehd.scot.nhs.uk/ahp/_documents/ ahpworkloadmeasureandmanage.pdf

Sen, A. (2002). Why health equity? *Health Economics*, *11*(8), 659–666. doi:10.1002/hec.762 PMID:12457367

Sibbald, S. L., Singer, P. A., Upshur, R., & Martin, D. K. (2009). Priority setting: What constitutes success? A conceptual framework for successful priority setting. *BMC Health Services Research*, *9*(1), 43. doi:10.1186/1472-6963-9-43 PMID:19265518

Soares, M. O. (2012). Is the QALY blind, deaf and dumb to equity? NICE's considerations over equity. *British Medical Bulletin*, *101*(1), 17–31. doi:10.1093/bmb/lds003 PMID:22331197

Stacey, D., Murray, M. A., Legare, F., Sandy, D., Menard, P., & O'connor, A. (2008). Decision coaching to support shared decision making: A framework, evidence, and implications for nursing practice, education, and policy. *Worldviews on Evidence-Based Nursing*, *5*(1), 25–35. doi:10.1111/j.1741-6787.2007.00108.x PMID:18266768

Thomas, W. J. (1993). The Oregon Medicaid Proposal: Ethical Paralysis, Tragic Democracy, and the Fate of a Utilitarian Health Care Program. *Oregon Law Review*, *72*, 47.

Towle, A., Godolphin, W., Greenhalgh, T., & Gambrill, J. (1999). Framework for teaching and learning informed shared decision making. *BMJ: British Medical Journal*, *319*(7212), 766–771. doi:10.1136/bmj.319.7212.766 PMID:10488010

Tsuchiya, A., & Dolan, P. (2009). Equality of what in health? Distinguishing between outcome egalitarianism and gain egalitarianism. *Health Economics*, *18*(2), 147–159. doi:10.1002/hec.1355 PMID:18484571

Turnbull, C., Grimmer-Somers, K., Kumar, S., May, E., Law, D., & Ashworth, E. (2009). Allied, scientific and complementary health professionals: A new model for Australian allied health. *Australian Health Review*, *33*(1), 27–37. doi:10.1071/AH090027 PMID:19203331

Victoria State Government. (n.d.). *Allied health therapy and science disciplines: Position Paper*. Melbourne: Health and Human Services. Retrieved from https://www2.health.vic.gov.au/about/publications/policiesandguidelines/allied-health-categories-position-paper

Whitehead, M. (1991). The concepts and principles of equity and health. *Health Promotion International*, *3*(6), 217–228. doi:10.1093/heapro/6.3.217

Wilson, R. D., Lewis, S. A., & Murray, P. K. (2009). Trends in the Rehabilitation Therapist Workforce in Underserved Areas: 1980-2000. *The Journal of Rural Health*, *25*(1), 26–32. doi:10.1111/j.1748-0361.2009.00195.x PMID:19166558

Yancey, A. K., Cole, B. L., & McCarthy, W. J. (2010). A graphical, computer-based decision-support tool to help decision makers evaluate policy options relating to physical activity. *American Journal of Preventive Medicine*, *39*(3), 273–279. doi:10.1016/j.amepre.2010.05.013 PMID:20709260

Chapter 4
Inherent Requirements and Social Work Education:
Issues of Access and Equity

Steve Boucher
RMIT University, Australia

ABSTRACT

The aim of this chapter is to contribute to addressing issues of access and equity in social work education for people with mental health disabilities. The objective is to carefully consider the introduction of inherent requirements in universities, and particularly in relation to social work education, in Australia. A targeted review of relevant literature including legislation, policy, and practice standards frameworks identifies the parameters of inherent requirements and possible areas of discrimination. Consideration of the use of inherent requirements in social work education is from a human rights social justice perspective that acknowledges the strength and resources of people and communities and actively advocates for the protection of disability rights.

INTRODUCTION

The generation of knowledge through research is not a neutral activity. What is investigated, how and by whom is intrinsically political and invites the question, what is the purpose of this inquiry? This is particularly true when it comes to studies which serve to delineate the terms on which historically oppressed groups are to be granted access to mainstream activities. As I consider literature relating to the participation of "mad" students in tertiary education I believe that it is essential for me to clearly state my own experience, position and purposes.

I am a person whose life and perspectives have been fundamentally shaped by the experience of disability, both physical and psychological. Furthermore, I have worked as an advocate within the tertiary sector and in an organisation which has encouraged me to dedicate myself to actively fighting against discrimination alongside students with disability. My approach to research comes from an originally Marxist understanding of how experience is shaped through social processes of class based oppression,

DOI: 10.4018/978-1-5225-7402-6.ch004

deepened by the application of critical disability studies to understand how the material experience of living within a 'disabled' body/mind is mediated by discourses, physical and social structures which serve to limit and marginalise the participation (and perspective) of those who deviate from a medicalised 'norm'. For me, the purpose of scholarship is to take a side and consciously work to develop tools for change.

The management of disability within the western tertiary sector is a complex and contested space (Bessant, 2012). Despite the rights of students with disabilities being protected by legislation, critical authors have noted that university practices focus on short term individualised accommodation, within existing educational practices, at the expense of change towards a more truly inclusive system (Jung, 2003; Meacham, Tandy, Giddings, Vodde, Curington, Morris, & Holliman, 2004). From a disability rights perspective, disability is tolerated on the proviso that individual students comply with institutionalised rituals and norms within a system which often considers 'it' to pose a threat to underlying academic and professional standards (Poole, Jivraj, Arslanian, Bellows, Chiasson, Hakimy, Pasini, & Reid, 2012; Price, 2011; Quinn, Wilson, MacIntyre, & Tinklin, 2009).

A growing trend with Australian universities has been to articulate statements of 'inherent requirements' in order to help programs define their standards in relation to disability (Brett, Harvey, Funston, Spicer, & Wood, 2016). To date these statements have received little critical scrutiny despite their apparently pivotal significance in drawing boundaries to inclusion (McNaught, 2013). Whether these statements will act as a platform for more inclusive practice or create further rationales for limiting the participation of students with disabilities remains to be determined.

The literature review in this chapter provides a background for an investigation into the potential impact of the statements in social work, a discipline with both a long history of managing 'unsuitable' behaviour and an active commitment to inclusive and empowering practice (Meacham, Tandy, Giddings, Vodde, Curington, Morris, & Holliman, 2004). It provides an overview of disability accommodation within the Australian university sector with a particular focus on the experience of students with depression and anxiety, amongst the most prevalent disabilities on campus, which are also often unaccommodated by disability support systems due to low disclosure rates and structural barriers to support (Markoulakis, 2014; Martin, 2010). The review concludes by examining social work's literature on professional suitability and critiques of its practices regarding mental health.

BACKGROUND

The Australian Tertiary Education Sector

The preceding three decades have been a time of significant structural change in Australian higher education (Watts, 2016). Reforms have caused an expansion in student enrolments and the number of public universities (Harvey, Burnheim, & Brett, 2016). Public providers now face direct competition from private colleges and within a globalised marketplace, for fee paying international student enrolments necessary to maintain institutional budgets in the face of reductions in government funding (Marginson, 2006). A key reform has been to link tertiary education to labour market outcomes and universities have refocused teaching away from disciplines such as liberal arts into vocational and professionally focused programs (Watts, 2016). This can add another level of regulatory complexity as programs also have to teach towards accreditation standards set by professional qualifying bodies (Harvey, Burnheim, & Brett, 2016; McNaught, 2013).

Universities are heavily regulated (Probert, 2015). Public universities' primary source of government funding are commonwealth grants through the Higher Education Support Act which are linked to enrolled student load and which require compliance with external quality frameworks, particularly the *Threshold Standards for Higher Education Providers* and the *Australian Quality Framework* which respectively set mandatory standards for facilities, staffing and administration and the educational levels of qualifications (DIISRTE, 2011; Watts, 2016).

Universities are required to meet equitable performance targets. First elaborated by the Commonwealth in *A Fair Chance for All* (1990), targeting focuses on recruitment of students with characteristics which have traditionally been underrepresented in higher education, including people with disability (Harvey, Burnheim, & Brett, 2016). This regime has succeeded in increasing both participation and completion rates for students with disability (Brett, 2014). The increased participation of these students adds another significant regulatory overlay to higher education, anti-discrimination law (Varnham & Kamvounias, 2009).

DISABILITY RIGHTS IN UNIVERSITIES

Although universities are covered by state equal opportunity legislation (Varnham & Kamvounias, 2009), government funding and service agreements stipulate compliance with the Disability Discrimination Act, 1992, (Cth) (DDA) (Urbis, 2015). Section 22 of the DDA prohibits discrimination in education, including by refusing to accept or placing unreasonable conditions on admission, denying access to benefits or services, expelling a student and/or by developing or accrediting criteria which will have these effects (DDA, 1992). The Act also applies to bodies which regulate professional qualifications (s19). The definition of 'disability' in the Act is broad and is explicitly based on a social model of disability (Howe & Duffy, 1992). Similar to disability rights legislation in other English-speaking countries, such as Britain, Canada and the United States (Harvey, Burnheim, & Brett, 2016), the foundational assumption is that discrimination occurs as the product of an interaction between an individual's impairment and social conditions ranging from policies and standardised expectations through to aspects of the built environment (Howe & Duffy, 1992). Section 6 of the DDA has the effect of requiring adjustments to be made to requirements placed on people with disability where reasonable alternatives can be identified (Australian Human Rights Commission, 2011).

A legislative instrument, the *Disability Standards for Education, 2005*, (DSE) provides detailed guidance on how the Act is to be implemented across schools, vocational education providers and universities. Standard 3 establishes processes for making adjustments and is generally considered to be the most critical standard in higher education (AHRC, 2011). There is not an automatic right for the impact of a disability to be accommodated (AHRC, 2011). Education providers must balance a number of factors, including the nature of a disability's impacts on particular requirements, the views of the affected party and the broader impact of making an adjustment including costs and benefits (DSE, 2005, Part 3). An additional significant proviso is that:

In assessing whether an adjustment to the course or program in which the student is enrolled, or proposes to be enrolled, is reasonable, the provider is entitled to maintain the academic requirements of the course or program, and other requirements or components that are inherent in or essential to its nature (DSE, 2005, 3.4(3)).

In universities, reasonable adjustments are typically recommended by specialised units located outside of academic programs (Jung, 2003; Timmerman & Mulvihill, 2015). The system requires students to provide medical documentation to verify their status as disabled and only captures students who are prepared to disclose their condition (Jung, 2003). Although common adjustments to assessment have been demonstrated to have high validity (Konur, 2002), their implementation is at the discretion of academic staff who sometimes refuse to make accommodations (Fuller, Healey, Bradley, & Hall, 2004). Studies of the system of seeking accommodations have documented that students find it time consuming and difficult to navigate (Markoulakis, 2014).

INHERENT REQUIREMENTS IN HIGHER EDUCATION

Despite a significant early judgement, W v Flinders University, which considered inherent requirements in relation to a teaching practicum (Dickson, 2012), inherent requirements in education have received very little attention in academic publications until recently (McNaught, 2013). Borrowing from principles established for considering claims of discrimination in employment, Watts and colleagues at Curtin University first enunciated a framework for Australian university programs to define inherent requirements in the year 2000. Although the term still has no universally accepted definition it is commonly understood that inherent requirements should be explicitly based on fundamental requirements for learning and practice as distinct, for instance, from the methodologies used situationally to teach or assess these requirements (Bialocerkowski, Johnson, Allan, & Phillips, 2013; Dickson, 2012).

Watts and colleagues' (2000) central arguments were that universities need to define inherent requirements in order to assist prospective students to make informed choices before enrolment and to facilitate determining which adjustments were reasonable. This position was strongly advocated by a number of universities during the 2010 and 2015 reviews of the DSE (DSERT, 2012; Urbis, 2015). The reviews found that greater clarification of the relationship between inherent requirement statements and the Standards was required with the 2015 review concluding that the application of inherent requirements in the vocational education context was inconsistent and contested (Urbis, 2015). Brett and colleagues (2016) identified the University of Melbourne as the first to publish statements across all programs but noted that these were typically brief and generic. Despite notes of concern, universities have begun to publish increasing numbers of statements (Bialocerkowski, Johnson, Allan, & Phillips, 2013). More significant to the process of developing statements was the introduction of Western Sydney University's Inherent Requirements of Nursing Education (IRONE) project in 2010-11 (McNaught, 2013). IRONE set out a detailed framework of domains for requirements which is now being applied to other health disciplines across Australia (Bialocerkowski, Johnson, Allan, & Phillips, 2013).

Brett's (2016) study is the first large scale attempt to map statements in Australian tertiary education. Conducted in 2015 its targeted search located a total of 78 unique statements. The authors noted that methodological difficulties with the search, which focussed primarily on fields of education where it was known that statements existed together with its time limited rather than longitudinal nature, meant that this figure underestimates the likely true number of statements. Statements themselves vary considerably in detail, 17 are of less than 500 words and 30 are 2000+ (p. 21). There are differing frequencies with which statements are encountered by university grouping and field of education (pp. 22-3) with the greatest prevalence being in health, where 59% of programs surveyed had a statement. In social work and community welfare the figure was 9 out of 31 or 29% of sampled programs (p. 24).

Table 1. Frequency of common domains in inherent requirement statements (reproduced from Brett, 2016)

Category	Number of inherent requirement statement including category	Percentage of inherent requirement statement including category
Verbal and non-verbal	73	93.6
Behavioural stability	66	84.6
Cognition	65	83.3
Written	52	66.7
Motor skills	51	65.4
Ethical behaviour	48	61.5
Literacy	44	56.4

While the statements show a degree of borrowing from other institutions they do not all cover the same categories. Brett provides a Table (p. 24), reproduced below, of the general categories employed to group requirements together with their frequency.

These broader categories are split into sub-domains which contain specific statements of requirements. Exemplars given by Brett (pp. 30-2) include:

Verbal and Non-Verbal Communication: *"Effective and efficient verbal communication, in English, is an essential requirement to provide safe delivery of care."*

Behavioural Stability: *"Students will be exposed to highly complex human situations and will be required to have behavioural stability to manage these events competently and professionally."*

Cognition: *"Consistent and effective knowledge and cognitive skills must be demonstrated."*

Motor Skills: *"Tasks that include fine motor skills include being able to grasp, press, push, turn, squeeze and manipulate various objects and individuals."*

Brett found that only nine statements provided information about their legal basis. None included explanatory case studies or reference to complaint processes and the rights individuals could rely on to seek accommodations (p. 25).

The lack of contextual information accompanying the individual requirements suggest that the statements will be problematic for both people with disabilities and the universities. The DSE requires that adjustments be made to requirements to avoid discrimination with universities currently providing students with adjustments such as Auslan interpreters, rest and recovery breaks in assessments and participation aids to assist with motor tasks (Konur, 2002). Performance requirements such as the manipulation of equipment falls into an additional legal dimension of adjustment; whether an institution (or future employer) has an obligation to provide modified equipment (AHRC, 2011). Such decisions require consideration of whether modifications will result in 'unreasonable hardship' by placing a strain on overall resources (Waldeck & Guthrie, 2004). That a university can undertake a greater level of expense than a small employer is uncontroversial but raises the question of how universities should manage the boundary between education and preparation for future employment (Brett, 2014; Harvey, Burnheim, & Brett, 2016).

There has been little analytical scholarship on the potential impacts of statements. In the context of a case study regarding a visually impaired physiotherapy student's participation in professional placement, the authors noted that statements of inherent requirements may have a discriminatory effect by not taking adequate account of personal factors such as a student's adaptability and resilience (Johnston, Mackintosh, Alcock, Conlon-Leard, & Manson, 2016). Noting that several of the common domains of requirements will potentially impact on the participation of students with mental health issues, McNaught (2013) questions whether the statements, in potential combination with requirements for mandatory reporting of impaired health, will deter students from disclosing these conditions to their universities.

PARTICIPATION OF STUDENTS WITH DEPRESSION AND ANXIETY

Students with mental health problems are participating in tertiary studies in increasing numbers. College counselling services in the United States have reported increases both in the number of students seeking help and the severity of their symptoms (Wyden, 2007); a trend which has been reported across English speaking countries. Although higher levels of distress in students are often reported (Larcombe, Finch, Sore, Murray, Kentish, Mulder, & Williams, 2016), these increases have been found to be reflective of broader societal trends which include the common age of onset of disorders, more widespread awareness and diagnosis and improved treatment regimens (Cvetkovski, Jorm, & Reavley, 2012; Hunt & Eisenberg, 2010; Stallman, 2010). Retrospectively analysing files from an English university counselling centre, Schwartz (2006) found that the underlying prevalence and degree of student distress was relatively stable over the period from 1992 to 2002. Exactly identifying the prevalence of mental health problems amongst students has been complicated by different studies employing different methodologies and cut off points for identifying serious levels of distress (Buchanan, 2012). If, it is accepted that the mental health of the Australian student body is reflective of that of the broader community, the yearly prevalence rate of depression alone is 11% (APS, 2012). This makes the accommodation of mood disorders is a serious issue for universities. Large scale studies of the impact of disease by the Australian Institute of Health and Welfare (2016, pp. 38-9) have estimated that mood and substance abuse disorders contribute 24% of the non-fatal burden of disease, and that the contribution of depression and anxiety is greater within the age groups traditionally entering university:

Study can be a stressful experience and students have been shown to be at heightened risk of developing depression and anxiety while at university (Hunt & Eisenberg, 2010). Students experience greater stress during first year (Cooke, Bewick, Barkham, Bradley, & Audin, 2006) and distress across their degrees

Table 2. Contribution of depression and anxiety to non-fatal burden of disease by age and gender

		Depression	Anxiety
15-24 year olds	Males	8.3%	7.1%
	Females	11%	14%
25-44 year olds	Males	8.5%	7.5%
	Females	10%	12%

with one Australian study of over 6000 students finding that 19.2% of students demonstrated clinical symptoms of anxiety and depression (Stallman, 2010). Compounding these issues are low disclosure rates and significant delays between the onset of mental health problems and treatment (El Ansari & Stock, 2011; Kessler, Olfson, & Berglund, 1998; Laidlaw, McLellan, & Ozakinci, 2015; Olfson, Kessler, Berglund, & Lin, 1998; Thompson, Hunt, & Issakidis, 2004; Wang, Berglund, Olfson, & Kessler, 2004). Although there is a generally decreasing trend over time in help-seeking delays these remain significant (Christiana, Gilman, Guardino, Mickelson, Morselli, Olfson, & Kessler, 2000).

Many students do not seek assistance from campus services (Hunt & Eisenberg, 2010; Julal, 2015; Kerns, 2013; Rosenthal & Wilson, 2008). A large-scale study of six colleges in Pennsylvania found that 73% of student in distress were not seeking help (Popple, 2013). Reasons for not seeking assistance have been linked to a lack of awareness of services and the existence of stigmas around mental illness (Laidlaw, McLellan, & Ozakinci, 2015; Lustig, Madon, Hyun, & Quinn, 2006; Rickwood, Deane, Wilson, & Ciarrochi, 2005; Thompson, Hunt, & Issakidis, 2004). Studies which spanned students and graduate practitioners in law and medicine students have confirmed the existence of high levels of perceived public stigma together with reluctance to seek help (Chew-Graham, Rogers, & Yassin, 2003; Di Stefano, 2010). More recent general scholarship has found that attitudinal factors are the primary barriers to seeking assistance (Hunt & Eisenberg, 2010). Psychological research into mental health stigma with students has tended to explore the difference between internalised feelings of shame and perceived public stigma towards the condition. Although heightened levels of concern about public stigma are reported (Eisenberg, Downs, Golberstein, & Zivin, 2009), it is commonly found that internal factors more critically influence disclosure and help-seeking decisions (Golberstein, Eisenberg, & Gollust, 2009; Hunt & Eisenberg, 2010).

Qualitative studies provide a rich insight into the lived experiences of students with mental health conditions illustrating reasons for not disclosing and experiences following disclosure. While most participants report positive experiences these are not universal (Martin, 2010; Timmerman & Mulvihill, 2015). In a meta-synthesis of existing studies of students who had disclosed Ennals, Fossey and Howie (2015) found that a common theme was of encountering difficulties negotiating appropriate support. Negotiating adjustments can be complex and time consuming for students with mental health problems (Markoulakis, 2014) and students with disability employ scripts in order to downplay their needs and avoid potential negative judgements (Barnard-Brak, Lechtenberger, & Lan, 2010; McCarthy, 2007). Participants interviewed by Andrade (2015) described frequent experiences with mental health stigma from other students, and prior to commencing study, with one respondent likening their experience to being "subjected to a hate crime" (p. 82).

These student experiences point to the ongoing presence of negative attitudes towards mental illness in the academy. Lack of exposure to students with disability has been found to be associated with negative attitudes amongst graduate students, who are frequently employed as tutors (McAllister, Wynaden, Happell, Flynn, Walters, Duggan, Byrne, Heslop, & Gaskin, 2014). Negative faculty attitudes about the participation of students with mental health problems have been reported by Thomas (2015) who found that:

- 31.5% of staff felt uncomfortable dealing with a student exhibiting mental health symptoms in the classroom;
- 12.4% did not feel secure in these circumstances, and;
- 10.9% felt that these students were dangerous.

Thomas' study was conducted in the United States of America, where portrayals of violence on campus have been reported to reinforce stereotypes by focussing on perpetrators' mental health status (Price, 2011). While Australia has lower levels of lethal violence on campus, incidents at Monash and Latrobe did lead to similar coverage and to Victorian universities adopting tribunal style processes for managing students with challenging mental health issues (Preiss, 2013).

Issues, Controversies, Problems: Social Work Students With Mental Health Problems

Social work students have been found to show elevated levels of depressive symptoms, with over 50% of students surveyed by Ting (2011) being over the cut off point for clinical levels of depression. Commenting on similar findings in social work and other caregiving professions, authors have posited that occupying such a role places professionals at higher risk for untreated distress (Pooler, 2008; Sherman, 1996; Strozier & Evans, 1998). A similar survey to Ting's in the United States by Horton, Diaz and Green (2009), found evidence of depression in 34% of respondents. Ting (2011) found that a mix of concerns about stigma, together with resource implications and a distrust of the mental health system, were contributing to low disclosure and treatment rates.

As a profession, social work influences and is influenced by mental health issues (Meacham, Tandy, Giddings, Vodde, Curington, Morris, & Holliman, 2004). Social workers play a pivotal role in mental health treatment systems and community support for underprivileged groups, including those with or at risk of mental health diagnoses (Scheyett, 2005). The profession's emphasis on the critical application of self as part of its signature process creates a situation where workers' unresolved personal difficulties can negatively affect clients (Collins, 2006; Gillis & Lewis, 2004; Watkinson & Chalmers, 2008).

In Australia, the profession employs three main devices to regulate professional conduct and the standard of graduating students; a code of conduct, accreditation standards for education programs and practice standards (AASW, 2010; AASW, 2012a; AASW, 2013). The Code of Ethics requires constructive and reflective practice and for students and professionals to seek adequate support when their performance may be impacted by personal factors, matters which may be impacted by mood disorders (AASW 2010). A search of the Education Standards and supporting documents reveals that the Association does not specify a direct requirement for programs to make adjustments for students with disability, except in the Guideline for Field Education Programs, where disability is treated an as 'extenuating circumstance' which may justify waiving the requirement for continuous five-day blocks of placement (AASW, 2012b, pp. 3-4). The lack of information about legal requirements to provide adjustments is extraordinary, given that bodies which accredit programs fall under the ambit of the DDA and DSE (Brett, 2014; DDA, 1992, S19; DSE s1.5(g)ii-iii). Social work must balance the imperative to ensure safe and effective practitioners with its historical commitments to social justice and inclusive practice without specific guidance from the professional accrediting body, the Australian Association of Social Workers (AASW), creating tensions for academics charged with responsibility for judging professional suitability (Adams, 2011; Sowbel, 2012).

The establishment of academic standards alone does not guarantee suitable graduates and significant attention has been devoted to how educators should manage issues of students' professional suitability. While some authors suggest that the primary site for gatekeeping should be within the application process (Collins, 2006; Tam & Coleman, 2009), application statements do not reliably predict future problems

(Regehr, Stalker, Jacobs, & Pelech, 2001). These difficulties are illustrated by legal action in Canada which resulted in damages against social work educators for an admission decision made on grounds of perceived suitability (Redmond & Bright, 2007). Once a student is admitted, social work programs tend to have low failure rates making the primary sites for screening out unsuitable students informal counselling and field practicums (Adams, 2011; Barlow & Coleman, 2003; Urwin, Soest, & Kretzschmar, 2006). It is logical to expect that statements of inherent requirements will be used within these processes to guide students and educators on the expected standards of the program with anecdotal reports suggesting this is happening (Adams, 2011; Elpers & FitzGerald, 2013; Mazza, 2015; McNaught, 2013).

While management of students with mental health problems is a common theme in social work's gatekeeping literature, discussion tends to be under-developed and problematic (Meacham, Tandy, Giddings, Vodde, Curington, Morris, & Holliman, 2004). It is common for articles to refer to errors with managing the impact of a student's mental health problem as a starting point for a discussion of gatekeeping issues, without providing any analysis of how shortcomings could have been addressed (Collins, 2006; Watkinson & Chalmers, 2008). When referring to legal issues, authors often devote considerable space to explaining the courts' traditional deference in matters of academic judgement without informing readers of rights and processes for making reasonable adjustments (Currer & Atherton, 2008; Wayne, 2004). Other articles report the development of gatekeeping policies without any specific discussion of disability rights (Barlow & Coleman, 2003; Urwin, Soest, & Kretzschmar, 2006). One notable exception is Valdosta State University whose social work program took the lack of clarity in the literature as a prompt for a sweeping review of their practice with students with disability (Meacham, Tandy, Giddings, Vodde, Curington, Morris, & Holliman, 2004).

Meacham commented that management of disability in practicum courses can be made more difficult by lack of knowledge and discriminatory attitudes amongst field supervisors and agencies (2004). This reflects a critique of social work by critical disability scholars and some faculty who contend that the profession has paid insufficient attention to disability rights (Dupre, 2013; Poole, Jivraj, Arslanian, Bellows, Chiasson, Hakimy, Pasini,& Reid, 2012). Acrey (2004) has documented social work scholarship's focus on medicalised models of mental health at the expense of empowerment and Scheyett (2005) notes that social work has made little contribution to the discussion of mental health stigma. Drawing these themes together, authors have begun to call for the discipline to thoroughly review its approach to mental health (Meekosha & Dowse, 2007; Poole, Jivraj, Arslanian, Bellows, Chiasson, Hakimy, Pasini,& Reid, 2012; Reid & Poole, 2013).

Social work has a significant role in mental health services and its current students have been demonstrated to have heightened risk of experiencing these problems. It has been the subject of justifiable criticism for its uncritical approach to the education and inclusion of students with mental health conditions. While professional standards apply these do not specifically address students with disability's rights. The discipline has a strong interest in screening out potentially unsuitable students and its approach to articulating inherent requirements will directly shape this practice. How social work programs frame their statements in regard to common hidden disabilities is therefore a critical issue for its currently enrolled students and requires further investigation.

SOLUTIONS AND RECOMMENDATIONS

Social work academy and professional accreditation bodies need to focus on the personal and political aspects related to inherent requirements. Disability rights are inherent in social work mission statements on social justice and human rights and this includes the disability rights of prospective and current social work students. Prejudicial, often covert, attitudes and practices of academic staff regarding 'personal views on suitability for social work practice' need to be openly named – for discriminatory practices to be addressed so that students feel safe in the knowledge they will be provided with appropriate adjustments in a supportive and non-judgmental environment. Open discussion is required amongst social workers on what is a very contentious topic with strong views on either side. However, a sign of a truly mature profession is in its ability to engage with and openly discuss controversial topics particularly where issues of human rights and discrimination are involved. Education is a main facilitator of life opportunities leading to increased employment opportunities, affordable housing options and socialisation. If inherent requirements are to be adopted by universities and social work programs, it is imperative that these do not become another vehicle for discriminatory practice by social work academics and practitioners who believe that people with certain disabilities are more suited to client and not worker roles. Recent developments in the consumer movement with the co-design and co-production of mental health services, and the rapid growth of the peer mental health workforce, suggest that a focus needs to be on student's strengths and capabilities and not a narrow and limited view of disability from a deficits perspective.

FUTURE RESEARCH DIRECTIONS

Further research is required on the implementation and impacts of inherent requirements, particularly in relation to the health and human services disciplines. This includes impacts on student disclosure and help-seeking for initial entry into a degree program as well as when problems develop post enrolment. This is in relation to different mental health issues as stigma and discrimination vary according to diagnosis. Further research is required on discriminatory attitudes amongst staff and students toward students with disabilities and issues of social inclusion and exclusion in the university environment. Research that considers roles and responsibilities of universities, professional accreditation and registration bodies and practitioner communities in determining suitability for practice would be useful.

CONCLUSION

The introduction of inherent requirements in social work education requires careful consideration of the mission of social work and the personal and political aspects of the profession. Universities need to carefully consider whose responsibility it is to determine a person's suitability for enrolment to study in a particular discipline. The limits of such decisions need careful consideration. For instance, does a university simply decide on a person's capacity to effectively engage in and complete a program of study, or does this extend to deciding on a person's suitability to practice in a particular profession? Universities take a different view on this and in disciplines and countries, such as Australian social work, that do not have a professional registration body, pressure is placed on universities to be the gatekeepers for the profession. Any actions taken by universities need to uphold disability rights and to acknowledge the strengths and capabilities of students with mental health issues. Prejudicial attitudes and discriminatory practices need to be eliminated and staff held to account if students are to feel truly safe and supported and to have their rights upheld at university and in practice during field practicum.

ACKNOWLEDGMENT

This thesis was undertaken as a social work honours thesis with thanks expressed to Dr Sharlene Nipperess for her supervision.

REFERENCES

Acrey, P. L. (2004). *Social work research and disability: Does research emphasize strengths or deficits?* (Unpublished master's thesis). University of Texas, Arlington, TX.

Adams, M. P. J. (2011). *Social work field instructors' perceptions of core attributes. Implications for leadership and gatekeeping* (Unpublished doctoral dissertation). Bowling Green State University, Bowling Green, OH.

Andrade, A. (2015). *Community college students' experiences of mental-health stigma: A phenomenological study* (Unpublished doctoral dissertation). Colorado State University, Fort Collins, CO.

Australian Association of Social Workers (AASW). (2012a). *Australian Social Work Education and Accreditation Standards (ASWEAS) V1.4.* Canberra: Australian Association of Social Workers.

Australian Association of Social Workers (AASW). (2012b). *Australian Social Work Education and Accreditation Standards (ASWEAS) 2012: Guideline 1.2: Guidance on field education programs.* Canberra: Australian Association of Social Workers.

Australian Association of Social Workers (AASW). (2013). *Practice Standards.* Canberra: Australian Association of Social Workers.

Australian Human Rights Commission (AHRC). (2011). *Federal Discrimination Law - Chapter 5. The Disability Discrimination Act.* Australian Human Rights Commission. Retrieved 16 May, 2016, from https://www.humanrights.gov.au/sites/default/files/content/legal/FDL/2011/5_DDA.pdf

Australian Institute of Health and Welfare (AIHW). (2016). *Australian Burden of Disease Study: Impact and causes of illness and death in Australia 2011. Australian Burden of Disease Study Series no. 3. BOD 4.* Canberra: Australian Institute of Health and Welfare.

Australian Psychological Society (APS). (2012). *Stress and Wellbeing in Australia in 2012: A State-of-the-Nation Survey.* Melbourne: The Australian Psychological Society.

Barlow, C., & Coleman, H. (2003). Suitability for practice guidelines for students: A survey of Canadian social work programmes. *Social Work Education, 22*(2), 151–164. doi:10.1080/0261547022000058206

Barnard-Brak, L., Lechtenberger, D., & Lan, W. Y. (2010). Accommodation strategies of college students with disabilities. *Qualitative Report, 15*(2), 411.

Bessant, J. (2012). 'Measuring Up'? Assessment and students with disabilities in the modern university. *International Journal of Inclusive Education, 16*(3), 265–281. doi:10.1080/13603116.2010.489119

Bialocerkowski, A., Johnson, A., Allan, T., & Phillips, K. (2013). Development of physiotherapy inherent requirement statements–an Australian experience. *BMC Medical Education, 13*(1), 1. doi:10.1186/1472-6920-13-54 PMID:23590219

Brett, M. (2014). Equity policy and knowledge in Australian higher education. In T. Fitzgerald (Ed.), *Advancing Knowledge in Higher Education: Universities in Turbulent Times: Universities in Turbulent Times, 44*. Hershey, PA: IGI Global. doi:10.4018/978-1-4666-6202-5.ch004

Buchanan, J. L. (2012). Prevention of depression in the college student population: A review of the literature. *Archives of Psychiatric Nursing, 26*(1), 21–42. doi:10.1016/j.apnu.2011.03.003 PMID:22284078

Chew-Graham, C. A., Rogers, A., & Yassin, N. (2003). 'I wouldn't want it on my CV or their records': Medical students' experiences of help-seeking for mental health problems. *Medical Education, 37*(10), 873–880. doi:10.1046/j.1365-2923.2003.01627.x PMID:12974841

Christiana, J., Gilman, S., Guardino, M., Mickelson, K., Morselli, P., Olfson, M., & Kessler, R. (2000). Duration between onset and time of obtaining initial treatment among people with anxiety and mood disorders: An international survey of members of mental health patient advocate groups. *Psychological Medicine, 30*(03), 693–703. doi:10.1017/S0033291799002093 PMID:10883723

Collins, S. (2006). Mental health difficulties and the support needs of social work students: Dilemmas, tensions and contradictions. *Social Work Education, 25*(5), 446–460. doi:10.1080/02615470600738809

Currer, C., & Atherton, K. (2008). Suitable to remain a student social worker? Decision making in relation to termination of training. *Social Work Education, 27*(3), 279–292. doi:10.1080/02615470701381343

Cvetkovski, S., Jorm, A. F., & Reavley, N. J. (2012). The prevalence and correlates of psychological distress in Australian tertiary students compared to their community peers. *The Australian and New Zealand Journal of Psychiatry, 46*(5), 457–467. doi:10.1177/0004867411435290 PMID:22535294

Di Stefano, G. (2010). Courting the Blues: Attitudes towards depression in Australian law students and legal practitioners. *Bulletin, 32*(4), 18.

Dickson, E. (2012). The assessment of students with disabilities: The Australian law as to reasonable adjustment and academic integrity. *International Journal of Law & Education, 17*(2), 49–61.

Disability Discrimination Act, 1992 (Cwth).

Disability Standards for Education. (2005). *Attorney General*. Canberra: Author.

Disability Standards for Education Review Team (DSERT). (2012). *Report on the Review of Disability Standards for Education 2005*. Retrieved 14 May, 2016, from https://docs.education.gov.au/system/files/doc/other/report_on_the_review_of_disability_standards_for_education_2005.pdf

Dupre, M. E. (2013). *Social work education and disability: a multicase study of approaches to disability in core and specialized curricula in three Bachelor of Social Work programs* (Unpublished doctoral dissertation). University of Manitoba, Manitoba.

Eisenberg, D., Downs, M. F., Golberstein, E., & Zivin, K. (2009). Stigma and help seeking for mental health among college students. *Medical Care Research and Review*, *66*(5), 522–541. doi:10.1177/1077558709335173 PMID:19454625

El Ansari, W., Stock, C., Snelgrove, T. U. K. S. H. G. S., Hu, X., Parke, S., Davies, S., ... Mabhala, A. (2011). Feeling healthy? A survey of physical and psychological wellbeing of students from seven universities in the UK. *International Journal of Environmental Research and Public Health*, *8*(5), 1308–1323. doi:10.3390/ijerph8051308 PMID:21655121

Elpers, K., & FitzGerald, E. A. (2013). Issues and challenges in gatekeeping: A framework for implementation. *Social Work Education*, *32*(3), 286–300. doi:10.1080/02615479.2012.665867

Ennals, P., Fossey, E., & Howie, L. (2015). Postsecondary study and mental ill-health: A meta-synthesis of qualitative research exploring students' lived experiences. *Journal of Mental Health (Abingdon, England)*, *24*(2), 111–119. doi:10.3109/09638237.2015.1019052 PMID:25915818

Fuller, M., Healey, M., Bradley, A., & Hall, T. (2004). Barriers to learning: A systematic study of the experience of disabled students in one university. *Studies in Higher Education*, *29*(3), 303–318. doi:10.1080/0307507041000l682592

Gillis, H., & Lewis, J. S. (2004). Addressing the issue of psychiatric disability in social work interns: The need for a problem-solving framework. *Journal of Social Work Education*, *40*(3), 391–402. doi:10.1080/10437797.2004.10672295

Golberstein, E., Eisenberg, D., & Gollust, S. E. (2009). Perceived stigma and help-seeking behavior: Longitudinal evidence from the healthy minds study. *Psychiatric Services (Washington, D.C.)*, *60*(9), 1254–1256. doi:10.1176/ps.2009.60.9.1254 PMID:19723742

Harvey, A., Burnheim, C., & Brett, M. (2016). Towards a fairer chance for all: Revising the Australian student equity framework. In A. Harvey, C. Burnheim, & M. Brett (Eds.), *Student Equity in Australian Higher Education: Twenty-five Years of A Fair Chance for All*. Singapore: Springer. doi:10.1007/978-981-10-0315-8_1

Howe, B., & Duffy, M. (1992). *Disability Discrimination Bill, Explanatory Memorandum*. Canberra: Parliament of Australia. Retrieved 20 May, 2016, from http://www.humanrights.gov.au/disability-discrimination-bill-1992-explanatory-memorandum

Hunt, J., & Eisenberg, D. (2010). Mental health problems and help-seeking behavior among college students. *The Journal of Adolescent Health*, *46*(1), 3–10. doi:10.1016/j.jadohealth.2009.08.008 PMID:20123251

Johnston, K. N., Mackintosh, S., Alcock, M., Conlon-Leard, A., & Manson, S. (2016). Reconsidering inherent requirements: A contribution to the debate from the clinical placement experience of a physiotherapy student with vision impairment. *BMC Medical Education*, *16*(1), 74. doi:10.118612909-016-0598-0 PMID:26922499

Julal, F. S. (2015). Predictors of undergraduate students' university support service use during the first year of university. *British Journal of Guidance & Counselling*, 1–11.

Jung, K. E. (2003). Chronic illness and academic accommodation: Meeting disabled students' unique needs and preserving the institutional order of the university. *Journal of Sociology and Social Welfare*, *30*, 91.

Kerns, C. M. (2013). *The influence of social norms on attitudes toward help seeking behavior of college undergraduates at a major midwestern university* (Unpublished doctoral dissertation). Ohio University, Athens, OH.

Kessler, R. C., Olfson, M., & Berglund, P. A. (1998). Patterns and predictors of treatment contact after first onset of psychiatric disorders. *The American Journal of Psychiatry*, *155*(1), 62–69. doi:10.1176/ajp.155.1.62 PMID:9433340

Konur, O. (2002). Assessment of disabled students in higher education: Current public policy issues. *Assessment & Evaluation in Higher Education*, *27*(2), 131–152. doi:10.1080/02602930220128715

Laidlaw, A., McLellan, J., & Ozakinci, G. (2015). Understanding undergraduate student perceptions of mental health, mental well-being and help-seeking behaviour. *Studies in Higher Education*, 1–13.

Larcombe, W., Finch, S., Sore, R., Murray, C. M., Kentish, S., Mulder, R. A., & Williams, D. A. (2016). Prevalence and socio-demographic correlates of psychological distress among students at an Australian university. *Studies in Higher Education*, *41*(6), 1074–1091. doi:10.1080/03075079.2014.966072

Lustig, S., Madon, T., Hyun, J. K., & Quinn, B. C. (2006). Graduate student mental health: Needs assessment and utilization of counseling services. *Journal of College Student Development*, *47*(3), 247–266. doi:10.1353/csd.2006.0030

Marginson, S. (2006). Dynamics of national and global competition in higher education. *Higher Education*, *52*(1), 1–39. doi:10.100710734-004-7649-x

Markoulakis, R. (2014). *The social relations of accessibility: Explicating the work of accommodation for students with mental health problems in university* (Unpublished doctoral dissertation). University of Toronto, Toronto, Canada.

Martin, J. M. (2010). Stigma and student mental health in higher education. *Higher Education Research & Development*, *29*(3), 259–274. doi:10.1080/07294360903470969

Mazza, E. T. (2015). Working with students with psychiatric disabilities or other emotional problems. *Journal of Teaching in Social Work*, *35*(4), 425–448. doi:10.1080/08841233.2015.1066916

McAllister, M., Wynaden, D., Happell, B., Flynn, T., Walters, V., Duggan, R., ... Gaskin, C. (2014). Staff experiences of providing support to students who are managing mental health challenges: A qualitative study from two Australian universities. *Advances in Mental Health*, *12*(3), 192–201. doi:10.1080/18374905.2014.11081897

McCarthy, D. (2007). Teaching self-advocacy to students with disabilities. *About Campus: Enriching the Student Learning Experience*, *12*(5), 10–16. doi:10.1002/abc.225

McNaught, K. (2013). The potential impacts of 'Inherent Requirements' and 'Mandatory Professional Reporting'on students, particularly those with mental health concerns, registering with university disability support/equity services. *Journal of the Australia and New Zealand Students Services Association*, *42*, 25–29.

Meacham, M., Tandy, C., Giddings, M., Vodde, R., Curington, A., Morris, B., & Holliman, D. (2004). The thorny dilemma of gatekeeping versus inclusion for students with disabilities. *Journal of Social Work in Disability & Rehabilitation*, *3*(4), 69–88. doi:10.1300/J198v03n04_05

Meekosha, H., & Dowse, L. (2007). Integrating critical disability studies into social work education and practice: An Australian perspective. *Practice*, *19*(3), 169–183. doi:10.1080/09503150701574267

Olfson, M., Kessler, R. C., Berglund, P. A., & Lin, E. (1998). Psychiatric disorder onset and first treatment contact in the United States and Ontario. *The American Journal of Psychiatry*, *155*(10), 1415–1422. doi:10.1176/ajp.155.10.1415 PMID:9766774

Perlin, M. L. (1999). Half-wracked prejudice leaped forth: Sanism, pretextuality, and why and how mental disability law developed as it did. *Journal of Contemporary Legal Issues*, *10*(3).

Poole, J., Jivraj, T., Arslanian, A., Bellows, K., Chiasson, S., Hakimy, H., ... Reid, J. (2012). Sanism, 'mental health' and social work/education: A review and call to action. *Intersectionalities: A Global Journal of Social Work Analysis. Research, Polity, and Practice*, *1*(1), 20–36.

Preiss, B. (2013). RMIT students slam 'invasive' mental health test. *The Age*. http://www.theage.com.au/national/tertiary-education/rmit-students-slam-invasive-mental-health-test-20130624-2osy1.html

Price, M. (2011). *Mad at School: Rhetorics of Mental Disability and Academic Life*. Ann Arbor, MI: University of Michigan Press. doi:10.3998/mpub.1612837

Probert, B. (2015). *The Quality of Australia's Higher Education System: How it Might be Defined, Improved and Assured*. Canberra: Office for Learning and Teaching.

Quinn, N., Wilson, A., MacIntyre, G., & Tinklin, T. (2009). 'People look at you differently': Students' experience of mental health support within higher education. *British Journal of Guidance & Counselling*, *37*(4), 405–418. doi:10.1080/03069880903161385

Redmond, M., & Bright, E. (2007). Gatekeeping in the academy: lessons for Canadian social work educators from Young v. Bella. *Canadian Social Work Review/Revue canadienne de service social*, 167-181.

Regehr, C., Stalker, C. A., Jacobs, M., & Pelech, W. (2001). The Gatekeeper and the Wounded Healer. *The Clinical Supervisor*, *20*(1), 127–143. doi:10.1300/J001v20n01_10

Reid, J., & Poole, J. (2013). Mad students in the social work classroom? Notes from the beginnings of an inquiry. *Journal of Progressive Human Services*, *24*(3), 209–222. doi:10.1080/10428232.2013.835185

Rickwood, D., Deane, F. P., Wilson, C. J., & Ciarrochi, J. (2005). Young people's help-seeking for mental health problems. *Australian e-Journal for the Advancement of Mental Health*, *4*(3), 218–251. doi:10.5172/jamh.4.3.218

Rosenthal, B., & Wilson, W. C. (2008). Mental health services: Use and disparity among diverse college students. *Journal of American College Health*, *57*(1), 61–68. doi:10.3200/JACH.57.1.61-68 PMID:18682347

Scheyett, A. (2005). The mark of madness: Stigma, serious mental illnesses, and social work. *Social Work in Mental Health*, *3*(4), 79–97. doi:10.1300/J200v03n04_05

Schwartz, A. J. (2006). Are college students more disturbed today? Stability in the acuity and qualitative character of psychopathology of college counseling center clients: 1992-1993 through 2001-2002. *Journal of American College Health*, *54*(6), 327–337. doi:10.3200/JACH.54.6.327-337 PMID:16789648

Sowbel, L. R. (2012). Gatekeeping: Why shouldn't we be ambivalent? *Journal of Social Work Education*, *48*(1), 27–44. doi:10.5175/JSWE.2012.201000027

Stallman, H. M. (2010). Psychological distress in university students: A comparison with general population data. *Australian Psychologist*, *45*(4), 249–257. doi:10.1080/00050067.2010.482109

Tam, D., & Coleman, H. (2009). Defining criteria on professional suitability for social work practice. *The Journal of Baccalaureate Social Work*, *14*(2), 105–121.

Thomas, L. Y. (2015). *Faculty on the frontline: Faculty attitudes toward mental illness in 2-year college students* (Unpublished doctoral dissertation). Mercer University, Atlanta.

Thompson, A., Hunt, C., & Issakidis, C. (2004). Why wait? Reasons for delay and prompts to seek help for mental health problems in an Australian clinical sample. *Social Psychiatry and Psychiatric Epidemiology*, *39*(10), 810–817. doi:10.100700127-004-0816-7 PMID:15669662

Timmerman, L. C., & Mulvihill, T. M. (2015). Accommodations in the college setting: The perspectives of students living with disabilities. *Qualitative Report*, *20*(10), 1609.

Urbis. (2015). *Report on the Review of Disability Standards for Education 2005*. Retrieved 16 May, 2016 from http://auspeld.org.au/wp-content/uploads/2012/08/Report_on_the_Review_of_DSE.pdf

Urwin, C. A., Soest, D. V., & Kretzschmar, J. A. (2006). Key principles for developing gatekeeping standards for working with students with problems. *Journal of Teaching in Social Work*, *26*(1-2), 163–180. doi:10.1300/J067v26n01_10

Varnham, S., & Kamvounias, P. (2009). Unfair, unlawful, or just unhappy: Issues surrounding complaints of discrimination made by students against their universities in Australia. *International Journal of Law & Education*, *14*(5).

Waldeck, E., & Guthrie, R. (2004). *Disability Discrimination in Education and the Defence of Unjustifiable Hardship*. School of Business Law, Curtin University of Technology.

Wang, P. S., Berglund, P. A., Olfson, M., & Kessler, R. C. (2004). Delays in initial treatment contact after first onset of a mental disorder. *Health Services Research*, *39*(2), 393–416. doi:10.1111/j.1475-6773.2004.00234.x PMID:15032961

Watkinson, A. M., & Chalmers, D. (2008). Disability, professional unsuitability and the profession of social work: A case study. *Social Work Education*, *27*(5), 504–518. doi:10.1080/02615470701379974

Watts, O., Stickels, C., Fraser, C., Carroll, R., Stewart, N., & Radloff, A. (2000). *Guidelines and Procedures to assist Universities to Examine the Inherent Requirements of their Courses*. Curtin University of Technology. Retrieved 28 April, 2016, from http://www.adcet.edu.au/download/attachment/5200%E2%80%901/

Watts R. (2016). *Public Universities, Managerialism and the Value of the University*. Palgrave-McMillan.

Wayne, R. H. (2004). Legal guidelines for dismissing students because of poor performance in the field. *Journal of Social Work Education*, *40*(3), 403–414. doi:10.1080/10437797.2004.10672296

Wyden, R. G. (2007). *Administrative perceptions of mental health trends and college counseling services* (Unpublished doctoral dissertation). University of North Florida, Jacksonville, FL.

Chapter 5
Mental Health Access Issues by People of Refugee Backgrounds in Australia

Ndungi wa Mungai
Charles Sturt University, Australia

Jeanette Ninnis
Service for Treatment and Rehabilitation of Torture and Trauma Survivors, Australia

Ruth (Isobel) Bailey
Charles Sturt University, Australia

ABSTRACT

This chapter presents a critical discussion on the understanding and access of mental health services by people from diverse refugee backgrounds delivered in a Western cultural setting. Mental health services are heavily influenced by a biomedical approach, but there is a growing understanding of the importance of culture and biopsychosocial approaches. This chapter highlights some of the institutional and cultural issues that need to be addressed for the services to be effective. Practical approaches that have worked in different places are explored and critically discussed. A recovery-oriented model that recognizes that the individual is part of the community and the importance of spirituality are canvassed.

INTRODUCTION

Mental health work with migrant and refugee communities settling in developed countries like Australia is both challenging and rewarding for the wide range of professionals involved. While all the professional knowledge in mental health is important, the biggest challenges are presented by the diversity of cultures, diversity of prior experiences, settlement challenges, social and political dynamics and the negotiation of divergent worldviews. While cross-cultural mental health work would include working with a wide range of cultures, in this chapter only migrants and refugees are considered, while other cultural groups such as Indigenous people or Lesbian, Gay, Bisexual, Transgender, Queer and Inquiring (LGBTQI) are not considered except in passing where necessary.

DOI: 10.4018/978-1-5225-7402-6.ch005

Regular migrants and forced migrants including refugees, asylum seekers and undocumented migrants, have radically different issues on arriving at their destination. However, they also face similar issues such as displacement and dislocation, discrimination and a desire to rebuild disrupted lives. A study of migrants in Europe identified eight types of problems: language-based problems, lack of health insurance cover, poverty and trauma experience, lack of knowledge about services, divergent notions of diseases and treatment, unhelpful attitudes among both migrants and staff and missing medical history (Priebe, Sandhu, Dias, Gaddini, Greacen, Loannidis, … Bogic, 2011). Weiss (2015) has noted that in Switzerland migration worsens physical and mental health risks because migrants encounter cultural barriers. At the same time clinicians also experience challenges related to the complicated circumstances of their patients. Considering this is important due to the rapidly growing numbers involved in international migration. The number of international migrants globally reached 244 million in 2015, an increase of 41 per cent compared to 2000, and includes 20 million refugees (UN Sustainable Development Goals, 2016). The main direction is from developing to developed countries but there is also movement of refugees from developing to developing countries; indeed, most refugees are located in developing countries like Pakistan, Lebanon and Uganda. Turkey is the exception, as a European country with very high numbers of refugees.

In Australia, a wide range of disciplines including social workers, psychologists, nurses and psychiatrists assist patients suffering from mental health disorders. For that reason, the dynamics could be described as both multidiscipline and multicultural interaction. Experience with clients of ethnic Arabic people has shown that mental health services may be viewed by migrants with mistrust and suspicion and because of the stigma associated with mental illness, mental health services may be viewed negatively and therefore underused (Al-Krenawi & Graham, 2000). Building trust in this situation is a high priority. Defining mental illness and what is normal or abnormal varies between cultures and a cultural understanding is therefore critical in any mental health intervention (Kleinman, 1988; Weiss, 2015). Migration is stressful and migrants have been reported to be at higher risk of developing mental health disorders. Cultural factors, for example, affect the care-seeking behaviours and attitudes of older Iranian migrants in the United States (Martin, 2009). These older Iranians are reported to mistrust prescribed medication, hold a holistic view about mind body and spirit and their conceptualisation of mental health, including the language used, is at variance with that of service providers.

A recovery-oriented framework is currently supported by the government in Australia. The *National Standards for Mental Health Services* (2010) defines the principles of recovery oriented mental health practice and notes:

From the perspective of the individual with mental illness, recovery means gaining and retaining hope, understanding of one's abilities and disabilities, engagement in an active life, personal autonomy, social identity, meaning and purpose of life, and a positive sense of self. (State of Victoria Department of Health, 2013, p. 7)

Recovery is not the same as cure but rather puts the recovering person at the centre of what they want in life. The framework recognises the importance of partnerships between different professionals in supporting the recovering person to achieve their goals.

The aim of this chapter is to critically discuss the challenges of working with refugee groups experiencing mental health problems. It highlights the important role played by social workers and advocates a strength-based community development approach that forms a recovery partnership with people with refugee backgrounds. The barriers that stand in the way of such partnership such as individualism and boundaries set by codes of ethics are explored. The strength-perspective based on acceptance of the cultural worldviews of people from non-Western backgrounds are noted as important starting points.

SOCIAL WORK ROLE IN CROSS-CULTURAL MENTAL HEALTH

In the multidisciplinary care for people experiencing a mental health disorder, social work plays a fundamental role in engaging, motivating, advocating, counselling and supporting individuals, families and communities. This is consistent with the internationally agreed definition of the role of social work:

The social work profession promotes social change, problem solving in human relationships and empowerment and liberation of people to enhance wellbeing. Utilising theories of human behaviour and social systems, social work intervenes at the point where people interact with their environments. Principles of human rights and social justice are fundamental to social work. (Australian Association of Social Workers [AASW], 2010, p. 7)

Given the vulnerability of people experiencing mental health disorders, the ethical commitment to human rights and social justice is critical and all professionals are expected to operate in an ethical manner and uphold human rights. World Health Organisation (WHO) defines mental health as 'a state of wellbeing in which every individual realizes his or her own potential, can cope with normal stresses of life, can work fruitfully and productively, and be able to make a contribution to her or his community' (WHO, 2017, para. 1). This broad view is consistent with WHO constitution definition of health that is considered wellbeing and not just merely absence of disease: 'health is a state of complete physical, mental and social well-being and not merely the absence of disease or infirmity' (WHO, 2017, para. 2). These definitions show clearly that social work is philosophically well positioned to play a key role in both physical and mental health and underscores the bio-psychosocial dimensions in the ideal approach to mental health. It is well documented that in Western countries gender and power relations are rooted deeply within the dynamics of medical and mental health and are systemic in nature. Social workers often experience ethical strain in balancing the biomedical view of psychiatry against their commitment to non-hierarchical and genuinely collaborative processes, culturally informed and respectful practices and human rights perspectives (Probst, 2012). But social workers ought to develop, refine and use their collaborative skills and standpoint to bring these issues to the table in the interdisciplinary context of the medical and mental health care of migrants and refugees, rather than capitulating to or avoiding their effects. Social workers in mental health care have a responsibility to meaningfully collaborate, with integrity and a clear purpose, with other health professionals as well as other service providers and networks to ensure the wellbeing of their clients:

The purpose of practice is to promote recovery, restore individual and family wellbeing, to enhance the development of each individual's self-determination and to advance principles of social justice. (AASW, 2014)

Among the allies in achieving these goals are the cross-cultural psychiatrists who also realise the limitations of a biomedical modal in meeting the mental health needs of multicultural communities, or anyone else for that matter.

Cross-Cultural Psychiatry

Cross-cultural psychiatry is also known as transcultural psychiatry or cultural psychiatry and refers to psychiatry that is concerned with the cultural context of mental health. What is considered as 'new transcultural psychiatry' is traced back 40 years ago in the work of Arthur Kleinman (Kleinman, 1977; Krimayer, 2006). The approach demonstrated clearly the critical cultural dimension of mental health. Krimayer identifies some key features for ongoing development in transcultural psychiatry: that it is multidisciplinary and integrative and views culture as a key feature of human biological theory; psychological processes are important in understanding the individual but social factors are equally fundamental; and, local and global systems of knowledge need to be critically examined in the context of a globalizing world (Krimayer, 2006). In practical terms psychiatrists engage their migrant patients in an open way about their understanding of their problem in order to understand the meaning the problem has to the patient and how they might have approached it in their cultural setting (Weiss, 2015).

The increasing number of refugees and migrants in Western countries has renewed an interest in cross cultural and cultural psychiatry. It is considered that being able to appreciate the patient's background and develop rapport with patients and their families or communities will enhance the treatment and recovery (Bracken, Thomas, Timimi, Asen, Behr, Beuster, ... & Downer, 2012; Bracken & Thomas, 2001; Double, 2002; Wintrob, 2010). A study with Chinese migrants in Australia found that communication about mental health was hampered by lack of understanding of cultural norms and values and this affected diagnosis (Blignault, Ponzio, Rong, & Eisenbruch, 2008). Communication, however, was only one aspect affecting awareness and access to services, as stigma, quality of services and lack of trust are also factors. A focus on the social context avoids the pitfall of a narrow view of mental health and brings to the fore important but complex social problems that demand political, social and economic solutions (Krimayer, 2006).

The challenge remains then for psychiatrists and other professionals as to how they apply diagnostic tools like the DSM V to people from other cultures who may not conform to the Western formulation of mental health symptoms. How symptoms are perceived and manifested is governed by both culture and context (Fried, Bockting, Ajard, Borsboom, Amshoff, Cramer, … Carr, 2015; Krimayer, Gomez-Carrillo & Veissiére, 2017). This concept challenges the notion of a universal human biology and argues for an understanding of the dynamic interaction between culture and biology. Simply adding the extra observed symptoms to a diagnostic manual is not considered good enough, as a completely different approach is called for:

Unfortunately, simply adding more symptoms to the ontological category does not rid the process of Western cultural bias and might make it worse by over-extending the category to include syndromes or patterns of distress that are better conceptualized in other terms. (Krimayer, Gomez-Carrillo, & Veissiére, 2017, p. 167)

A biopsychosocial approach in mental health takes into consideration the wide range of issues that contribute to wellbeing including biological and social factors. A variety of approaches then that take into consideration cultural and community factors would be preferable to a narrow focus on a specific disorder (Fried, Bockting, Ajard, Borsboom, Amshoff, Cramer, … Carr, 2015; Jordans, Tol, Komproe & de Jong, 2009; Krimayer, Gomez-Carrillo, & Veissiére, 2017). This would also be consistent with a social work approach to mental health.

COMMUNITY DEVELOPMENT AND CROSS-CULTURAL MENTAL HEALTH

The concept of individual autonomy pervades Western thinking and approaches and informs the bio-medical model of mental health. The biomedical model of mental health is the dominant approach to mental health and is based on the belief that mental disorders are brain diseases that are treatable through pharmacological interventions to correct specific biological abnormalities (Deacon, 2013). The biopsychosocial alternative is less established and regarded as not evidence-based to the same level as the biomedical or biological model. The biopsychosocial model has been in development over the last four decades and suggests that biological, psychological processes are integrated and how the processes interact is important in understanding both physical and mental health (Suls & Rothman, 2004; Wade & Halligan, 2017). That mental health involves more than chemical imbalances in the brain is gaining more acceptance in the west and hopefully moving closer to the more holistic view in traditional societies.

Traditional societies tend to view the individual as part of a larger group rather than a solitary and autonomous unit. Many non-Western communities prefer to seek solutions to mental health within the family, extended family or community rather than focusing on the individual autonomy favoured in the West. That is claimed to be the case within Arabic communities for example, where it is noted that:

Contrary to a Western therapeutic emphasis on the individual, all interventions with Arab clients need to be couched in the context of the family, extended family, community, or tribal background (Al-Krenawi & Graham, 2000, p. 13).

The African communities also identify with this communal approach as the best way to address problems faced by members of their communities. This communal approach is underpinned by the concept of Ubuntu that posits that individuals exist within a web of interconnection with others and the world and the wellness of one is dependent on the wellness of the whole (Mungai, 2017). The community development approach has been used by Foundation House trauma counsellors to address the issues of torture and trauma within the Sudanese community resettled in Melbourne (Mungai, 2014; Mitchell, Kaplan & Crowe, 2007). Kenny (2011) supports the community development approach with communities with collectivist cultures because group and individual decisions tend to be made in consultation with the group. Failure to recognise this process can be detrimental to social work intervention as well as psychiatric treatment.

The WHO comprehensive mental health action plan 2013-2020 clearly shows the broad view necessary in addressing metal health through 'six cross-cutting principles' identified as: universal health coverage, human rights, evidence-based practice, life course approach, multisectoral approach and empowerment of persons with mental disorders (WHO, 2013). This broad approach is consistent with a community development approach. Empowerment in particular aligns with a community development approach and it calls for involvement of people with mental disorders in advocacy, and all possible activities relating to research, policy and services delivery that affect them. Ife (2010) argues that community development is intricately associated with human rights and identifies seven dimensions underpinning community development as: social development, economic development, political development, cultural development, environmental development, spiritual development and survival-based development. At different times, and for different programs, these dimensions would apply rather than assuming that they would all be there in every community development program.

Mental illness is often accompanied by multiple problems including stigma and isolation. WHO (2013) points out that mental disorders put people at risk of poverty and homelessness, imprisonment and other forms of vulnerability. A community development approach would be a suitable way to address the issues of marginalisation, isolation and stigma while promoting a sense of belonging (Francis, Pulla & Goel, 2014). Communities may be people who share a common identity such as nationality, ethnicity or religion or live in a common geographical area (Kenny, 2011). Community development is therefore appropriate to address mental health disorder issues given the major implications for the lives of individuals and their families and communities. Medication alone could never address all the implicated social and biological issues adequately. Focusing on the strengths of the individual and community is regarded as the starting point in recovery and rebuilding lives that are affected by mental health disorder (Francis, Pulla, & Goel, 2014).

Community development is not the answer to all problems related to mental disorder but an important part of the response. There are people who may not identify with a particular community or even family and would prefer to be treated as individuals and that has to be respected. Communities can be wonderful and nurturing but can also be a source of stress when they impose conformity. Traditional cultures cannot be assumed by virtue of people's ethnicity as other influences including religion, education, globalisation, colonisation, migration and the media have their impact on these cultures. Experiences such as war, systematic state based violence and insecurity during refugee displacement can rupture community trust bonds and cultural norms. It has also been argued that both past and current indigenous knowledge concepts could be hard to ascertain as history is contested and the indigenous knowledge that is unaltered by modernity could be an illusion (Bar-On, 1999). The Africans, for example, have a culture that has been described as based on a triple heritage: indigenous cultures; European capitalism and religions imposed through colonialism; and, Islam imposed through jihad and evangelism (Mazrui, 1986). This diversity underscores the importance of allowing people to define themselves and the best way to work with them. Williams (2018) notes the importance of checking the relevance of culture to the issue at hand and suggests letting people determine their cultural identity and what it means to them should be standard practice.

Community Trauma

A model of healing communities after trauma suggests that linking individuals, families and communities to rediscover their resilience and collective resources, is far more effective than working with individuals. It also argues that the resilience of families and communities is inseparable and therefore the role of the worker or therapist is to assist in rekindling this connectedness that is disrupted by grief, loss, trauma and other stressors that negatively impact on individuals, families and communities. This model known as LINC and developed by Linking Human Systems LLC trains communities to help themselves:

The LINC Model as a means of extending social support systems to help empower individuals, families, and communities to bind their own wounds by leveraging their collective power to overcome adversity and sustain long-term change with minimum of time and effort on the part of outside professionals (Landau, 2007; Landau-Stanton, 1986). (Landau, 2010, p. 517)

The model has evolved from Transitional Family Therapy and focuses on strengths, rather than deficits, of families and communities. It is a whole system approach focused on change and elimination of guilt and shame while mobilising resources for the healing process. The model has been applied with good results in: Buenos Aires, Argentina in a province afflicted with violence and HIV/AIDS; in Kosovo after the war with a whole country focus on general health and mental health including trauma, grief and loss; and, a Romanian border village with child welfare, gang violence-related issues and social inequalities (Landau, 2010). The outside professionals do not impose their culture. They start by identifying the cultural strengths in the community and train and resource the local people that the communities can trust and are seen as the key to success of the programs.

True to its origin in family therapy, the LINC model is based on the importance of connection to the family and community. In Kosovo, the connection to the family and culture of origin has been found to be correlated with reduced risk-taking behaviour, sexual risk-taking and a reduction in a range of mental health disorders (Agani, Landau & Agani, 2010). Agani and colleagues (2010) found that closeness to the family, whether, emotional, physical or spiritual (shared stories), was beneficial while distance was detrimental. An effective community-wide intervention then had to involve all the systems and have the people design the content and priorities that would contribute to trauma recovery, healing and resilience.

FRIENDS AND PROFESSIONALS DILEMMA

The concept of 'professionals' can sometimes be alien to people from non-Western backgrounds who are used to seeking help from friends and relatives. It can be confusing enough in Western cultures too but in cross-cultural contexts it can be more complex. In some professions like medicine it is easier to identify the boundaries of friendship and professional relationship than in social work where establishing good rapport is critical to the helping process. In medicine, the idea of the physician as friend can be traced back to ancient Greece but the consensus now is that friendship can help in the healing process but there are also ethical, practical and institutional barriers that suggest a healing relationship is the better option (Davis, 2000). In social work the concept of setting boundaries is emphasised in codes of ethics for legal and practical reasons but there is a need to review the impact this has on social work and cross-cultural social work in particular (O'Leary, Tsui & Ruch, 2013).

It can be confusing as to where one draws the line between friendship and professional engagement with the objective to help. Summers (2010) suggests that there is a clear distinction between professional relationships and friendship. One notable distinction is that the professional has a formal legal and ethical relationship with the client while friends generally have informal relationships and could be intimate and could also involve exchanging gifts. This still does not show where the clear boundaries are, as a worker and a client could still exchange small gifts, for example. One way of understanding boundaries is considering situations where the worker may have interests that are outside the working relations and is hence considered to have 'dual relationships'. However, even that may be unavoidable in small communities where interaction between a worker and a client in multiple roles is unavoidable as the client could be the worker's child's school teacher or both worker and client sing in the church choir. The main boundary issue then would be whether there is anything harmful or illegal occurring between the worker and client:

Boundary crossings are harmful when the dual relationship has negative consequences for the social worker's client or colleague and, possibly for the social worker as well. For example, a clinical social worker who discloses to a client personal, intimate details about his or her own life, ostensibly to be helpful to the client, ultimately may confuse and compromise the client's mental health because of complicated transference issues produced by the social worker's self-disclosure. (Reamer, 2003, p. 123)

O'Leary and colleagues (2013) argue that the notion of boundaries in the social work relationship is derived from a situation that has relevance for professions such as medicine and law, but has a restrictive application for social work relationships, where aspects of the relationship share many of the qualities of friendship (Beresford, Croft, & Adshead, 2008; Doel, Allmark, Conway, Cowburn, Flynn, Nelson, & Tod, 2010). Commonly, effective social work relationships are built through the practitioner's expertise and skills in establishing connection through informal conversations and contacts. Very often, these relationships establish an atmosphere in which highly personal information and feelings are shared (O'Leary, Tsui, & Ruch, 2013). The realities and philosophy of social work practice demands connection rather than separation, mutuality rather than hierarchy, and Western conventions and understandings of a professional boundary create restrictive artificial barriers that are not in keeping with the profession's values (O'Leary, Tsui, & Ruch, 2013).

There can be no argument against avoiding anything that could be harmful to the client, if that can be predicted. The problem here is predicting the outcome as even self-disclosure could be therapeutically helpful if applied properly and could help normalise the client-worker relationship (Reamer, 2001). The literature and codes of ethics clearly suggest having an awareness of the boundaries and workers should avoid clear issues such as intimate relationships, criminal activities or other exploitative relationships (Reamer, 2003; 2001). There are also grey areas on issues such as touching, hugging, accepting gifts, accepting food or drinks and friendship after ending therapeutic relationships.

When working with clients from diverse refugee backgrounds, there are many situations where friendship is assumed or expected in the helping relationship. Many social workers are asked to be friends in real life or in social media. Food is also offered during home visits and refusal could be regarded as rude and could potentially ruin the relationship. The worker then has to consider the issues that could enhance or threaten trust. A fundamental virtue is therefore creating an environment of trust – trusting self, client, institutions and clients – and reflective practice (O'Donovan, 2000). Making an effort to understand the client's cultural expectation and the worker also explaining their expectation is one way of minimising the risk of misunderstanding. Reflection is therefore needed both at the individual level and discipline level on the ontological basis of practice in order to establish relevance to clients served by social work (Bell, 2012). Acknowledging that boundaries can become walls between social workers and clients and clarifying what the clients mean when they want to be friends with the social workers is a starting point.

To be a friend may also mean more than a personal friend to one client in a collective culture but being accepted and trusted by the community. In this situation, to reach the individual the social worker has to reach the community. This is well known by workers with Aboriginal Australians but it is also suggested as the case with ethnic Arab communities:

Individual's interests unite with those of their group of allegiance, and the general good supersedes the personal. Individual problems draw the members of the group in common pursuit of solutions. Individuals in trouble do not choose, in isolation from others among the alternative courses of action. (Al-Krenawi, 2000, p. 13)

This can make the work frustratingly slow but it is important to take the time to understand what works best for the individual client and the community. It is equally important to bear in mind the diversity between and within ethnic communities and even within one family. Factors like age, education, religion, acculturation, size of the community, gender and migration status have significant impact on the culture of origin. Recognising this heterogeneity is important to avoid oppression through stereotyping and generalising:

The practitioner's lens must be clear to recognise heterogeneity among groups, patterns that may be responses to years of indifference or oppression, and other underlying factors that impact perceptions. It is through the sensitivity of the ethnic lens that barriers associated with ethnicity can be removed. (Cox & Ephross, 1998, p. 158)

Appreciating the common issues faced by ethnic groups and at the same time taking time to understand the specific individuals and communities with their particular lived experience, background, history and culture, makes for effective practice. This is achieved through respect and genuine curiosity. In addition, the principles of inclusion, participation and building credibility and trust between the worker and the client as well as the community and institutions.

The ideal to the question of friendship or professionalism remains ambiguous in social work and other professional codes of ethics. Schiele (1996) suggests, from an Afrocentric perspective, to do away with boundaries between the helper and the helped and practice engaged relationships for an emotional, trusting and transformative connection. This radical approach assumes that the worker identifies with the client's problem and collaborates to find a solution as equal interested parties.

Challenges of Serving Own Community

There is not much literature on social workers working in their own ethnic communities. There can be both advantages and disadvantages. Cox and Ephross (1998) suggest that families with ethnic identities may prefer workers from their own ethnic group but competence may be valued more and, at the other extreme, members of the same ethnicity may be mistrusted. Ethnicity alone is clearly not enough for one to be accepted. However, for those who are accepted and can be regarded as part of the community they can be integral part of their community's endeavours at self-help in addressing a wide range of issues such as mental health and housing. This is articulated in the Afrocentric paradigm that notes that:

Black self-help from an Afrocentric perspective is politically and economically necessary to guard African Americans against both the planned and capricious forces of continued racism and Eurocentric oppression (Karenga, 1993; Shujaa, 1994; Wilson, 1993). (Schiele, 2000, p. 148).

There is therefore a need to decolonise social work and therapeutic practices so that non-European clients are not seen through Eurocentric perspectives. Akinyela (2014) calls for cultural democracy in therapeutic work. That means moving beyond multiculturalism and inclusion to actually having knowledge produced by non-Western cultural groups. Attempting to fit non-Western cultural groups into therapies produced within a Eurocentric worldview only entrenches the domination over the 'other'. What is needed, then, is that 'other voices are being identified as world communities speak on behalf of their own healing in their own cultural languages with their own cultural meanings' (Akinyela, 2014, p. 49).

This will mean that Indigenous healing practices from around the world can speak between themselves and with Western practices as equals and learn from each other.

Social workers use anti-oppressive practices to address oppression experienced by their clients. Anti-oppressive practice acknowledges the diverse forms of oppression within societies and the harmful effects of inequality (Connolly & Healy, 2013). In this sense, social work takes a political position against oppression and rejects such oppressive practices as sexism, racism and ageism and other generalisations that lead to stereotypes and oppression. Schiele (1996) argues that while these practices raise awareness about the problems faced by minority groups, they fall short of embracing their worldview and cultural values.

THE ROLE OF CULTURAL RITUALS AND DANCES IN HEALING

The biological basis of mental health problems like depression are well understood in the Western cultures and the treatments that include both medication and counselling are well-established. How other cultures understand and treat depression is far less understood. Solomon (2001) has reported that other cultures have different ways and the rituals and community-approach in Senegal, West Africa, are examples of the different approaches. The Senegalese, despite the Islamic faith, exhibited a belief in sprits and the role of blood rituals and communal dancing movements to exorcise the spirits that caused depression. Solomon notes that different practices were also found in Rwanda (Solomon, 2015). It was clear from the experience in Rwanda that if Western-trained practitioners did not take the cultural differences into consideration they could be ineffective or rejected in Rwanda as an informant suggested to Solomon in regard to Western therapists after the genocide:

Their practice did not involve being outside in the sun, like you're describing, which is, after all, where you begin to feel better. There was no music or drumming to get your blood flowing again when you are depressed, and you're low, and you need to have your blood flowing. There was no sense that everyone had taken the day off so that the entire community could come together to try to lift you up and bring you back to joy. There was no acknowledgment that the depression is something invasive and external that could actually be cast out of you again.

Instead they would take people one at a time into these dingy little rooms and have them sit around for an hour or so and talk about bad things that had happened to them. We had to get them to leave the country. (Solomon, 2015, p. 41)

Not all communities in Africa continue to perform these rituals as the major religions have tended to discourage cultural practices which they see as satanic and contrary to modern religions and enlightenment-inspired science. Nevertheless, it would be worthwhile checking what people's beliefs are and how they interpret the causes of their illness. It is not unusual for people to be educated, Christian or Muslim and still use traditional healers alongside Western medicine. Western practices, including medication and counselling, can play a role but they have to be adapted to the cultures of the people.

Culture as a Strength

Where people are able to reconnect with their culture, they can begin to regain their self-esteem and rediscover their strengths. Successful programs that have helped people to reconnect with their culture also help them to find their strength even after the program ends. Work with American Indian and Alaska Native (AI/AN) has demonstrated this view in a culturally grounded program that also focused on skills to address problems of substance abuse among the tribal youth (Donovan, Thomas, Sigo, Price, Lonczak, ... Bagley, 2015). This educational program grounded on cultural practices demonstrated the effectiveness of the approach to increase connection to the tribe and prevent important issues such as suicide, substance abuse and behavioural health issues:

Community-derived, culturally grounded prevention curricula represent promising practices. Integrating evidence-based components of positive youth development and tribal-specific culture, traditions, and values, the curricula have the potential of reducing substance use; increasing hope, optimism, and self-efficacy; and facilitating cultural identity. (Donovan, Thomas, Sigo, Price, Lonczak, ... Bagley, 2015, p. 67)

The challenge is taking time to work with the concerned people and identifying what is significant to them, what can be adapted to address the problem being experienced and making it work positively for the people. The canoe journey in this case was based on long traditions that people could easily identify with so the community participation, the dancing and the celebrations reconnected people to those traditions and rekindled pride in their heritage and the motivation to live better and purposeful lives.

Dance, songs and storytelling are part of the important cultural expressions that communities use to promote cohesion and explore culturally appropriate ways of healing. A good example of this is the native dance called Danza Azteca in the United States as practised by the Chicanos/Mexicans. Yañez (2014) found that the dance was a powerful means of reclaiming political space, spiritual awakening and healing from colonisation trauma that was the root cause of many mental health issues:

At its most fundamental level enacting "your culture" and promoting community cohesion is a political act because it disrupts narratives that have been essential to the nation-state and Euro-American values such as the idealization of individuality verses community well-being and the accumulation of capital and resources with little regard for communities of color, group cohesion, or spiritual wellness. (Yañez, 2014, pp. 36-37)

The role of the social worker is assisting people to identify what cultural activity would be ideal in their healing process. It is empowering for the participants to get involved in the selection of activities that work well for them and the worker can assist in accessing the resources needed and how to embed the intervention into the activities. Where people might not have a cultural identity to fall back on they could choose to have modern dances like rap or opt for sporting activities like soccer matches. These activities can go a long way in addressing issues like isolation and break the barriers between the worker and the clients. Crafts and gardening are other activities that are possible and could have other benefits like generating income or food.

Hip Hop and Rap

The health benefits of music and dance for mental health and general wellbeing are well established. A relatively new area of interest is using rap music particularly with youth who are marginalised. Rap music in therapy has been used for listening, performing, composition and improvising. Hip hop is a culture that young people identify with as their own and is particularly identified with young African Americans.

Hip hop as an urban culture evolved in the streets of the Bronx, New York, in the 1960s and early 1970s. Its roots are the oral expression traditions from Africa maintained and promoted by poor black youth but has since become part of a popular global youth urban culture and a visible subset of it is rap music (Price, 2006). Rap represents a powerful form of storytelling. Its power arises from the Bantu notion of Nommo, the African belief in the power of the spoken word to change and reconstruct reality. Stories are formed by reality and they also form and shape reality (Yancy & Hadley, 2011). Crooke and Travis (2017) note it is now being taught in mainstream universities, such as Melbourne University, as a therapeutic tool for healing when working with young people. They suggest it is important to recognise more than the profanity in some rap music and note the core of it is a struggle for social justice, peace, respect, self-esteem, community and simply a good time. There are genres that range from feminist to anti-drugs and violence and reject homophobia (Rine, 2013). In Brazil, hip hop is regarded as an artistic movement of social protest to claim recognition and social citizenship (Alves, Oliveira & Chaves, 2016). Rap music has been found to be an effective culturally specific form of therapeutic individual and group intervention with vulnerable or at-risk young people (Tyson, 2011; Yancy & Hadley, 2011).

Religion and Spirituality

Religion and spirituality are very fundamental to the way people understand the world and in particular how they understand mental health. The importance here is for social workers to pay attention to how the individual or community interpret their reality. The workers also need to have an awareness of their own religious beliefs including not having any. Minority groups, like Muslims, have experienced problems in the Western counrties and these may make them wary of the workers. There is a history of 'Christian West' and 'Muslim East' being in conflict dating back to the crusades, the holy wars between the Christians and Muslims starting about 900 years ago. But the more relevant history is the current issues with terrorism that is associated with a small but violent radical group within the Muslim faith that destroyed some buildings in America on 11 September 2011 (or 9/11):

Next to the people who lost their life [sic], Muslims were the worst sufferers of the 9/11 attack on the Twin Towers. Although some Muslim fanatics accomplished the terrible task of destroying the towers, the entire Muslim community had to suffer for this. They suffered immediately from the hate-crimes and discrimination although these were initially sporadic. Later, because of the US government's social, local and foreign policy, the Muslim community started to suffer from what can be labelled as "institutional discrimination." (Abdullah, 2015, p. 58)

What this demonstrates is that even though faith and spirituality can be regarded as personal issues, there are also political, social, identity and even economic implications. Given the implication of discrimination on oppression and mental health, workers cannot afford to ignore the role religion plays in people's lives and life-chances. Religious beliefs can also be a source of strength as conveyed in the word the Muslims use when committing to a future action, inshallah, meaning if Allah wills or God willing.

In traditional African and Eastern traditional belief systems, spirituality is not separate from mind and body or even the material world, as it is in the Western empiricist view of the world. In the Eastern traditions, everything and every aspect of life is linked to spirituality which is the web that links all beings. Religion and spirituality in African traditions is inseparable from other aspects of life such that "religion permeates into all departments of life so fully that it is not easy or possible to isolate it" (Mbiti, 1989). Spirituality in traditional societies is also linked to morality and ethics and it has been argued that in social work this can have a role in addressing problems such as mental health problems, alienation, drug use and violence (Belgrave, Cherry, Cunningham, Walwyn, Letlaka-Rennert, & Phillips, 1994; Schiele, 2000). Social workers therefore need to take these spiritual factors into consideration:

The spiritual factors for social workers will involve the notion of identity and the sense of being. There will be consideration of hope and optimism, consideration of the sense of aesthetics, consideration of the sense of purpose, understanding of religion and consideration of ontological and existential issues. The social worker ought to have a well-considered position on these issues. (Pawar & Anscombe, 2015, p. 53)

Spirituality is not emphasised in social work, but Hay (2012) suggest that it would be beneficial to have a spiritual component in the social work curriculum. Even when a social worker does not believe in the existence of a spiritual dimension, they need to understand the significance of the spirit world and its influence on the people they work with. For the people who believe in the spirit world then there could be symbolic ways of appeasing the spirits. When something is considered evil or taboo, it is considered a threat, not only to the individual but to the entire community, so some ritual cleansing is important for the stability of the community and avoidance of shame (Ekeke, 2011). The Igbo people of Nigeria, for example, had a substitute for the community in the form of an animal or a human being dragged through the polluted places in the community so they could symbolically absorb the uncleanliness, then the soiled victim is thrown away (Ikenga-Metuh, 1985).

The healing power of rituals is important for those who subscribe to it and this is consistent with the ethical basis of social work, which respects people's belief systems. Research has shown that Congolese and Somalis settled in the United States turn to traditional healers and religious leaders in times of distress before they consider accessing western mental health services (Piwowarczyk, Bishop, Yusuf, Mudymba & Raj, 2014). This in part could explain the low utilization of mental health services among different African refugee groups, despite rates of posttraumatic stress disorder that are higher than the general population (Kinzie, 2006; Piwowarczyk, Bishop, Yusuf, Mudymba, & Raj, 2014). The traditional and religious rituals approach to mental health are based on a worldview that accepts the existence of a spirit world. Complications could arise where the rituals to address mental health may contradict the laws for example, in terms of cruelty to people or animals and where the human rights of others may be impinged upon. The duty of the social workers then is to explain to the individual or community why there might be objections to their practises outside of their place of origin.

CONCLUSION

This critical review of cross-cultural social work in mental health has demonstrated the challenges that social workers and other professionals working in the field face. The authors have underlined that awareness of own culture and making effort to understand the cultural worldview of the mental health service user is important for engagement. Understanding of seemingly ordinary issues such as friendship and what that means in other cultures, may prevent misunderstanding. While codes of ethics and organisational codes of practice may have good reasons for proscribing against expression of friendship, it is important to review the implications for the helping professions.

The important aspects of culture like collective orientation and spirituality have been identified as critical in understanding why people with refugee backgrounds may not utilise services even when their symptoms suggest such services are needed. Respecting how people define their understanding of mental health is consistent with a recovery-oriented framework that the Australian government promotes. While there are inevitable generalizations in the discussion, it is important to understand the unique situations for individuals and communities and hence the importance of maintaining a genuine curiosity and an open mind at all times. There is need for research to continue informing how mental health services can be made more responsive to people from minority cultures.

REFERENCES

Abdullah, Md. A. S. (2015). Muslims in pre- and post-9/11 contexts. *International Journal of Comparative Literature & Translation Studies*, *3*(3), 52–59.

Agani, F., Landau, J., & Agani, N. (2010). Community-building before, during, and after times of trauma: The application of the LINC Model of community resilience in Kosovo. *The American Journal of Orthopsychiatry*, *80*(1), 143–149. doi:10.1111/j.1939-0025.2010.01017.x PMID:20397999

Akinyela, M. M. (2014). Narrative therapy and cultural democracy: A testimony view. *Australian and New Zealand Journal of Family Therapy*, *35*(1), 46–49. doi:10.1002/anzf.1041

Al-Krenawi, A., & Graham, J. R. (2000). Culturally sensitive social work practice with Arab clients in mental health settings. *Health & Social Work*, *25*(1), 9–22. doi:10.1093/hsw/25.1.9 PMID:10689599

Alves, H.C., de Oliveira, N.P., & Chaves, A.D. (2016). "We want to show our face, man": Hip hop helping to build identity, awareness and social participation of young people in a socially vulnerable situation. *Cadernos de Terapia ocupacional*, *24*(1), 39-52. doi: 10.4322/0104-4931.ctoAO0637

Australia Human Rights Commission (AHRC). (2010). *In our own words: African Australians: A review of human rights and social inclusion issues*. Retrieved October 20, 2017 from https://www.humanrights.gov.au/our-work/race-discrimination/projects/our-own-words-african-australians-review-human-rights-and

Australian Association of Social Workers (AASW). (2010). *Code of Ethics*. Canberra, Australia: AASW.

Australian Association of Social Workers (AASW). (2014). *Practice standards for mental health social workers*. Retrieved October 20, 2017 from https://www.aasw.asn.au/document/item/6739

Bar-On, A. (1999). Social work and the 'Missionary zeal to whip up the heathen along the path of righteousness'. *British Journal of Social Work, 29*(1), 5–26. doi:10.1093/oxfordjournals.bjsw.a011440

Belgrave, F. Z., Cherry, V. R., Cunningham, D., Walwyn, S., Letlaka-Rennert, K., & Phillips, F. (1994). The influence of Afrocentric values, self-esteem, and Black identity on drug attitudes among African American fifth graders: A preliminary study. *The Journal of Black Psychology, 20*(2), 143–156. doi:10.1177/00957984940202004

Bell, K. (2012). Towards post-conventional philosophical base for social work. *British Journal of Social Work, 42*(3), 408–423. doi:10.1093/bjsw/bcr073

Beresford, P., Croft, S., & Adshead, L. (2008). 'We don't see her as a social worker': The importance of the social worker's relationship and humanity. *British Journal of Social Work, 38*(7), 1388–1407. doi:10.1093/bjsw/bcm043

Blignault, I., Ponzio, V., Rong, Y., & Eisenbruch, M. (2008). A qualitative study of barriers to mental health services utilisation among migrants from mainland China in South East Sydney. *The International Journal of Social Psychiatry, 54*(2), 180–190. doi:10.1177/0020764007085872 PMID:18488410

Bracken, P., & Thomas, P. (2001). Postpsychiatry: A new direction for mental health. *British Medical Journal, 322*(7288), 724–727. doi:10.1136/bmj.322.7288.724 PMID:11264215

Bracken, P., Thomas, P., Timimi, S., Asen, E., Behr, G., Beuster, C., ... Downer, S. (2012). Psychiatry beyond the current paradigm. *The British Journal of Psychiatry, 201*(6), 430–434. doi:10.1192/bjp.bp.112.109447 PMID:23209088

Connolly, M., & Healy, K. (2013). Social work practice theories and frameworks. In M. Connolly & L. Harms (Eds.), *Social work: Context and Practice* (pp. 19–33). South Melbourne, Australia: OUP.

Cox, C. B., & Ephross, P. H. (1998). *Ethnicity and social work practice*. Oxford, UK: Oxford University press. doi:10.1093/acprof:oso/9780195099317.001.0001

Crooke, A., & Travis, R. (2017). *Hip Hops healing power*. Retrieved October 20 from https://pursuit.unimelb.edu.au/articles/hip-hop-s-healing-power

Curtice, M. J., & Exworthy, T. (2010). FREDA: A human rights-based approach to healthcare. *The Psychiatrist, 34*(4), 150–156. doi:10.1192/pb.bp.108.024083

Daniel Davis, F. (2000). Friendship as an ideal for the patient-physician relationship: A critique and an alternative. In D. C. Thomasma & J. L. Kissell (Eds.), *The health care professional a friend and healer: Building on the work of Edmund D. Pellegrino* (pp. 24–34). Washington, DC: Georgetown University Press.

Deacon, B. J. (2013). The biomedical model of mental disorder: A critical analysis of its validity, utility, and effects on psychotherapy research. *Clinical Psychology Review, 33*(7), 846–861. doi:10.1016/j.cpr.2012.09.007 PMID:23664634

Doel, M., Allmark, P., Conway, P., Cowburn, M., Flynn, M., Nelson, P., & Tod, A. (2010). Professional boundaries: Crossing a line or entering the shadows? *British Journal of Social Work, 40*(6), 1866–1889. doi:10.1093/bjsw/bcp106

Donovan, D. M., Thomas, L. R., Sigo, R. L. W., Price, L., Lonczak, H., ... Bagley, L. (2015). Healing of the canoe: Preliminary results of a culturally grounded intervention to prevent substance abuse and promote tribal identity for native youth in two Pacific Northwest tribe. *American Indian and Alaska Native Mental Health Research*, *22*(1), 42–76. doi:10.5820/aian.2201.2015.42 PMID:25768390

Double, D. (2002). The limits of psychiatry. *British Medical Journal*, *324*(7342), 900–904. doi:10.1136/bmj.324.7342.900 PMID:11950743

Ekeke, E. C. (2011). African traditional religion: A conceptual and philosophical analysis. *LUMINA*, 22(2). Retrieved from https://ejournals.ph/article.php?id=7341

Francis, A. P., Pulla, V., & Goel, K. (2014). Community development and mental health promotion. In K. Goel, V. Pulla, & A. P. Francis (Eds.), *Community work: Theories, experiences & challenges* (pp. 162–180). Bangalore, India: Niruta Publications.

Fried, E. J., Bockting, C., Ajard, R., Borsboom, D., Amshoff, M., Cramer, O. J., ... Carr, D. (2015). From loss to loneliness: The relationship between bereavement and depressive symptoms. *Journal of Abnormal Psychology*, *124*(2), 256–265. doi:10.1037/abn0000028 PMID:25730514

Hay, J. (2012). Considering the spiritual dimension of human life and its relevance to social work education: Social workers', educators' and students' views. *Advances in Social Work and Welfare Education*, *14*(1), 52–66.

Ife, J. (2010). *Human rights from below: Achieving rights through community development*. Cambridge, UK: Cambridge University Press.

Ikenga-Metuh, E. (1985). Ritual dirt and purification rites among the Igbo. *Journal of Religion in Africa. Religion en Afrique*, *15*(1), 3–24. doi:10.1163/157006685X00020

Jordans, M. J. D., Tol, A. W., Komproe, I. H., & de Jong, J. V. T. M. (2009). Systematic review of evidence and treatment approaches: Psychosocial and mental health care for children in war. *Child and Adolescent Mental Health*, *14*(1), 2–14. doi:10.1111/j.1475-3588.2008.00515.x

Kenny, S. (2011). *Developing communities for the future* (4th ed.). South Melbourne, Australia: Thomson.

Kessler, R. C., Gaxiola, S. A., Alonso, J., Chatterji, S., Lee, S., Ormel, J., ... Wang, P. S. (2009). The global burden of mental disorders: An update from the WHO World Mental Health (WMH) surveys. *Epidemiologia e Psichiatria Sociale*, *18*(1), 23–33. doi:10.1017/S1121189X00001421 PMID:19378696

Kinzie, J. D. (2006). Immigrants and refugees: The Psychiatric perspective. *Transcultural Psychiatry*, *43*(4), 577–591. doi:10.1177/1363461506070782 PMID:17166947

Kleinman, A. (1977). Depression, Somatization and the new cross-cultural psychiatry. *Social Science & Medicine*, *11*(1), 3–9. doi:10.1016/0037-7856(77)90138-X PMID:887955

Kleinman, A. (1988). *Rethinking psychiatry: From cultural category to personal experience, cross-cultural comparison, psychiatry, psychopathology, socioeconomic factors*. New York, NY: The Free Press.

Krimayer, L. J. (2006). Beyond the 'new cross-cultural psychiatry': Cultural biology, discursive psychology and the ironies of globalization. *Transcultural Psychiatry*, *43*(1), 126–144. doi:10.1177/1363461506061761 PMID:16671396

Krimayer, L. J., Gomez-Carrillo, A., & Veissiére, S. (2017). Culture and depression in global mental health: An ecosocial approach to the phenomenology of psychiatric disorders. *Social Science & Medicine*, *183*, 163–168. doi:10.1016/j.socscimed.2017.04.034 PMID:28478959

Landau, J. (2010). Communities that care for families: The LINC Model for enhancing individual family, and community resilience. *The American Journal of Orthopsychiatry*, *80*(4), 516–524. doi:10.1111/j.1939-0025.2010.01054.x PMID:20950292

Martin, S. S. (2009). Illness of the mind or illness of the spirit? Mental health-related conceptualization of and practices of older Iranian immigrants. *Health & Social Work*, *34*(2), 117–126. doi:10.1093/hsw/34.2.117 PMID:19425341

Mazrui, A. A. (1986). *The Africans: A triple heritage*. London, UK: Little Brown.

Mbiti, J. S. (1989). *African religions and philosophy* (2nd ed.). Johannesburg, SA: Heinemann.

Mitchell, J., Kaplan, I., & Crowe, L. (2007). Two cultures: One life. *Community Development Journal: An International Forum*, *42*(3), 282–298. doi:10.1093/cdj/bsl016

Mungai, N. W. (2014). Ubuntu approaches to working with immigrant communities. In K. Goel, V. Pulla & A.P. Francis (Eds.), Community work: Theories, experiences & challenges (pp. 214-235). Bangalore, India: Niruta Publications.

Mungai, N. W. (2017). Community development: Is it coming back? *New Community*, *15*(1-2), 57–58.

O'Donovan, L. J. (2000). A profession of trust: Reflections on a fundamental virtue. In D. C. Thomasma & J. L. Kissell (Eds.), *The health care professional a friend and healer: Building on the work of Edmund D. Pellegrino* (pp. 1–10). Washington, DC: Georgetown University Press.

O'Leary, P., Tsui, M., & Ruch, G. (2013). The boundaries of the social work relationship revisited: Towards a connected, inclusive and dynamic conceptualisation. *British Journal of Social Work*, *43*(1), 135–153. doi:10.1093/bjsw/bcr181

Pawar, M., & Anscombe, B. (2015). Reflective social work practice: Thinking, doing and being. Sydney, Australia: Cambridge.

Piwowarczyk, L., Bishop, H., Yusuf, A., Mudymba, F., & Raj, A. (2014). Congolese and Somali beliefs about mental health services. *The Journal of Nervous and Mental Disease*, *202*(3), 209–216. doi:10.1097/NMD.0000000000000087 PMID:24566506

Price, E. G. (2006). *Hip-Hop culture*. Santa Barbara, CA: ABC-CLIO.

Priebe, S., Sandhu, S., Dias, S., Gaddini, A., Greacen, T., & Loannidis, E. … Bogic, M. (2011). Good practice in health care for migrants: Views and experiences of care professionals in 16 European countries. *BMC Public Health*, *11*(187). Retrieved October 20, 2017 from https://www.ncbi.nlm.nih.gov/pmc/articles/PMC3071322/

Probst, B. (2013). "Walking the tight rope": Clinical social workers' use of diagnostic and environmental perspectives. *Clinical Social Work Journal*, *41*(2), 184–191. doi:10.100710615-012-0394-1

Reamer, F. G. (2001). *Tangled relationships: Managing boundary issues in human services*. New York, NY: Columbia University Press. doi:10.7312/ream12116

Reamer, F. G. (2003). Boundary issues in social work: Managing Dual relationships. *Social Work*, *48*(1), 121–133. doi:10.1093w/48.1.121 PMID:12564713

Rine, C. M. (2013). Therapeutic uses of rap and hip-hop. *Health & Social Work*, *38*(1), 59–62. doi:10.1093/hsw/hls061

Schiele, J. H. (1996). Afrocentricity: An emerging paradigm in social work practice. *Social Work*, *41*(3), 284–294. PMID:8936084

Schiele, J. H. (2000). *Human services and the Afrocentric paradigm*. New York, NY: Haworth Press.

Solomon, A. (2001). *The noonday demon: An anatomy of depression*. London, UK: Chatto & Windus.

Solomon, A. (2015). Notes on an exorcism. In C. Burns & A. Gopnik (Eds.), *The moth: This is a true story* (pp. 34–42). London, UK: Serpent's Tail.

State of Victoria Department of Health. (2013). *National Practice Standards for the mental health workforce*. Retrieved 04 December 2017 from http://www.health.gov.au/internet/main/publishing.nsf/Content/5D7909E82304E6D2CA257C430004E877/$File/wkstd13.pdf

Suls, J., & Rothman, A. (2004). Evolution of the biopsychosocial model: Prospects and challenges for health psychology. *Health Psychology*, *27*(2), 119–125. doi:10.1037/0278-6133.23.2.119 PMID:15008654

Summers, N. (2010). *Managing social service staff for excellence: Five keys to exceptional supervision*. Hoboken, NJ: John Wiley & Sons. doi:10.1002/9781118270004

Tyson, E. H. (2011). Hip-Hop healing: Rap music in grief therapy with an African American adolescent male. In S. Hadley & G. Yancy (Eds.), *Therapeutic uses of rap and hip hop* (pp. 293–306). New York, NY: Routledge.

United Nations Sustainable Development Goals. (2016). *244 million international migrants living abroad worldwide, new UN statistics reveal*. Retrieved October 20, 2017 from http://www.un.org/sustainabledevelopment/blog/2016/01/244-million-international-migrants-living-abroad-worldwide-new-un-statistics-reveal/

Veltre, V. J., & Hardley, S. (2011). Hip-Hop: A Hip-Hop feminist approach to music therapy with adolescent females. In S. Hadley & G. Yancy (Eds.), *Therapeutic uses of rap and hip hop* (pp. 79–98). New York, NY: Routledge.

Wade, D. T., & Halligan, P. W. (2017). The biopsychosocial model of illness: A model whose time has come. *Clinical Rehabilitation*, *31*(8), 995–1004. doi:10.1177/0269215517709890 PMID:28730890

Weiss, R. (2015). *Confronting cultural challenges for migrant healthcare in Switzerland. Independent Study Project (ISP) Collection, PAPER 2104*. Retrieved October 20, 2017 from http://digitalcollections.sit.edu/isp_collection/2104

Williams, C. (2018). Revisiting cross-cultural practice. In M. Connolly, L. Harms & J. Maidment (Eds.), Social work: Contexts and practice (pp. 64-80). South Melbourne, Australia: Oxford.

Wintrob, R. (2010, January). Cross-cultural psychiatry: Introduction. *The Psychiatric Times.*

World Health Organisation (WHO). (2013). *Mental health Action Plan.* Retrieved October 20, 2017 from http://www.who.int/mental_health/action_plan_2013/bw_version.pdf?ua=1

World Health Organisation (WHO). (2017). *Mental health: A state of well-being.* Retrieved October 20, 2017 from http://www.who.int/features/factfiles/mental_health/en/

Yancy, G., & Hadley, S. (2011). Introduction: Give 'em just one mic: Therapeutic agency of rap and hip hop. In S. Hadley & G. Yancy (Eds.), *Therapeutic uses of rap and hip hop (pp. xxiii-xlii).* New York, NY: Routledge.

Yañez, A. M. (2014). *"Think with your feet": The cultural politics of Native Dance* (Unpublished doctoral dissertation). University of California, San Diego, CA

KEY TERMS AND DEFINITIONS

Afrocentricity: This refers to scholarship on African people and people of African descent that treats them as subjects, rather than objects. African history, culture, and philosophy is put at the center while a Eurocentric approach, by contrast, would use a European lens that marginalizes the African people.

Hip Hop: Hip hop or hip-hop refers to the African American urban culture that evolved in the streets of Bronx, New York, in the 1960s and early 1970 and the practices within that culture. Rap music and its sub-genres are one component of that hip hop culture that has now spread around the world. In therapy, it is used to engage young people who identify with that culture or art form.

Nommo: *Nommo* comes from Bantu languages in Africa and represents the power of the spoken word to create harmony and balance. This is power of the spoken word suggests that language is important for the community and change and healing can be generated from speaking if it is done well.

Chapter 6
Individual Funding for People With Mental Health Issues:
Opportunities, Tensions, and Outcomes

Christina David
RMIT University, Australia

Carmel Laragy
RMIT University, Australia

Elizabeth Hudson
RMIT University, Australia

ABSTRACT

This chapter outlines the key features of individual funding programs and examines their suitability for people with mental illness. This is a contested area with some writers concerned that mental illness is different from other types of disability and unsuitable for individual funding. The recovery model and the episodic nature of mental illness are seen as conflicting with individual funding eligibility criteria for consistent and permanent disability. The counter view is that flexible individual funding is ideally suited to meeting the fluctuating needs of people with mental illness: its key principles of empowerment and self-direction being consistent with the recovery paradigm. Evidence from Australian and international studies is reviewed, suggesting that successful outcomes can be achieved if the necessary supports and resources are available to meet people's needs.

INTRODUCTION

The past four decades have seen a marked increase in individual funding models internationally and in Australia, particularly in disability and aged care. Individual funding aims to shift choice and control to people using services through flexible budgets in a services market, with the option to self-direct arrangements if preferred. This chapter explores the implications of these approaches for people with mental illness. Factors influencing choice, control and access to services will be considered, given the

DOI: 10.4018/978-1-5225-7402-6.ch006

episodic nature of mental illness and principles of the recovery paradigm. The authors consider key debates, opportunities and risks for people with mental illness and the ensuing challenges for individual funding policy, implementation, and practice. These challenges have been scrutinised in Australia as the National Disability Insurance Scheme (NDIS) rolls out and grapples with ways to respond to the needs of people with mental illness. This major reform offers important lessons for Australia and elsewhere regarding mental health service and support systems. The chapter concludes with recommendations for policy, practice and further research.

BACKGROUND

Individual funding is linked to the broader personalisation agenda in disability and aged care, seeking to promote greater choice and control for people using services in a competitive market model. Individual funding has emerged in response to the shortcomings of previous block funding models where service users were tied to one provider, restricted to services the provider offered, and did not know the budget allocated for their support. From a government's perspective, the previous model provided limited accountability for public funds, as service providers had discretion to distribute funds between running costs and participants' supports.

Individual funding was seen as a mechanism for overcoming these limitations; giving people with disability more choice and control over services, and therefore in their lives. Disability advocates, particularly from the field of physical disability, lobbied for its introduction, as did western governments interested in potential cost savings and finding a way of meeting their obligations to give rights to people living with disability (Dickinson, 2017). Individual funding was seen as a mechanism to encourage creative planning and provide a wider range of supports to meet individual needs and preferences. People with reduced decision-making capacity would be assisted by family or professionals as appropriate. Importantly, individual funding was to place the person at the centre of the decision-making process: to choose their supports and give them greater independence and improved quality of life (Alakeson, 2008; Croft & Parish, 2016).

Individual funding programs reportedly commenced in the 1960s and 1970s when parents of children with disabilities in Canada (Hutchison, Lord, & Salisbury, 2006), and Vietnam veterans with disabilities in the US (Yeandle & Ungerson, 2007) lobbied for community living. Subsequently an array of individual funding programs has emerged in disability and aged care services, with many different structures, administrative arrangements and names. Self-directed support (SDS) has emerged as the most common name being used in Scottish legislation (2013), by the United Kingdom (UK) advocacy group *In Control* (2017), and by the *Cash and Counseling* program in the US (RWJF 2010). Under the umbrella term of self-directed support, the UK has personal budgets and direct payments (Hamilton, Tew, Szymczynska, Clewett, Manthorpe, Larsen, & Pinfold, 2016). Other terms are used elsewhere with some European countries referring to 'cash-for-care' (Da Roit & Le Bihan, 2010) and Australian aged care using the term 'consumer directed care' (CDC).

These programs have core features in common despite their various names and configurations. An assessment of personal needs is undertaken, a budget is allocated to purchase services and supports, and the person has a degree of control over what is purchased. There is an important difference between programs that expect the person with individual funding to self-direct their budget by arranging their supports, employing staff and managing their accounts, and programs that offer support to assist or undertake all these tasks. The UK Direct Payments program is an example of the former, and the US *Cash & Counseling* program an example of the latter.

Much research demonstrates positive outcomes for people with mental illness in the US programs; the strongest evidence of the benefits of individual funding for this group coming from the *Cash & Counseling* program. Evidence based on randomised controlled studies with large numbers of people across 15 states showed that people could self-direct their budget with appropriate support, achieving a wide range of positive outcomes (Barczyk & Lincove, 2010; Shen, Smyer, Mohoney, Simon-Rusinowitz, Shinogle, Norstrand… del Vecchio, 2008).

Other research identifying positive outcomes includes an Australian study that looked in depth at the experience of 16 people using individualised funding who had consistent contact with managers in positive person-centred relationships. This study found there were practical and psychological benefits for consumers and that consistent support for self-direction enabled their growth and capacity to build hopeful lives (Peterson, Buchanan, & Falkmer, 2014).

In a systematic review of the international literature Laragy, Sanders, and Brophy (2015) also found positive outcomes for people with mental illness using individual funding models. These included less time in psychiatric hospitals and criminal justice settings, creative use of funding to facilitate independent living, continued education or work, more personal relationships, and improved social life. Importantly there were no adverse outcomes for participants when they were given appropriate support (Laragy, Sanders, & Brophy, 2015).

These international findings suggest that individual funding programs have the potential to give people with mental illness more choice and control. Better outcomes are achieved if adequate support for planning and management is provided and appropriate support services are available (Croft & Parish, 2016; Simon-Rusinowitz, Croft, Loughlin, & Mahoney, 2013).

Other studies have identified mixed outcomes. In particular, the National Direct Payments Survey (NDPS), a collaborative project of three UK research teams, highlights a range of challenges for mental health users as well as reports of direct payments significantly improving lives (Glasby & Littlechild, 2016). In their summary of the NDPS, Glasby and Littlechild (2016, p. 54), identify a number of barriers for people with mental illness in the program. These include:

- The underuse of advance directives (a statement which outlines the person's treatment preferences should they become unwell) to support people with episodic mental illness when planning for crisis situations;
- Limited resources to meet people's needs as care packages for mental health fail to delineate financial responsibilities between the clinical, mental health and social care sectors;
- Lack of specific mental health expertise in those providing support to people in establishing or managing direct payments.

The differences in program outcomes raises the question: do program characteristics impact on their outcomes? While this is an emerging field and more research is needed, the evidence to date suggests they do.

It has been difficult to produce a rigorous evidence base regarding the effectiveness of individual funding models because they are so diverse (Dickinson, 2017). Despite the limitations, studies have identified a range of factors that appear to impact on outcomes. An important and recurrent theme is that the way a model is implemented has an impact on the outcomes achieved (Dickinson, 2017; Laragy

& Ottmann, 2011). Evidence suggests that well designed self-directed support models, when properly implemented and resourced, have the potential to facilitate consumer control and produce better outcomes for all participants, including people with mental illness (Alakeson, 2008; Barczyk & Lincove, 2010).

Two systematic reviews have identified the following as necessary conditions to achieve positive outcomes in individual funding programs:

- Choice to participate in self-management or traditional service delivery;
- Provision of appropriate cognitive, physical and cultural supports for active participation in planning, choice making, and support co-ordination;
- Flexible and adequate funding to meet needs and goals;
- Flexible and responsive review mechanisms and processes;
- Culturally appropriate, accessible and targeted information about program policies, spending guidelines, and services;
- Culturally appropriate services;
- Support to manage administrative demands;
- Peer support;
- Organisations and staff working from an empowerment and rights-based approach;
- Adequate workforce conditions;
- Support and oversight to manage risks;
- Access to a developed market which can offer appropriate services (Dickinson, 2017; Laragy & Ottmann, 2011).

An important debate relating to the conditions in which individualised funding takes place concerns access and equity and the limits of market approaches to provide adequate social supports for marginalised and disadvantaged groups (Fawcett & Plath, 2014). In particular, there are concerns that individual funding approaches do not invest in the collective structural reforms required to address deeply embedded social inequality. There are concerns that this will reproduce disadvantage for vulnerable groups, particularly in the absence of adequate supports to engage and participate (Dodd, 2013). Related to this critique are concerns regarding 'thin' markets where services do not exist to meet diverse and complex needs (Croft & Parish, 2016). These risks are likely to be particularly high in rural and remote areas. There are concerns for marginalised groups, including those with mental illness, and those with limited social supports and/or capacity to advocate for their needs when required supports are not available (Bigby, 2013; Miller & Hayward, 2017).

Despite these debates, Australia reflects international trends in adopting individual funding as a central component of the NDIS reform. It is suggested that Australia's experience can offer key insights into the particular needs of people with mental illness and how individual funding models can best respond. The following section describes key features of the NDIS and the integration of mental health.

THE NATIONAL DISABILITY INSURANCE SCHEME

The NDIS is based on individual funding in a fee for service market based model (Productivity Commission, 2017). The scheme was introduced in trial sites around Australia in 2013, full transition began in July 2016, and by 2019 it is expected to support 456,900 people with disability, referred to as 'participants'

(NDIA 2015). The scheme has 64,000 participants identified by the NDIS as having a psychosocial disability (Joint Standing Commitee, 2017). The *NDIS Act 2013* is based on rights and principles outlined in the United Nations Convention on the Rights of Persons with Disabilities (UN General Assembly, 2007). It stipulates that participants have choice and control in the pursuit of their goals, and the planning and delivery of their supports. The legislation uses the term 'psychosocial disability' when referring to mental health issues that result in 'severe effects and social disadvantage' (Joint Standing Commitee, 2017, p. 3). The introduction of the NDIS received bi-partisan political endorsement, support from the disability and community services sectors and significant support and commitment from people with disabilities and their carers (Bonyhady, 2014). It is widely considered to be having a significant social and economic impact nationally.

Prior to the NDIS, state based disability individual funding programs offered varying levels of choice and control through different options for funds administration (Purcal, Fisher, & Laragy, 2014). Some allowed participants to hold the funds, employ their own support workers, purchase support from a wide range of sources and account for spending. Others were individual funding in name but were little different from traditional block funded services (Laragy, Fisher, Purcal, & Jenkinson, 2015).

The NDIS model of support is based on a plan being developed with a facilitator, approved and funded by NDIS administrators. The support and choice model offers participants three options for controlling and administering their individual package. These are full self-management, management through a financial intermediary, or management through the NDIA. The person's capacity and their interest in having administrative responsibility and greater choice and control determines the model used. In June 2017, 8% of NDIS participants fully self-managed; 10% partially self-managed; 13% had their plan managed by a paid service; and 68% had their plan managed by the National Disability Insurance Agency (NDIA 2017, p. 21).

Integration of Mental Health Into the NDIS

Representatives of the physical and intellectual disability sectors lobbied for reform in disability funding and services and the establishment of the NDIS. Some commentators argue that the design of the NDIS is better suited to people with a physical or intellectual disability than those with mental health problems (McGorry & Matthew, 2016; Mental Health Australia, 2016; Williams & Smith, 2014). Contentious issues include the fact that people with psychosocial disability face barriers accessing the NDIS because they do not identify as having a disability; and because the concept of permanence, a key eligibility criterion for an individual funding package, conflicts with key principles of the recovery model (Bonyhady, 2014; Brophy, Bruxner, Wilson, Cocks, Stylianou, & Mitchell, 2015; O'Halloran, 2014). Other arguments suggest that programs such as the NDIS continue to promote a biomedical model and 'categorise' people with disabilities through clinical diagnosis (Davies & Gray, 2015; Slade & Longden, 2015).

These concerns about supports and outcomes for people with mental health issues in the NDIS have been reflected in initial reviews and studies. The NDIS has commissioned an extensive evaluation and has released its *Intermediate Report* (Mavromaras, Moskos, & Mahutea, 2016). The findings are based on quantitative data and interviews in the five trial sites with participants, family members and carers (N=62), NDIS registered disability service providers (N=25), senior personnel in workforce organisations (N=15) and NDIS staff (N=46). While the quantitative and qualitative evidence indicated improvements in the choice and control NDIS participants experience and better outcomes overall, this was not the case for people with mental illness. People with mental illness and psychosocial disability reported that the portal used to communicate with the NDIS was difficult to navigate, they had less choice and control over their supports since becoming NDIS participants and some received fewer supports.

Similar findings for NDIS participants with mental illness were reported in a smaller study conducted in one of the trial sites (see Warr, Dickinson, Olney, Hargrave, Karanikolas, Kasidis, . . . Wheeler, 2017). After conducting 47 interviews with participants they reported:

- Participants with diverse needs and circumstances, including people with mental illness and those from socioeconomic disadvantaged backgrounds need more support;
- Plans are not sufficiently flexible to meet people's fluctuating needs, including people with mental illness, and 'contingency plans' are needed to purchase services, equipment and support on an ad hoc basis;
- Services were 'thin' in some areas and did not meet diverse needs, especially in rural areas;
- Rural participants spent a significant portion of their funding allocation in travelling to services;
- When participants were unable to access services listed in their plan, the item was deemed to be unnecessary and it was removed at the next review.

These findings highlight some early deficiencies in the NDIS model for supporting people with mental illness. The findings are also reflected in submissions to two public enquiries into the NDIS, both of which raised concerns about the eligibility criteria and the lack of support to engage with planning and choice. One enquiry dealt specifically with the provision of services to people with psychosocial disability (Joint Standing Commitee, 2017) while another examined Costs (Productivity Commission, 2017). Despite these early implementation issues however, reports from both enquiries agreed that the NDIS presents significant opportunities for people with mental illness if the necessary supports are provided.

TENSIONS AND DEBATES

This section reviews the experience of the NDIS transition and the international literature to better understand key debates and tensions for mental health consumers, advocates and services providers in the context of individual funding reform. Consideration is given to the principles of choice, control, access and equity and the policy and practice implications of enacting these principles for those experiencing episodic mental illness.

Choice, Control, and Episodic Mental Health

Self-directed approaches have been described by some commentators as consistent with personal recovery principles (Davies & Gray, 2015). However, there are also well documented concerns regarding the limits of market forces in promoting self-direction and equitably meeting diverse needs (Fawcett & Plath, 2014; Glendinning, 2008; Lymbery, 2014).

The recent NDIS experience shows that a range of barriers can limit choice, control, and self-direction for people with mental illness (Joint Standing Commitee, 2017). Barriers include lack of mental health expertise among those in assessment and planning roles, barriers to engaging 'hard to reach' groups, and lack of appropriate mental health services including community based early intervention supports. The evidence highlights the point that choice and control is mediated by a person's circumstances, resources and capacity to advocate for needs, comprehend complex information and navigate complex information and service systems (Dickinson, 2017; Warr, Dickinson, Olney, Hargrave, Karanikolas, Kasidis, . . . Wheeler, 2017). This has significant implications for people with episodic conditions, fluctuating needs and capacity, and those who are socially isolated.

For people with mental health issues, fluctuating conditions and unpredictable change in needs can limit capacity to engage with complex systems and manage self-direction in a services market. The evidence suggests that support planning processes and review systems often fail to respond quickly or flexibly to fluctuating needs. The Joint Standing Commitee (2017) reported that the NDIS planning approach, established at the point of entry to the scheme, failed to sufficiently build in early intervention supports to help engagement and choice making and to prevent relapse (2017). Research into the experiences of NDIS participants in the Barwon trial site also found that people with fluctuating conditions, such as those with both physical and psychosocial disabilities, had 'no scope' for a 'contingency plan to purchase services, equipment and support on an ad hoc basis' (Warr, Dickinson, Olney, Hargrave, Karanikolas, Kasidis, . . . Wheeler, 2017, p. 8).

An evaluation of the UK direct payments model also found that mental health service consumers desire more accessible contingency funding to ameliorate mental health crises, in order to maintain their choice and control (Spandler & Vick, 2006). Furthermore, the authors of this study recommended advance directives as a possible mechanism for providing greater flexibility in payments and self-directed support during crises. This evidence supports recommendations that assessment, planning and delivery choices need to be flexible, giving due regard to the implications of episodic and fluctuating conditions and changes in people's needs (Glendinning, 2008; Mitchell, Bruxner, & Brophy, 2014).

Access, Eligibility and Recovery Principles

A key debate concerns the lack of fit between recovery principles and the language of permanent disability central to NDIS eligibility requirements. Recovery has been described as a self-defined, non-linear journey involving hope, social inclusion, and fostering psychological, physical, emotional, and spiritual wellness (Anthony, 1993). It has been argued that self-direction is a key tenet of recovery and that individual funding programs provide an opportunity to put 'recovery principles into practice' (Simon-Rusinowitz, Croft, Loughlin, & Mahoney, 2013, p. 5). However, the language of permanence central to individual funding eligibility across many programs has been described as being at odds with the concept of hope central to the recovery paradigm. Related to this is the requirement for a clinical diagnosis which reflects a medicalised approach focused on symptoms rather than a personal notion of recovery (Davies & Gray, 2015; Slade & Longden, 2015).

In their literature review on mental health and the NDIS, Nicholas and Reifels (2014) examined a cross-section of Australian and international health services to determine the language used to regulate eligibility. Their findings reveal that the term 'permanent' as an eligibility requirement is used in a range of jurisdictions including Australia, New Zealand, the UK and the US, whilst terms such as 'long-term', 'indefinite duration' or 'not expected to improve' are used in Canada.

People experiencing episodic disability who shift between periods of illness and recovery do not fit standard categories; consequently, disability classification becomes problematic (Fulcher, 1989; Lightman, Vick, Herd, & Mitchell, 2009). This episodic phenomenon is proving a barrier to service access for people with psychosocial disability in the NDIS. Submissions to the Joint Standing Commitee (2017) identified that many people experiencing 'severe and functionally disabling mental ill-health' were found to be ineligible for individual funding (2017). This included young people for whom it would 'not be possible (or clinically advisable) to diagnose the illness as a "permanent" condition' (Joint Standing Commitee, 2017, p. 11). The inquiry also described the reluctance of many medical professionals to diagnose symptoms as a 'particular illness' or to assess it as 'permanent or likely to be permanent' (p.11).

The requirement for a clinical diagnosis also fails to take into account negative identity issues associated with stigma and shame. Some people experiencing mental illness avoid the association with disability as the assignation of labels can compound the effects of stigmatisation (Forrester-Jones & Barnes, 2008; Goffman, 1963). Studies have found that people with mental illness can be 'trapped in unsatisfying situations in order to avoid [mental illness] disclosure' and fear of being 'found out' (Stuart, Arboleda-Flórez, & Sartorius, 2012, p. 9). Simon-Rusinowitz et al. (2013) concluded from their literature review of self-direction in mental health that these approaches require 'a paradigm shift from the medical model of illness and disability to the more holistic recovery model' (p. 10) and that critical principles of self-determination and person-centredness are at risk if funding and support models are compromised by eligibility limitations.

A contrasting position argues that diagnosis, particularly for those with invisible disabilities such as mental illness, is an important process for appropriating supports and obtaining medical acceptance (Shakespeare, 2014).

As noted previously, the way programs are implemented is critical. In Australia, the speed of NDIS implementation has impacted on the quality of assessment and planning with implications for people with mental illness (Hallahan, 2015). Pressure to meet targets has disadvantaged those who may require more time and support in the eligibility and planning process, who are least informed about their rights within funding systems, and who are least able to navigate complex service systems and choices (Productivity Commission, 2017).

NDIS participation rates indicate early problems with eligibility for this group with 19% of those with psychosocial disability who applied being rejected. This eligibility rate was the lowest compared to other disability categories such as people with intellectual disability who had an acceptance rate of 97.5%. Furthermore, during 2016-2017, the rejection rate of people with psychosocial disability increased compared to other primary disability groups (Joint Standing Commitee, 2017, pp. 15-16).

IMPLICATIONS FOR POLICY AND PRACTICE: SOLUTIONS AND RECOMMENDATIONS

The review of the NDIS and additional evidence presented above lead to the following policy and practice implications.

Promoting Choice, Control, Access and Recovery

The principles underpinning individualised and self-directed approaches are consistent with the self-determined and highly personal nature of the recovery paradigm. However, research indicates that there is sometimes a gap between policy intentions and implementation. To ensure that people with significant mental ill-health can enjoy greater choice and control in their lives, specialised supports are required to facilitate assessment, engagement with services, and to support choice making.

Clinical and symptom based assessment and eligibility criteria can act as a barrier to service access. A clinical conception of recovery can negatively impact on service participation and progress toward recovery goals. Concerns regarding the limits of clinical diagnoses to identify eligibility and inform planning may be addressed by assessment tools which focus instead on functional capacity. The Joint Standing Commitee (2017) recommended this approach for the NDIS, suggesting the development of a validated 'fit-for-purpose' assessment tool which would better accommodate the needs of people with psychosocial disability (Rec. 4).

Building the service sector capacity and knowledge of recovery principles is also key to the successful implementation of individual funding in a mental health context. Equipping authorities, decision makers and practitioners with the appropriate professional development, supervision and tools can be an effective means of creating a shared understanding. Examples include recovery learning modules via interactive webinars and websites such as those commissioned by the NDIS (Mental Health Coordinating Council, 2017).

Primary health professionals also need to be suitably informed about mental health services to ensure they can provide timely and accurate information about funding and support options. Specialised supports need to be provided by appropriately trained staff experienced in mental health.

It is evident that people who are better resourced and who can self-advocate, or who have someone who can advocate for them, do better in individualised funding programs where supports are purchased from a services market. People already marginalised or less able to negotiate and co-ordinate their supports are likely to be further disadvantaged in this context. They require appropriate and timely information and assistance to engage and make informed choices about market based supports.

Assertive outreach designed for people with mental illness is needed to support people with mental illness who may not identify as having a disability and who therefore will not access programs like the NDIS. This approach should include face to face contact and other strategies designed to engage 'hard to reach' groups. Outreach might also be needed to engage the person's supporters and family carers who are navigating services.

Community capacity building strategies have also been identified as important in building confidence, influencing community attitudes toward disability and mental health, and increasing access, inclusion, and choice. Strong evidence supports co-design approaches to capacity building and strategies which build on the lived experience of mental health consumers (Williams & Smith, 2014).

Giving people with mental illness choice and control also relies on access to a 'thick', diverse and mature market, ready and able to provide quality and culturally appropriate services across a continuum of needs. Historically, a funding and service gap in mental health has resulted in a distinct lack of meaningful choice. Many are doubtful that market approaches will be able to address complex and fluctuating mental health needs (Gooding, 2016). Governments may need to intervene strategically in market dynamics to ensure a minimum level of service in 'thin' market areas, such as rural and remote regions which have traditionally struggled to provide adequate mental health supports.

Optimising Opportunities to Promote Recovery

The individual funding model is an enabler to recovery if properly executed with adequate supports, and when aligned with the principles of person-centredness. Assisting the person to develop a plan appropriate to their needs has been shown to be important to the success of the self-direction process. In contrast to the traditional medical model, person-centered planning focuses on strengths and capabilities, integrating family and social network supports with mental health services. A team approach with all those involved working from an empowerment and person-centred perspective has been shown to be important. With these supports people with mental illness are better able to participate in decisions regarding provider and service choices.

Because eligibility criteria requiring the demonstration of permanent disability can be in tension with recovery principles of hope and optimism, there is a strong argument for review of this language and related policy. Such review would seek to better reflect recovery principles and reduce barriers to proving eligibility (Joint Standing Commitee, 2017). The Joint Standing Committee (2017) called for a review of the NDIS Act 2013 to revise permanence as an eligibility provision and consider if the term 'psychiatric condition' is required.

Finally, there is a need for more rigorous long term research into the experiences of people with mental illness using individual funding (Webber, Treacy, Carr, Clark, & Parker, 2014). Data needs to be collected showing the numbers of people experiencing mental illness who do not identify as such, and who need assistance to seek help. This data will highlight gaps and support positive change in policy and practice.

CONCLUSION

This review has shown that there is no simple answer to the question, 'do individual funding programs result in positive outcomes for people with mental illness'? This is because programs are complex, they have various designs, they provide different levels of support, they operate in diverse contexts, and they can be implemented to different standards. It is clear that successful outcomes can be achieved for people with mental illness if programs provide the necessary support and if required services are available. It was noted that the NDIS and other programs that use 'permanent disability' as eligibility criteria need to reconsider this approach. The concept of a permanent disability is misplaced because mental illness fluctuates and people work to a recovery model. The problems identified in the research are not insurmountable; programs that provide good support achieve positive outcomes. As individual funding programs are widely used to provide supports to people with mental illness, there is an imperative to ensure that issues are resolved and the rights of people with mental illness are upheld.

REFERENCES

Alakeson, V. (2008). Self-directed care for adults with serious mental illness: The barriers to progress. *Psychiatric Services (Washington, D.C.)*, *59*(7), 792–794. doi:10.1176/ps.2008.59.7.792 PMID:18586997

Anthony, W. A. (1993). Recovery from mental illness: The guiding vision of the mental health service system in the 1990s. *Psychosocial Rehabilitation Journal*, *16*(4), 11–23. doi:10.1037/h0095655

Barczyk, A. N., & Lincove, J. A. (2010). Cash and counseling: A model for self-directed care programs to empower individuals with serious mental illnesses. *Social Work in Mental Health*, *8*(3), 209–224. doi:10.1080/15332980903405298

Bigby, C. (2013). A National Disability Insurance Scheme—challenges for social work. *Australian Social Work*, *66*(1), 1–6. doi:10.1080/0312407X.2013.771602

Bonyhady, B. (2014, Summer). Tides of change: the NDIS and its journey to transform disability support. *Newparadigm: The Australian Journal on Psychosocial Rehabilitation*, 7-9.

Brophy, L., Bruxner, A., Wilson, E., Cocks, N., Stylianou, M., & Mitchell, P. (2015). People making choices: the support needs and preferences of people with psychosocial disability: project summary. *newparadigm*, 14-15.

Croft, B., & Parish, S. (2016). Participants' assessment of the impact of behavioral health self-direction on recovery. *Community Mental Health Journal*, *52*(7), 781–792. doi:10.100710597-016-9999-0 PMID:26911369

Da Roit, B., & Le Bihan, B. (2010). Similar and yet so different: Cash-for-care in six European countries' long-term care policies. *The Milbank Quarterly*, *88*(8), 286–309. doi:10.1111/j.1468-0009.2010.00601.x PMID:20860573

Davies, K., & Gray, M. (2015). Mental health service users' aspirations for recovery: examining the gaps between what policy promises and practice delivers. *British Journal of Social Work, 45*(suppl 1), i45-i61.

Dickinson, H. (2017, September). Individual funding systems: What works? *Evidence Base*, *2017*(3), 1–18. doi:10.21307/eb-2017-003

Dodd, S. (2013). Personalisation, individualism and the politics of disablement. *Disability & Society*, *28*(2), 260–273. doi:10.1080/09687599.2012.699283

Fawcett, B., & Plath, D. (2014). A National Disability Insurance Scheme: What social work has to offer. *British Journal of Social Work*, *44*(3), 747–762. doi:10.1093/bjsw/bcs141

Forrester-Jones, R., & Barnes, A. (2008). On being a girlfriend not a patient: The quest for an acceptable identity amongst people diagnosed with a severe mental illness. *Journal of Mental Health (Abingdon, England)*, *17*(2), 153–172. doi:10.1080/09638230701498341

Fulcher, G. (1989). *Disabling policies?: a comparative approach to education, policy, and disability*. New York: Falmer Press.

Glasby, J. a., & Littlechild, R. (2016). Direct payments and personal budgets: putting personalisation into practice (3rd ed.). Bristol, UK: Policy Press.

Glendinning, C. (2008). Increasing choice and control for older and disabled people: A critical review of new developments in England. *Social Policy and Administration*, *42*(5), 451–469. doi:10.1111/j.1467-9515.2008.00617.x

Goffman, E. (1963). *Stigma: notes on the management of spoiled identity*. New York: Simon & Schuster.

Gooding, P. (2016). From deinstitutionalisation to consumer empowerment: Mental health policy, neoliberal restructuring and the closure of the 'Big bins' in Victoria. *Health Sociology Review*, *25*(1), 33–47. doi:10.1080/14461242.2015.1134261

Hallahan, L. (2015). Disability policy in Australia: A triumph of the scriptio inferior on impotence and neediness? *The Australian Journal of Social Issues*, *50*(2), 191–209. doi:10.1002/j.1839-4655.2015.tb00344.x

Hamilton, S., Tew, J., Szymczynska, P., Clewett, N., Manthorpe, J., Larsen, J., & Pinfold, V. (2016). Power, choice and control: How do personal budgets affect the experiences of people with mental health problems and their relationships with social workers and other practitioners? *British Journal of Social Work*, *46*(3), 719–736. doi:10.1093/bjsw/bcv023

Hutchison, P., Lord, J., & Salisbury, B. (2006). North American approaches to individualised planning and direct funding. In J. Leece & J. Bornat (Eds.), *Developments in Direct Payments* (pp. 49–62). Bristol, UK: The Policy Press, University of Bristol. doi:10.2307/j.ctt1t898xj.8

Joint Standing Commitee. (2017). *Joint Standing Committee Report on the National Disability Insurance Scheme, Provision of services under the NDIS for people with psychosocial disabilities related to a mental health condition*. Retrieved from http://www.aph.gov.au/Parliamentary_Business/Committees/Joint/National_Disability_Insurance_Scheme/MentalHealth/Report

Laragy, C., Fisher, K. R., Purcal, C., & Jenkinson, S. (2015). Australia's individualised disability funding packages: When do they provide greater choice and opportunity? *Asian Social Work and Policy Review*, *9*(3), 282–292. doi:10.1111/aswp.12068

Laragy, C., & Ottmann, G. (2011). Towards a framework for implementing Individual Funding based on an Australian case study. *Journal of Policy and Practice in Intellectual Disabilities*, *8*(1), 18–27. doi:10.1111/j.1741-1130.2011.00283.x

Laragy, C., Sanders, F., & Brophy, L. (2015). *Implications for family carers when people with psychosocial disability have individualised funding packages - literature review*. Retrieved from Melbourne: https://www.mindaustralia.org.au/sites/default/files/publications/Implications_for_family_carers_literature_review.pdf

Lightman, E., Vick, A., Herd, D., & Mitchell, A. (2009). 'Not disabled enough': Episodic disabilities and the Ontario Disability Support Program. *Disability Studies Quarterly*, *29*(3). doi:10.18061/dsq.v29i3.932

Lymbery, M. (2014). Understanding personalisation: Implications for social work. *Journal of Social Work*, *14*(3), 295–312. doi:10.1177/1468017313477326

Mavromaras, K., Moskos, M., & Mahutea, S. (2016). *Evaluation of the NDIS Intermediate Report*. Retrieved from National Institute of Labour Studies (NILS) Flinders University Adelaide: https://www.dss.gov.au/sites/default/files/documents/11_2016/final_intermediate_report_wcag_compliant_24_nov_2016.pdf

McGorry, P., & Matthew, H. (2016). Stepwise expansion of evidence-based care is needed for mental health reform. *The Medical Journal of Australia*, *204*(9), 351–353. doi:10.5694/mja16.00120 PMID:27169969

Mental Health Australia. (2016). *Letter to Disability Reform Council on 2017 Productivity Commission review on the NDIS*. Author.

Mental Health Coordinating Council. (2017). *Reimagine, mental health, my recovery and the NDIS*. Retrieved from http://reimagine.today/

Miller, P., & Hayward, D. (2017). Social policy 'generosity' at a time of fiscal austerity: The strange case of Australia's National Disability Insurance Scheme. *Critical Social Policy, 37*(1), 128–147. doi:10.1177/0261018316664463

Mitchell, P., Bruxner, A., & Brophy, L. (2014). *People making choices: The support needs and preferences of people with psychosocial disability*. Retrieved from http://dro.deakin.edu.au/view/DU:30079593

National Disability Insurance Agency. (2017). *Quarterly Report to COAG Disability Reform Council, 2016-17 Quarter 4, 30 June 2017*. Retrieved from https://www.ndis.gov.au/medias/documents/hac/h30/8803440066590/COAG-DRC-Report-2016-17-Q4.pdf

National Disability Insurance Agency (NDIA). (2015). *2015 – 2019 Corporate Plan*. Retrieved from https://www.ndis.gov.au/html/sites/default/files/NDIA Corporate Plan 2015 -19 FINAL_0.pdf

Nicholas, A., & Reifels, L. (2014). *Mental health and the NDIS: A literature review*. Melbourne: Centre for Mental Health, University of Melbourne.

O'Halloran, P. (2014). *About psychosocial disability and the NDIS, introduction to the concept of holistic psychosocial disability support*. Canberra, Australia: National Disability Insurance Agency. Retrieved from https://www.ndis.gov.au/html/sites/default/files/O'Halloran paper.pdf

Peterson, S., Buchanan, A., & Falkmer, T. (2014). The impact of services that offer individualised funds, shared management, person-centred relationships, and self-direction on the lived experiences of consumers with mental illness. *International Journal of Mental Health Systems, 8*(1), 1–14. doi:10.1186/1752-4458-8-20 PMID:24944564

Productivity Commission. (2017). *National Disability Insurance Scheme (NDIS) Costs, Study Report*. Retrieved from http://www.pc.gov.au/inquiries/completed/ndis-costs/report/ndis-costs.pdf

Purcal, C., Fisher, K. R., & Laragy, C. (2014). Analysing choice in Australian individual funding disability policies. *Australian Journal of Public Administration, 73*(1), 88–102. doi:10.1111/1467-8500.12063

Robert Wood Johnson Foundation (RWJF). (2010). *Developing and implementing self-direction programs and policies: A handbook*. Retrieved from USA: https://www.bc.edu/content/dam/files/schools/gssw_sites/nrcpds/cc-full.pdf

Scottish Parliament. (2013). Social Care (Self-directed Support)(Scotland) Act 2013. *Scottish Parliament.*

Shakespeare, T. (2014). *Disability rights and wrongs revisited*. Abingdon, UK: Routledge.

Shen, C., Smyer, M., Mahoney, K. J., Simon-Rusinowitz, L., Shinogle, J., Norstrand, J., ... del Vecchio, P. (2008). Consumer-directed care for beneficiaries with mental illness: Lessons from New Jersey's Cash and Counseling program. *Psychiatric Services (Washington, D.C.), 59*(11), 1299–1306. doi:10.1176/ps.2008.59.11.1299 PubMed

Simon-Rusinowitz, L., Croft, B., Loughlin, D., & Mahoney, K. (2013). *An environmental scan of self-direction in behavioral health: A review of the literature*. Chestnut Hill, MA: Human Services Research Institute and The National Resource Center for Participant-Directed Services.

Slade, M., & Longden, E. (2015). *The empirical evidence about mental health and recovery: how likely, how long, what helps*. Melbourne: MI Fellowship.

Spandler, H., & Vick, N. (2006). Opportunities for independent living using direct payments in mental health. *Health & Social Care in the Community*, *14*(2), 107–115. doi:10.1111/j.1365-2524.2006.00598.x PMID:16460360

Stuart, H. L., Arboleda-Flórez, J., & Sartorius, N. (2012). *Paradigms lost: fighting stigma and the lessons learned*. New York: Oxford University Press. doi:10.1093/med/9780199797639.001.0001

UN General Assembly. (2007). *Convention on the Rights of Persons with Disabilities: resolution adopted by the General Assembly, 24 January 2007, A/RES/61/106*. Retrieved from http://www.refworld.org/docid/45f973632.html

Warr, D., Dickinson, H., Olney, S., Hargrave, J., Karanikolas, A., Kasidis, V., & Wheeler, J. (2017). *Choice, control and the NDIS: Service users' perspectives on having choice and control in the new National Disability Insurance Scheme*. Melbourne: Social Equity Institute, University of Melbourne.

Webber, M., Treacy, S., Carr, S., Clark, M., & Parker, G. (2014). The effectiveness of personal budgets for people with mental health problems: A systematic review. *Journal of Mental Health (Abingdon, England)*, *23*(3), 146–155. doi:10.3109/09638237.2014.910642 PMID:24803221

Williams, T., & Smith, G. (2014). Can the National Disability Insurance Scheme work for mental health? *The Australian and New Zealand Journal of Psychiatry*, *48*(5), 391–394. doi:10.1177/0004867414530007 PMID:24671233

Yeandle, S., & Ungerson, C. (2007). Conceptualizing cash for care: The origins of contemporary debates. In C. Ungerson (Ed.), *Cash for Care in Developed Welfare States* (pp. 1–11). Basingstoke, UK: Palgrave Macmillan.

Chapter 7
Aboriginal Wellbeing:
A Culturally Safe, Trauma-Informed Framework for Health and Mental Health Services

Jennifer Martin
Swinburne University, Australia

Jenni White
Monash University, Australia

Susan Roberts
Swinburne University, Australia

Zac Haussegger
Swinburne University, Australia

Emily Greenwood
Swinburne University, Australia

Kellie Grant
Monash University, Australia

Terry Haines
Monash University, Australia

This content has been removed at the discretion of the publisher and the editors.

DOI: 10.4018/978-1-5225-7402-6.ch007

This content has been removed at the discretion of the publisher and the editors.

This content has been removed at the discretion of the publisher and the editors.

This content has been removed at the discretion of the publisher and the editors.

This content has been removed at the discretion of the publisher and the editors.

This content has been removed at the discretion of the publisher and the editors.

This content has been removed at the discretion of the publisher and the editors.

This content has been removed at the discretion of the publisher and the editors.

This content has been removed at the discretion of the publisher and the editors.

This content has been removed at the discretion of the publisher and the editors.

This content has been removed at the discretion of the publisher and the editors.

This content has been removed at the discretion of the publisher and the editors.

This content has been removed at the discretion of the publisher and the editors.

This content has been removed at the discretion of the publisher and the editors.

This content has been removed at the discretion of the publisher and the editors.

This content has been removed at the discretion of the publisher and the editors.

This content has been removed at the discretion of the publisher and the editors.

This content has been removed at the discretion of the publisher and the editors.

This content has been removed at the discretion of the publisher and the editors.

This content has been removed at the discretion of the publisher and the editors.

This content has been removed at the discretion of the publisher and the editors.

This content has been removed at the discretion of the publisher and the editors.

This content has been removed at the discretion of the publisher and the editors.

This content has been removed at the discretion of the publisher and the editors.

This content has been removed at the discretion of the publisher and the editors.

This content has been removed at the discretion of the publisher and the editors.

This content has been removed at the discretion of the publisher and the editors.

Chapter 8
Violence:
Mental Health, Family, and Media Reporting

Samuel Teague
Swinburne University, Australia

Peter Robinson
Swinburne University, Australia

ABSTRACT

This chapter explores the extent to which journalists draw on long-standing mental health narratives when telling their stories about the "mentally ill" and, in particular, their tendency to depict the mentally ill as violent and dangerous. The chapter is divided into three sub-categories based on the perpetrators of violent crime committed against members of their immediate family. These were "fathers," of which 24 articles were dedicated to the stories of 11 men; "mothers," where 22 articles documented the stories of 24 mothers who harmed their children; and finally, "progeny," where 58 articles presented 17 cases of sons or daughters who killed, or planned to kill, one or both of their parents. Despite differences in the way Australian journalists explain the violence depicted in these stories, particularly when the perpetrator was a female, they continually drew on mental health as an explanatory device to account for how and why these crimes took place. This provides evidence for a continuation of the confinement narrative presented in Chapter 1.

INTRODUCTION

The stories told in this chapter represent a continuation of the history of confining the mentally ill person, albeit in an invisible form presented in Chapter 1 of this text. In the years preceding the fifteenth century, the mentally ill were placed on boats and dumped on foreign lands. The seventeenth century saw institutions formerly built for lepers come to house the mentally ill and any other minority that threatened enlightened progress. The twentieth century witnessed the four-walls confinement of the asylum overtaken by the segregation of the doctor-patient relationship and medicalization. This chapter

DOI: 10.4018/978-1-5225-7402-6.ch008

illustrates the emergence of a complementary form of confinement – that of the stigmatized identity – reinforced through the telling of stories that use mental illness as an explanation for violent crime in the media. The purpose of this chapter is to assess the extent to which journalists draw on historically-derived mental health narratives when telling their stories about the mentally ill, and in particular, their tendency to depict the mentally ill as violent and dangerous. It is therefore a broad study focused on all types of mental disorder. Three cases involving fathers are presented followed by two cases involving mothers and four cases involving progeny. The chapter adopts Mindframe's guidelines for mental health reporting that recommend using language that separates an individual from their experience of mental illness (Hunter Institute of Mental Health, 2014). For example, describing a person as "having been diagnosed and treated for paranoid schizophrenia" is a more sensitive description than using the description "a paranoid schizophrenic". The authors have chosen to preserve the use of the phrase "the mentally ill" when it has been used by the journalist whose reporting is the subject of examination.

BACKGROUND

Author and journalist Sonya Voumard (2016) wrote about the intricacies of constructing news stories in her work entitled *The Media and the Massacre*. She wrote the following in regard to how journalists can use accounts provided by interviewees:

As a journalist you want something out of a subject: good quotes, insights, preferably controversial material. You must strike a rapport, conversationally win over the subject ... Back at the office, the reality hits that journalism is an inexact science with great limitations. Variables like space, time, objectivity, editors and other points of view mean you can never guarantee that you will tell the exact story the subject wants told ... you reject what you don't want, select and prioritize what you do.

Voumard's argument offers insight into the reality of assembling newspaper articles for print or online publication. Most revealing is the statement "you reject what you don't want, select and prioritize what you do". The analysis presented in this chapter offers support for this practice, evidenced in the way the mental health explanatory narrative was used differently across the mothers and fathers samples. It is remarkable how often journalists chose to select and prioritize mental illness in stories of violent crime and murder, and this was most evident in those articles devoted to mothers who killed their children.

This chapter is about storytelling, and in particular, the extent to which Australian journalists draw on mental health narratives when they tell their stories about the mentally ill. As explained in Chapter One, these narratives have changed over time, but still operate today in both subtle and overt ways. The authors conduct an analysis of the way journalists draw on and inform these narratives using discourse and narrative analysis techniques. The articles included in the analysis were collected from eight hard-copy Australian newspapers sourced through Factiva. Factiva was used to source articles published between November 2000 and May 2015. The analysis sourced those pieces containing both search terms "mental illness" and "mentally ill". Hard copy was chosen as it is considered a "trusted" source of news compared with online news mediums.

FATHERS

Case 1: Bribie Island, Queensland, Australia

The fathers sample contains eleven individual cases, three of which are addressed in this section. Five articles published between January 2008 and April 2009 told the story of a 39-year-old unemployed man who moved his family into a holiday home on Bribie Island and within days raped and murdered his 10-year-old daughter. Three of these articles were published in *The Courier-Mail* (Jan. 2008, Apl. 2009) and two in *The Australian* (Jan. 2008). The broad focus of this sub-sample was on a neglected health system and most representative of this narrative was Margaret Wenham's (2009) article entitled "System failure – warnings ignored before man raped and killed daughter". Wenham summarized the crime as follows:

The state's largest hospital was warned, so were police and a doctor, but no one stopped a mentally ill man from taking a family holiday which ended with him raping and killing his 10-year-old daughter.

Wenham reported that the unnamed father had been sole custodian of his four children since 2004 before he "ritualistically killed his daughter and spared her three younger siblings". Details of the graphic nature of this crime were a central component in the five articles that reported on this case, along with frequent mention of a "communications breakdown within the public sector" and persistent "underfunding"; descriptions which portrayed the rape and murder as the result of a neglected health system, one that failed to control a violent individual.

Co-authors Margaret Wenham and Janelle Mills argued in *The Courier-Mail* on 25 April 2009 that even an improved Queensland health system would not prevent a similar event from occurring again. This argument had been presented previously in an editorial published in *The Australian* in January 2008, which argued that "no system, however watertight, can prevent some dysfunctional individuals in fraught situations from harming those around them". The editors argued in this piece that "the frequent connection between mental health and violent crime [needs] to be addressed", and this statement was reinforced in four of the five articles that reported on the Bribie Island murder. While these articles explored some aspects of the broader social context that contributed to the murder of a 10-year-old girl, the journalists framed this broader context as relevant only in its ability to control a mentally ill man, who, without medication and/or involuntary admission to a mental health triage center, would be violent. Just one article addressed the reality of the link between mental illness and violence:

Crime and mental illness do not automatically go together. And anyone who does suffer from mental illness of whatever description has every right to be treated with compassion and sensitivity. (The Courier-Mail, 2008)

The effect of this statement is to remind the reader that while the crime was abhorrent, the case may not necessarily reflect the broader experience of mental illness. Short statements like this help to reduce the spread of stereotypes surrounding individuals with mental illness and their tendency to engage in violent criminal behaviour.

The editorial published in *The Australian* on 4 January 2008, entitled "Lessons must come from tragedy", shifted the focus from the publication's belief that a neglected health system led to this crime, to the safety of children who have mentally ill parents, and this relates to the principal argument of this section concerning the tendency for journalists to report abhorrent cases, and frame them as representative of broader social problems. The editors presented the Bribie Island murder alongside a number of other violent crimes, and in doing so, portrayed them as mental health cases. They wrote that "a report tabled in Queensland parliament in November [2007] revealed that 57 children known to the Department of Child Safety died in 2006-2007". It is unclear how many of these deaths were at the hands of parents being treated for mental illness. This detail was not mentioned and instead the editors continued with a discussion of how the problem was one that extended beyond Queensland's borders:

In Victoria in 2006, serial rapist William Craig Forde told a prison psychologist before he was released from jail that he would rape again. Three months later he took a young Ballarat mother captive at knife-point and raped her repeatedly during a 29-hour ordeal.

It is not clear how the actions of "serial rapist" William Craig Forde relate to the Bribie Island murder. Because the Bribie Island story is framed as a case of a mentally ill father raping and killing his daughter, one must assume that the additional stories and statistics presented by the editors are also related to mental illness and have been included to strengthen the claim that mental illness can help to explain violence. This point was not stated explicitly in the article, but was implied when the authors stated that "Prime Minister Kevin Rudd [would] inevitably need to look at care for the mentally ill". It is not unreasonable for a journalist to argue that a health system has been neglected, or an underfunded sector needs reform. But it harms the public's image of those being treated for mental illness to conflate mental illness and violence without an appreciation for the broader social context within which these crimes take place. Without consideration of other possible explanations for violent crime, the mental health narrative can continue to foster a belief in society, among lawyers, judges, journalists, academics, and the general public, that mental illness explains violent crime in domestic settings.

Case 2: Tyabb, Victoria, Australia

The second case that involved a father killing one or more of his children was no less graphic than the Bribie Island murder. In a summary of the death of 11-year-old Luke Batty, John Silvester portrayed Luke's father, Greg Anderson, as a man with motive. Silvester reported in *The Age* (2014) that after leaving his Frankston accommodation on 12 February 2014, Anderson "told fellow residents he would not be coming back". He concealed a knife in his backpack, caught public transport to Tyabb Recreation Reserve, and "it was there the mentally ill Anderson killed his son".

Silvester outlined some of the broader social circumstances involved in this case. He described Greg Anderson as "alone", "unemployed", and "unemployable". According to Silvester's account, jobs had dried up, Anderson's marriage to Rosie Batty had ended, and "he knew he would never be granted shared custody of his son or even allowed overnight visits". These details are important as they offer the reader a picture of the circumstances of Luke Batty's death, and, perhaps, the father's state of mind. Yet despite consistent reference to the social stressors involved, Silvester still asserted that the young boy's death was an outcome of mental illness. He explained that Anderson's plan was "borne from madness … he knew his tenuous links to his son were fraying [and] through the fog of his mental illness he saw it as the only possible release for both of them".

Silvester also portrayed Batty's death as reflective of a broader social problem concerning "the mentally ill", a method used by journalists who reported on the Bribie Island murder. Where the actions of the Bribie Island father were portrayed as the result of a neglected health system, John Silvester presented Greg Anderson as representative of other violent mentally ill individuals. He assumed a similar link between mental illness and violence as was assumed by the writers of *The Australian* when they tried to account for the Bribie Island murder:

The real issue is our inability to deal with the mentally ill, and the problem is getting worse. It is a massive problem, so much so that all police are being retrained to deal with the deeply disturbed. In 2009 the police dealt with 4798 people so disturbed they were taken to a mental health triage center.

By including these statistics, where 4798 individuals were involved in incidents so problematic they required intervention from law enforcement, Silvester implied that there is a casual link between mental illness and violence. Of the 4798 "deeply disturbed" individuals mentioned above, one could assume that their stories offer a deeper complexity than could be explained by a diagnosis of mental illness. Some individuals may be homeless, some addicted to illicit substances, some mentally ill, and any of these three in isolation would be incapable of explaining the malicious crime depicted in these articles. This lack of complexity illustrates the dangers present in relying on police testimony and court transcripts to construct stories for newspapers. While police have an important and often difficult role to play in incidents like the one that took place at Tyabb Recreation Reserve, where Luke Batty was murdered, they are not trained in diagnosing mental illness, and their appreciation for the broader contexts involved in crime often appears to be obscured by their tendency to make a layman's judgement about the mental state of male perpetrators of violent crime in domestic settings.

A similar pattern where journalists described an abhorrent event and portrayed it as representative of a broader social problem was present in *The Age* editorial published in February 2014, entitled "A bereft mother's insightful message". Its purpose was to commend Rosie Batty, who spoke to media less than 24 hours after the death of her son to explain that "no one loved Luke more than his father … I want to tell everybody that family violence happens to everybody, no matter how nice your house is, no matter how intelligent you are". If the editors had followed Rosie Batty's narrative, this article would have focused on the problem of family violence, yet two sub-sections, one that outlined family violence statistics and the other that paired these statistics with mental illness, dominated the 637-word editorial. In one paragraph, the authors explained that "family violence was involved in 80 per cent of child deaths … in 2013, up from 62 per cent in 2010". The following paragraph stated that "this year, 4 million Australians will have mental health problems … half of us will encounter such difficulty at some stage in our lives". The placement of these statistics can again have the effect of reinforcing a causal relationship between mental illness and family violence. The significance of this relationship, however, is dubious at best. While a large portion of Australians will deal with a personal experience of mental illness across their lifetime, the vast majority of this group will never engage in family violence. Is it not conceivable that the small percentage that do, do so for reasons beyond their mental illness? The murder of Luke Batty at the hands of his father might represent an intersection of family violence and mental illness, but the extent to which this story is reflective of most cases of family violence is questionable, and to reinforce the "mental illness-family violence" relationship is to offer an explanation to all perpetrators of abuse.

Case 3: Melbourne, Victoria, Australia

At 9.15am on 29 January 2009, Arthur Freeman threw his daughter Darcey from Melbourne's West Gate Bridge. The sample contained four articles which addressed varying aspects of this event (*The Age*, Mar. and May 2011, Aug. 2014; *The Herald Sun*, June 2010). In 2011, Andrea Petrie was the Supreme Court reporter for *The Age*. Her piece was a 1636-word summary of Darcey's death, and the discussion that took place in the Supreme Court two years later. Petrie's emotive opening sets the tone for the rest of the piece:

The only thing cold on the morning of January 29, 2009, was the heart of Arthur Phillip Freeman. But the nation felt a chill of horror when news broke that a little girl had been thrown off Melbourne's West Gate Bridge. Dozens of people in peak-hour traffic at 9.15am saw her tossed over the railing "like a rag doll". It was such a long way to fall: 58 meters. She sustained massive internal injuries and ultimately drowned.

In contrast with the sample that reported on mothers who took the lives of their children, explored in the following section of this chapter, Petrie's article represents an inclination of some reporters to provide multiple explanations for murders that are committed by fathers against their children. Where it appears unfathomable that a mother would knowingly and intentionally take the life of her child, Petrie presented an image of Freeman as possibly mentally ill, but more likely "cold" and "motivated by spousal revenge". This narrative is exclusive to the fathers sample.

Petrie began her analysis by quoting defence lawyer David Brustman, who asked in court whether Freeman was "mad" or "bad", and then argued that the father's actions were unintentional, unconscious, involuntary, and the result of a "highly disordered mind, a mind suffering mental illness". Petrie then contrasted this observation with the prosecution's claim that Freeman was "angry at his ex-wife" and "deliberately threw his daughter off the bridge because he was motivated by spousal revenge". The article underpinned this view with a quote from a relative of Arthur Freeman, who asked to remain unnamed:

A relative of Freeman's ... has told The Age of a comment the father-of-three made at a family dinner at the height of his custody concerns in 2008. "We were discussing the custody of his children, and Arthur said 'She [his ex-wife] would regret it if he lost custody of the children' ... it was only later that the comment began to play over and over in my mind".

This comment was representative of a broader stance the author took in this article. While even weight was given to all aspects of the trial, Petrie was transparent in her belief that Freeman acted knowingly when killing his daughter. This is significant as it contrasts with the central argument of this chapter; that mental illness is used as a default explanatory device to explain abhorrent events when no clear explanation is available to the journalist or the reader. In the case of Arthur Freeman, the presence of a mental illness was debated, and its relevance to the crime committed was obscured by a focus on "spousal revenge".

An interesting narrative that ran through the four articles that dealt with this case was the reputation of Professor Graham Burrows, described by Andrea Petrie as "the only one of six psychiatrists to conclude Freeman did not know what he was doing was wrong". According to Petrie, Professor Burrows had testified that the perpetrator "was suffering from a major depressive disorder at the time of the crime ...

was psychotic, out of touch with reality and was in a dissociative state". Yet the reputation of Burrows was questioned and then attacked in the next two articles, one published in *The Age* on 12 May 2011 and the other in *The Herald Sun* on 23 June 2011. *The Age* journalist Selma Milovanovic reported that a Liberal MP "accused Professor Graham Burrows of giving concocted evidence at the trial of Arthur Freeman". This article was titled "Expert witness in Freeman case should be sacked: MP". *The Herald Sun* provided additional evidence one month later, compounding this attack on Burrows. Lucie Van den Berg reported:

The Medical Board is monitoring allegations made by patients against high profile psychiatrist Professor Graham Burrows to determine what action may be necessary to protect the public. A Seven News Investigation raised a list of allegations against the doctor including over-medication of drugs, consultations of 30 seconds and a conflict of interest involving pharmaceutical companies.

The effect of these two articles, alongside Petrie's commentary on the event and the subsequent court case, was to discredit the defence witness in the Arthur Freeman trial. In contrast with the articles explored in the following section, there was an apparent reluctance on the part of the journalist to attribute Freeman's actions to mental illness. This is significant in its distinction with the rest of the sample, where consistently Australian journalists tend to draw on the mental health narrative as a means to explain abhorrent or abnormal behaviour. It would appear that in cases like that of Arthur Freeman, where a father has taken the life of a child, other explanations are likely to be explored and/or offered, and the mental illness explanation is not so readily the "default' stance". In the following section this trend is contrasted with 22 articles that reported on mothers who took the lives of their children.

MOTHERS

The articles that reported on mothers who killed their children are best considered in light of research relating to our constructed understanding of women and their role in western culture. American sociologist Arlie Hochschild's (1979) term for the unpaid domestic labour that falls predominantly on the shoulders of women is "emotion work", and George Levinger (1964) argued in his study on social behaviour in marriage that this work, which includes maintenance of family emotions and interpersonal relationships, has been an aspect of married life in the west since the middle of the twentieth century. Where this relationship has long been interpreted as a product of the "male breadwinner-female nurturer" model, today, women who are engaged in full time paid employment still take on the bulk of routine housework and childcare.

Rebecca Erickson (2005) argues that it is the socio-cultural construction of gender roles that informs this unequal division, meaning we generally come to see being an emotional caretaker as "something women *are* rather than something women *do*" (p. 349). A woman's performance in the household is interpreted as a "natural" expression of her love for her partner and her children, and Erickson (2005) explains that some women are driving this understanding:

Women themselves often discount the time and effort involved in caring work not only because it is expected to be a spontaneous expression of love but also because the illusion of effortlessness is part of doing the work well. (p. 338)

For many women, performing household labour with ease has become a core aspect of their identity construction. One must also consider the weight of traditional beliefs and theories of socialization that assert women continue to perform most of the work associated with "being female" because it is to these tasks that they are most suited (Erikson, 2005, p. 340). While this perspective is supremely archaic, some of this sentiment persists in the west.

It is in this context that 22 articles were examined, which documented the stories of 24 mothers who harmed their children. This is more than double the number of stories dedicated to fathers who killed their kids, of which there were eleven men in total. This group contained nine articles where mothers heard voices and/or messages from God compelling them to harm their children, while in all but three of the 22 articles the crime was murder. This section examines the reporting identified as unique to this sub-sample of articles that reported on mothers who murdered their children, and in particular, the tendency for journalists to portray mothers as psychotic and delusional, and to be more sympathetic to the plight of mentally ill mothers than fathers. Following is an analysis of those nine articles that involved mothers who reportedly heard voices that compelled them to kill their children.

Case 1: Houston, Texas, United States of America

On 20 June 2001, Andrea Yates drowned her five children in the bathtub of their home in Houston, Texas. The story gained national prominence across North America, and was overshadowed only briefly by the attacks on the World Trade Centre in New York City and the Pentagon in Washington on 9 September 2001. Journalist Andrew Cohen wrote in 2012 that a hearing to determine Yates's competency to stand trial for the murder of her five children was cancelled on September 11 because of the attacks. Two articles from the sample of eight east-coast Australian newspapers documented her crime (*The Australian*, 6 Dec. 2001; *The Herald Sun*, 20 Mar. 2002). *The Australian* ran the headline "Mama's deadly state of mind", and described the case as follows:

What police found inside the Yates's modest home shocked the nation. Neatly lined up under a sheet on a bed were the still-wet bodies of the couple's four youngest children: Mary, 6 months, Luke, 2, Paul, 3, and John, 5. Their eldest child, Noah, 7, was still in the bathtub in which Yates had drowned her children. Seeing what was happening to his siblings, Noah tried to run – but Yates chased and caught him.

Yates was described by the editors of *The Australian* as having suffered from "a bout of post-partum depression so devastating, so mind-altering, that she was incapable of judging right from wrong". She told psychologist Steven Rubenzer in one of eight interviews in Houston's Harris County Jail – where she was held and treated with anti-psychotic medication following her arrest – that she believed she was "Satan … George Bush will kill Satan", in the belief that the President at that time was still the governor of her home state. The editors portrayed Yates's actions as irrational, delusional, and the result of mental illness, and claimed "few would disagree that Yates is mentally ill. Her 1000-page medical record chronicles … a history of severe depression marked by delusional episodes". They then drew on statistics from "health experts" to support the link they were wanting to make between mental illness and the death of Yates's five children:

Health experts estimate about 40 per cent of women experience mood swings after having a baby ... However about two women in every 1000 ... can become delusional, have visions and hear voices urging them to harm themselves or their babies.

The Diagnostic and Statistical Manual of Mental Disorders (DSM-V) (APA, 2013) notes that depressive episodes that include psychotic features during pregnancy or following the birth of a child occur in 'from 1 in 500 to 1 in 1000 deliveries' (cited in Stone, 2013) and may be more common for women having their first child. Even though the statistics the editors cited were at odds with those from the DSM-V, they still portrayed the case as rare, and this appeared to be one moment in the article where the authors had the opportunity to emphasize and reiterate the extraordinary nature of Yates's crime in the broader story of mental illness. That Yates was severely mentally ill appears to be beyond dispute, but again, the fact is, the majority of severely mentally ill people would never contemplate a crime of this magnitude, and in the case of women who give birth, this story is exceptionally rare.

The editors that documented Yates's crime used mental illness as a default explanation for violence. The editorial published in *The Australian* in 2001 quoted Dianne Clements, from a Texas-based victims' rights group known as Justice For All, who argued that we "just can't conceive of someone in their right mind doing what [Yates] did". The previous analysis of the fathers sample showed that journalists can conceive of fathers committing the same acts in their "right mind". They seem to find it easier to imagine a father committing a similar act of violence deliberately and knowingly against his own children. Arthur Freeman, for example, was portrayed as someone "motivated by spousal revenge" when he threw his daughter Darcey off the West Gate Bridge. And journalist John Silvester framed Greg Anderson's "descent into homicidal madness" as calculated and deliberate. Anderson told fellow residents at his Frankston accommodation house that he "would not be coming back", and then took his son's life with a knife he had stowed in his backpack. Even the story of Robert Farquharson (Garner, 2014), the man who drove his three children into a dam between Geelong and Winchelsea on Father's Day in 2005, while not a mental health story in this sample, was still portrayed as a deliberate murderous act by an embittered and estranged father. Mothers from this sample, like Andrea Yates, are defined by contrast as psychotic, hearing voices, and out of control, and mental illness is presented as the only plausible explanation for their actions.

Case 2: Sydney, New South Wales, Australia

Shan Shan Xu was another mother who reportedly heard voices that compelled her to harm her child. She drowned her four-year-old son in 2003 and was later found not guilty by reason of mental impairment. John Stapleton followed Xu's trial in the NSW Supreme Court, and reported in *The Australian* on 19 February 2005 that after making suicide threats in 2002, Xu was admitted to the Caritas Centre, an acute-psychiatric unit in NSW. It was here that the hospital noted she had "thoughts of killing herself and her son ... and sees nothing wrong with this". An interesting aspect of this article is the way Stapleton presented evidence he sourced from the NSW Supreme Court trial. He portrayed Xu as having acted in a calculated manner when she drowned her son, and then overlooked any further discussion on the perpetrator's mental culpability in committing this crime. Stapleton (2005) reported that:

[Xu left] a note for her mother that said they would not be returning home to their western Sydney unit. "We are not coming back home. Please look after yourself. Just treat it as if we'd had an accident. I've really had enough", the note said.

Stapleton reported that Justice David Kirby oversaw this trial and accepted the evidence of two forensic psychiatrists that Xu "was suffering [from] a major depressive illness" at the time of the murder. This conclusion was reported by Stapleton but not given the subsequent analysis and discussion it deserved, and that I suspect it would have received had the perpetrator been a father. Instead of a debate about the mental health of the perpetrator, as was present in the case of Arthur Freeman, Stapleton concluded by using mental illness as an explanation for the crime. Stapleton did not point out that these sorts of crimes are extremely rare, and occur in roughly one in a thousand births. He also overlooked evidence that suggests when mothers do kill their children in circumstances like that presented in the cases of Andrea Yates, Christine Gifford, and Dena Schlosser, they often experience acute psychotic symptoms (Wondemaghen, 2013). One could argue that the scarcity of discussion presented in Stapleton's article reflects the Australian legal system's understanding of the killing of children by their parents. Section 6 of the Crimes Act (1958) (FindLaw Australia, 2017) defines infanticide as follows:

If a woman carries out conduct that causes the death of her child in circumstances that would constitute murder and, at the time of carrying out the conduct, the balance of her mind was disturbed because of: (a) her not having fully recovered from the effect of giving birth to that child within the preceding 2 years, or; (b) a disorder consequent on her giving birth to that child within the preceding 2 years.

This definition is significant because it provides for a defence of infanticide only in cases involving mothers. This suggests the disparate discussions surrounding mental culpability for mothers and fathers who kill their children could be reflective of the understandings of these crimes as they are presented in court.

While there were differences in the way journalists reported on mothers and fathers who took the lives of their children, some common reporting methods were evident across these two categories. The analysis showed that journalists who write about either mothers or fathers who have killed their children tend to use additional examples of what they perceive are cases of mental-health-related violence as a means of adding interesting or valuable content/context to an article. Andrea Yates's case is not used as an exemplar, or as evidence of a broader problem involving the mentally ill, but the authors of the editorial published in *The Australian* in 2001 did document other cases where mothers and/or spouses "got off" using a "not guilty by reason of mental impairment" defence. The editors reported:

Lorena Bobbitt, who cut off her husband's penis, got off. Susan Smith, who drowned her two sons by strapping them into the back seat of her car and rolling it into a lake, did not.

This technique was common across many articles in the family violence sample, with these stories seemingly used as a means to sensationalize and dramatize a story. Their purpose appears to be not to inform the reader, but to excite and incite (Uribe & Gunter, 2007).

Gendered Reporting

This analysis of cases where mothers heard voices that compelled them to harm or kill their children illustrates a clear distinction between two types of reporting: one involving fathers who murder their children, and the other involving mothers. While mental illness was the "default" position most frequently used by journalists to explain violent crime, the tendency to use this explanation was dependent on the identity of the perpetrator of the violent act. The notion of spousal revenge, preferable in cases involving fathers, was never used in the 22 articles that are the subject of this section of the chapter on mothers, as women were instead portrayed as generally psychotic, hearing voices, and in touch with a God who compelled them to kill their children. One could contextualize these reporting trends in the context of concrete social phenomena: first, that men are incapable of experiencing postpartum psychosis, and second, that men are more likely to be motivated by spousal revenge because they are more often rejected in their quests for custody of their children. But as feminist and writer Elaine Showalter (1987) argued in *The Female Malady*, attributing types of mental illness to some form of gendered psychology is a dangerous practice, one that has been common for many centuries and has disadvantaged women through the reinforcement of an "hysterical" woman narrative. What an analysis of this sample has shown is that journalists have overemphasized a very rare form of psychotic disorder, one that affects women giving birth at a rate somewhere between one in five hundred and one in one thousand. One could safely assume that the percentage of these mothers who act on voices that command them to harm their children is even more rare. Slightly less than half of the mothers sample accounted for women who heard voices. While these articles were accurate in their coverage of events, no piece contained a clear statement referring to the rarity of the case in question, or how it failed to reflect the broader reality of mental illness.

Mad or Bad

Concluding this section on mothers is an analysis of three newspaper articles that told the story of 31-year-old Louise Scotchmer, who killed her two-week-old son Shane in 1994 and 13-month-old daughter Melissa in 1996. Scotchmer was not charged with these murders until 2001, after she "drunkenly confessed" the crime to her husband. The three articles that reported on this crime were published in March 2003, two in *The Australian* and one in *The Herald Sun*. An account of this story contrasts with previous articles examined in this chapter, because while the three articles stated that Scotchmer committed the murders while in a "disassociated trance-like state", they explored the broader social circumstances involved in the crime, and so framed the killer as a victim.

Vanda Carson wrote in *The Australian* in March 2003 that Scotchmer's brother and husband planned to continue supporting the 31-year-old perpetrator because she had experienced "a horrible life and needed more support from mental health professionals". Scotchmer's younger brother, Anthony Gordon, was a central figure in both articles published in *The Australian*, and Carson used Gordon's commentary to structure a large portion of the piece:

Mr Gordon said the prison system had not been able to provide appropriate treatment for his sister's mental illness since she was detained in September last year [2002]. He said Scotchmer had been physically and sexually abused as a child and had been let down by the mental health system since her first counselling session as a five-year-old.

Vanda Carson also wrote the second article published in *The Australian*. The failing health system was the focus of this article, as the headline read: "Mental health system 'failed' mother jailed for killing babies". *The Herald Sun* focused on Scotchmer's husband in the same way *The Australian* made use of Scotchmer's brother, Anthony Gordon.

Mr Scotchmer, 49, said the sentence was unfair and he would support his wife, who engaged in acts of self-harm and was "quite fragile mentally". He said he was able to forgive her "because I don't believe she was in a normal frame of mind when she committed those acts". Mr Scotchmer said the surviving child, Jamie, visited his mother every fortnight.

The analysis presented here considers these three articles as an interwoven mosaic. The backdrop is the research presented to open this section concerning emotion work and traditional interpretations of women's "natural" role as nurturers and carers. These three articles, and their framing of the Scotchmer case, are placed within the context of that literature. It is difficult to comprehend a mother killing her children, but the framing in these articles is such that the mother, the killer, has become the only victim. A quantitative analysis of the type of language used in these three pieces showed that a total of 26 words were dedicated to the two children who died, two-week-old son Shane and 13-month-old daughter Melissa. This is a fraction of the 1055 words devoted to this story. We hear virtually nothing about the children and learn little of their short lives. The overwhelming majority of the content presented to the reader is instead devoted to Scotchmer's treatment, the support her family has and continues to provide her, her own history of physical and sexual trauma, and the fact she is "mentally fragile" and engaging in acts of self-harm.

In cases where a parent takes the life of his/her child, there are multiple victims, yet in the three articles examined above, Scotchmer appears as the sole victim, and the perpetrator is her mental illness. The children Scotchmer killed are mentioned infrequently and are secondary in the framing of this story. This contrasts with those pieces presented in the fathers sample, where the deceased are central figures, and they are remembered: Luke Batty, Darcey Freeman. The fathers are portrayed as lonely, unemployed, mentally ill, and often revenge-driven men with motive. The antithesis of a victim. In contrast, mental illness in women appears as tragic, and this would perhaps explain the "victim status" some have received in the articles explored in this chapter. The question "Was she mad or bad?" is rarely raised because our socio-cultural understanding of women and mothers tells us that no woman in her "right mind" could take the life of her child. This was most evident in the Scotchmer case, and also John Stapleton's account of Shan Shan Xu, who left a note for her family explaining that she would not return home as she intended to drown herself and her four-year-old son. The intention and calculation evident in this act did not prevent Stapleton from concluding that Shan Shan Xu was mentally ill at the time of the killing, and that this explains the crime. In men, mental illness is more appalling. Fathers are still described as mentally ill, but are portrayed as colder and more calculated killers, and are more often defined as "bad".

PROGENY

The final section of this chapter examines 58 articles that presented accounts of sons or daughters who killed their parents. A total of thirty-three articles from this progeny group were dedicated to four individual murder cases, suggesting that while this sub-sample is much larger than the fathers and mothers groups examined earlier in this chapter, its size is reflective of a more pronounced coverage of these four particular stories in Australian newspapers. These four cases are explored in this section, and they include the stories of Mark Briscoe, a "criminally insane killer" who took the life of his father "with a cane knife" and five years later escaped from a Brisbane mental health facility; Kylie Fitter, the 15-year-old girl who helped her older brother and father kill her mother in the New South Wales town of Glossodia in October 2001; Malcolm Robert Potts, a "paranoid schizophrenic" who killed his father following an argument over a birthday present; and Anthony Waterlow, another person reported as a "paranoid schizophrenic", who killed both his father and his sister.

Case 1: Brisbane, Queensland, Australia

Between January 2002 and February 2003, eight articles reported on "criminally insane killer" Mark Briscoe and his escape from a Brisbane mental health facility, with seven of these published in *The Courier-Mail*, and one in *The Australian*. Mark Briscoe went missing on 18 January 2002 for a total of 83 hours after being last seen eating lunch at Wolston Park mental health facility in Brisbane. Slightly short of a non-event, Briscoe never left the grounds of the facility. Wayne Smith reported for *The Courier-Mail* on 24 January 2002 that Briscoe appeared to have taken refuge in a cricket pavilion before he was found:

A fellow patient saw him there and telephoned The Hub ... where two registered nurses and an enrolled nurse were on duty. They immediately called the three rostered security staff who quickly made their way to Jacaranda House. Not finding Briscoe there, they looked outside and saw him about 100m away on a grassed area ... "Mark, where are you going?" one of them called. Briscoe stopped, turned, and then came over to them. There was no violence used by or against him and he walked meekly with nurses and security staff to the vehicle that took him to the high security unit. He told staff he was sorry he had caused them any concern but had wanted to spend some time alone.

Briscoe never left the 320 hectares hospital grounds, yet the coverage in response to this event was alarmist and fear inducing. Three articles published in the days following his "escape" and "recapture" described Briscoe as a "criminally insane killer", three as a "mentally ill killer", and two as "a paranoid schizophrenic", descriptions in stark contrast with *Mindframe's* guidelines for mental health reporting. To compound this prescribed identity were the descriptions of the crime committed by Briscoe in 1997, which lead to his admission to Wolston Park. Two articles published in *The Courier-Mail* in 2002 reported that "he beheaded his father with a cane knife", Chris Jones described Briscoe as "a paranoid schizophrenic who hacked off his clergyman father's head", while *The Australian* stated more plainly that "[Briscoe] killed his father with a cane knife". A cane knife is similar to a machete, and to be beheaded is to have one's head completely separated from his/her body. The effect of the language used by journalists reporting on this case is to convey a barbaric and brutal image of Briscoe's crime. A description of the brutality of the crime solidifies the legitimacy of the community safety narrative being presented in these articles; the more dangerous the man who committed the murder, the more reason to fear for public safety. The language used by journalists who reported on this case reinforced the supposed danger Briscoe posed to the general public.

And so, upon the descriptive foundations of a barbaric murder that took place five years earlier, the journalists framed their articles on Briscoe's escape from a Brisbane mental health facility around the issue of public safety. *The Courier-Mail* noted that "understandably, the community was alarmed by Briscoe's disappearance". Chris Jones drew on Premier Peter Beattie's response to the event, and framed his comments in the context of concerns for public safety, saying "Mr Beattie conceded there was no way to guarantee another criminally insane killer would not escape". Paula Doneman's response in *The Courier-Mail* (2002) mirrored Jones's:

While the Beattie Government has been using the soon-to-be implemented Mental Health Act as a shield to fend off criticism over the escapes, the truth is these provisions will not stop another determined killer from absconding.

This fear of determined killers undermining a neglected health system was drawn on and reinforced in articles examined earlier in this chapter, particularly in the cases of the unnamed Bribie Island father, who raped and murdered his daughter, and Greg Anderson, who killed his son. Wayne Smith's article published in *The Courier-Mail* in January 2002 reported that "from the community's viewpoint, the primary issue is not how such patients are returned but how they come to be in a position to go missing". The tone of all of these articles, coupled with descriptions of Briscoe's act as an "escape" and "recapture" situation, create a sense of an animal on the loose, one with the capability of inflicting indiscriminant violence on an unsuspecting public. The reality of this case is that Briscoe never left the grounds of Wolston Park. He was not violent, posed no threat, and hid in a cricket pavilion for the 83 hours he "went missing". Journalists took this event and turned it into a broader story about a crisis in Queensland, involving "determined killers" absconding from mental health facilities, and the danger they pose to an unsuspecting public.

Case 2: Sydney, New South Wales, Australia

The second case explored in this section of the chapter illustrates again how journalists tend to use mental illness to explain brutal crimes, even when this explanation appears insufficient. It also sheds light on the challenges journalists can face when constrained by sub-judice law. A particular crime is considered sub-judice when it is "before a judge", and sub-judice law is in place to prevent journalists publishing material that prejudices a fair trial, with punishment ranging from small fines to imprisonment (Pearson & Polden, 2011). In England and Wales, sub-judice law is applied when a case is "imminent", so when a crime has been committed but the suspect has not been apprehended, while in Australia the threshold is "pending", meaning that until an individual has been charged, journalists can report on a case and any relevant details without consequence. So, in the days before the apprehension of a suspect, journalists are free to document background information regarding the alleged offender and any additional details, such as criminal history or mental health status, identified as in the public's interest. As soon as that individual is charged, sub-judice law applies and journalists are restricted to documenting the facts of the case as they are presented in court.

If a case is before a judge, the journalist is restricted to reporting only on the facts presented within the courtroom. This constrains a journalist from engaging in deeper discussion and speculation about possible motives and likely causes of a crime. It restricts one from discussing the mental health history of an alleged killer if this is not a matter raised in court proceedings. It also allows for the identification of the accused as mentally ill, but then restricts the journalist from providing additional content if it was not raised before a jury.

The one newspaper article (*The Daily Telegraph,* 2 June 2001) that detailed the case of Malcolm Robert Potts contained similar reporting techniques to those that were described in the analysis of the Mark Briscoe case. Brad Clifton reported for *The Daily Telegraph* in 2002 that "an argument over a son's failure to buy his father a worthwhile birthday present ended with one of the men being stabbed to death". The accused, Malcolm Robert Potts, was described by Clifton as a "paranoid schizophrenic". After giving his father an unsatisfactory birthday present, and being insulted for doing so, Potts "threw a shopping trolley at [him]" and sprayed him with a can of insecticide.

The language used in this particular article published in *The Daily Telegraph* was detailed and unambiguous. The purpose of describing the shopping trolley and can of insecticide as weapons is unclear, but the effect was to dramatize the event that took place. The fact the argument preceding the murder was based on a birthday present trivializes the death of the father, encouraging the reader to view the event as abnormal and exceedingly violent given the circumstances. The assertion is that the killer must have been insane. The article concludes that "the jury would be satisfied that Mr Potts [the perpetrator] was suffering from an abnormality of mind at the time of the killing". Mr Potts took the life of his father and was clearly very angry, potentially psychotic. But whether he suffered from a mental illness at the time of the killing, and whether his story is representative of the broader experience of most mentally ill Australians, must certainly be questioned.

What is clear from the article is that more information about the circumstances surrounding the murder is required. As was evident in the articles detailing the murders of Luke Batty and Darcey Freeman, the inclusion of one alleged diagnosis of mental illness does little to explain the extreme events that took place. In the case of Mr Potts, Brad Clifton offers a description of the trigger for the event – a disappointing birthday present – and two of the weapons involved in the attack, these being a shopping trolley and a can of insecticide. What these details suggest is a complex and tempestuous relationship between a father and his son, perhaps living on the margins of society. Certainly, the presence of a shopping trolley in the family home indicates some issues within the relationship that may have class origins. More contextual information is required, and this is something lacking in Clifton's account, one suspects as a result of the restrictions placed on journalists by sub-judice law. Clifton quoted Crown Prosecutor Terry Thorpe, who stated "Malcolm Potts is mentally ill … and has been since 1985". The presence of a mental illness that had persisted since 1985 is insufficient to explain the death of a father at the hand of his son.

The story of Malcolm Robert Potts illustrates both the need for improvement in some reporting methods, but also the constraints that are placed on journalists telling mental health stories that are also the subject of criminal proceedings in courts. Clifton's description of Potts as a paranoid schizophrenic reinforces the public's misunderstanding of mental illness as a life sentence. A more suitable choice of words might have been to describe Potts as "an individual being treated for, or diagnosed with, paranoid schizophrenia"; a description that separates the individual from their illness. Setting aside these concerns with language, Brad Clifton was clearly restricted in reporting only those facts that were subject to scrutiny within the court. Sub-judice law constrained Clifton's ability to provide these additional details and explore this case in-depth. While the article was still sensationalized, and the focus on a birthday present trivialized the murder of a father by his son, Clifton reported the facts of the case as they were presented in court.

Case 3: Glossodia, New South Wales, Australia

The third progeny case explored in this section is detailed in six articles published between August 2002 and March 2009 describing the murder of Fiona Fitter by her "estranged husband and two teenaged children". Two of these articles were published in 2002 in the months immediately following the killing, while the other four articles were published between 2006 and 2009, and shifted the focus from the circumstances surrounding the crime to the rights of Fiona's daughter, Kylie, who was involved in the murder and had been a resident of a mental health facility since her mother's death.

Fiona Fitter's death took place in the town of Glossodia in New South Wales on 16 October 2001. Both articles published in 2002, in the months immediately following the killing, presented mental illness as an explanation for the violent crime. Lorna Knowles's description of the event, published in *The Daily Telegraph*, is representative of both articles:

The victim came home from work. Neighbours said they saw her run screaming across the road, with her son in pursuit. She sought refuge in a neighbour's house but the two men – her son holding two carving knives in the shape of a cross – kicked the front door in and chased her outside. Witnesses said they saw the trio kick her on the ground ... the daughter held both her mother's legs, while the husband and son bashed and stabbed her.

Knowles explained that the mother was killed because her husband and two children "believed she was a devil-worshipping witch", and all three would later plead not guilty "by reason of mental illness" in the NSW Supreme Court. The husband was described as a 40-year-old "cannabis dependent paranoid schizophrenic", his son, 18 years of age, "had attention deficit hyperactivity disorder and drug-induced psychosis", and his daughter "had learning difficulties and suffered depression".

It is unclear how relevant or reliable these diagnoses are. In considering the unnamed daughter's contribution to her mother's death, depression and learning difficulties are entirely insufficient to explain such actions. One has to wonder the effect of the association of this crime with the diagnoses offered by Knowles on those who suffer from clinical depression. For the victim's son, a diagnosis of attention deficit hyperactivity disorder could never legitimately explain or justify an individual's propensity for violence, and yet mental illness was still used by Knowles to explain the murder. The last line of the 384-word piece reads "the hearing will continue on Thursday", suggesting Knowles faced the same restriction as was faced by Brad Clifton, who reported on the murder committed by Malcolm Robert Potts, described in the previous section. This is a clear example of the restrictions of sub-judice law hindering a journalist from exploring the broader social circumstances involved in a crime. Knowles alludes to the fact that both the father and the son had been abusing drugs and that this could have induced a psychosis that led to the killing.

Like those journalists who reported on the Mark Briscoe case, Lorna Knowles made the decision to include details of the murder weapons and how they were used by the perpetrators in the murder. These were a "large carving knife" held by the son in the shape of a cross, and "a pair of surgical scissors", which were inserted up the victim's nose and "into her brain". How useful these details are for the reader's understanding of the event is unclear and their inclusion has only added to the sense of horror and terror that this story conveys. The four articles published between April 2006 and March 2009 shift the focus away from the horrific murder, and focus on the rights of Kylie Fitter, the 20-year-old daughter of the deceased victim. All four of these pieces were published in *The Sydney Morning Herald*, with three written by Adele Horin and one by health reporter Louise Hall. Unrestrained by the sub-judice restrictions faced by Lorna Knowles when she reported on this case in 2002, Horin's three articles described some of the broader circumstances involved in Fiona Fitter's murder, and campaigned for the rights of one of her killers, her youngest daughter. Two of Horin's articles were significant in length; one was 1162 words and the other was 2506. Both described Kylie Fitter as a "prisoner", both of her "past" and of "the state". They also portrayed the young woman as a victim:

Kylie was as much a victim as her beloved mother. A victim three times over: of an upbringing that made her unfit for the world, of a psychotic father and brother, and now of political expediency.

Throughout the article, Horin provided the details that Knowles was unable to offer when she reported on this case during the Supreme Court trial in 2002. She explained that Kylie Fitter's father was the primary source of her anguished upbringing, and had filled "her head with extreme Christian beliefs". He was described by Horin as "passionate about God and his family", and had "suffered mild psychosis" at different points during his life. Unrestrained by sub-judice restrictions, Horin was then able to present a fuller account of the challenges Kylie faced as a child:

Both Kylie's parents suffered abuse as children. Out of love for their children, they kept them close and fiercely protected. They moved a lot; there were several schools, and charismatic churches. By 13 Kylie was on Prozac. She left school at 14, a social misfit, believing she was stupid, and in isolation filled her days with computer games. Her brother was spiraling into schizophrenia, hearing "demons' voices" and becoming fixated on harming his mother.

A significant portion of the article was also dedicated to the challenges faced by Kylie's father, who was portrayed as having the greatest responsibility for the murder of Fiona Fitter, his former wife. Horin explained that the unnamed father lost his job in 1999 because of a back injury and that the resulting pain lead to him self-medicating with the use of cannabis. Horin stated that "for a devout Christian his heavy drug use was bizarre and it triggered outlandish behavior". He was known to share joints in the back shed of their home with his son, and he began to collect knives (though for what purpose is not made clear by the journalist). To consolidate the portrayal of Kylie as another victim of this crime, Horin concluded that "there were good days and bad … [Kylie's] father and brother lived in their shared world of demons, angels and paranoid delusions".

In a shorter piece, she wrote for *The Sydney Morning Herald* on 18 September 2006, Horin described Fitter as being "held prisoner by politics", and gave attention in the article to Ms Fitter's advocate, Bob Johnston, who stated that "Kylie is a virtual political prisoner because of the minister's concern that releasing her would damage the Government in the [upcoming] election". In March 2009, Louise Hall reported for *The Sydney Morning Herald* that the laws surrounding this issue had changed, and that "people who are declared unfit for trial or not guilty because of mental illness will no longer be detained or released 'at the Governor's pleasure', following widespread concern that patients' detention was being continued unfairly for populist or political reasons". Adele Horin interviewed Kylie and described her in an article published on 29 April 2006 in *The Sydney Morning Herald* as follows:

She is so gentle and polite as she offers tea and biscuits in a child-like voice that it defies imagination Kylie Fitter helped kill her mother in a crime of biblical proportions. Seated in the living room of an inner-city terrace, the willowy, 20-year-old spun-sugar blonde, sweetness itself, is out on weekend leave from jail. But in the view of her many supporters, Kylie is a political prisoner.

Remember that in later descriptions of the brother and father, also published by Horin in 2006, the two "lived in a shared world of demons, angels and paranoid delusions". According to Adele Horin, Kylie "lost capacity for rational thought and came to share the delusions of her father and brother" who believed Fiona Fitter was evil, and that she "drank babies' blood". Kylie was presented in these articles as separate to her delusional brother and father, and the victim of their paranoid thinking.

The purpose of this analysis has been two-fold. First, it offers insight into the potentially negative consequences of the constraints placed on journalists by sub-judice law. In contrast, the four articles published between 2006 and 2009 were not constrained by sub-judice law, and so engaged in broader questioning of the social circumstances that lead to Fiona Fitter's murder, in particular, the links between religion, the abuse of illicit drugs and alcohol, and paranoid and delusional thinking. While the articles still described the perpetrators as mentally ill, the reader was presented with a more complex (and more thorough) account of how such a horrific murder could take place. Second, the four articles published between 2006 and 2009 portray Kylie Fitter as a victim of multiple circumstances: a victim of her father's delusional thinking, a victim of her upbringing, and a victim of the state. This reinforces a pattern identified earlier in the chapter, where mental illness in women is portrayed as tragic, whereas in men it is abhorrent and despicable. Certainly, Fiona Fitter's son and father are portrayed as psychotic, drug dependent, paranoid schizophrenics who acted coldly and brutally. Kylie Fitter is presented as the 15-year-old who was seduced and hypnotized by their delusional thinking.

Case 4: Sydney, New South Wales, Australia

On 9 November 2009, Sydney-based curator, gallery director, and academic Nick Waterlow was killed by his son Anthony, described as a 43-year-old man "suffering from paranoid schizophrenia". A total of eighteen newspaper articles reported on this case and were published between 12 November 2009 and 7 November 2014; eleven in *The Sydney Morning Herald*, four in *The Australian*, two in *The Daily Telegraph*, and one in *The Courier-Mail*. This is the fourth case explored in this section of the chapter and the purpose of the analysis that follows is to explore the tendency for journalists to document explanations for violent crime that reside outside the individual. I examine the case of Anthony Waterlow and the eighteen newspaper articles devoted to the murders he committed in 2009, and assess the extent to which journalists were willing or able to explore some of the broader social circumstances involved in violent crime committed by individuals described as mentally ill.

Jodie Minus presented a full account of the two murders committed by Anthony Waterlow in a piece published in *The Australian* on 13 April 2011. Minus explained that despite the son killing both his father and sister, there was love in the Waterlow family, and a deep care for the suffering Anthony that persisted "to the very end":

Just moments before his mentally ill son came lunging at him with a 34cm kitchen knife, the 68-year-old cried out "I love you". Anthony, suffering from paranoid schizophrenia, then turned the knife towards his sister, Chloe, who pleaded, "No, don't – stop," as her three young children screamed and cried. Silence descended on the Randwick house, in Sydney's east, for a brief spell as Waterlow, his shirt soaked in blood, walked out the front door ... leaving Nick and 37-year-old Chloe on the floor.

A piece published just three days after the killings, at a time when Nick Waterlow had still not been apprehended by police, and so sub-judice restrictions were not applicable, sought to reduce mental health stigma by making it clear that there are no inherent links between violence and mental illness. Rick Feneley reported for *The Sydney Morning Herald* that the revelation that Waterlow "is a schizophrenic has raised concerns that people with mental illness will be demonized". Feneley explored some of the structural factors involved in the murders, and so looked beyond a simple explanatory link between mental illness and violence common to many of the articles explored in this chapter. He drew on SANE Australia's deputy director at the time, Paul Morgan, who explained that "when tragic cases do occur, it perhaps leads people to a mistaken impression that people with mental illness are more violent than they are". Feneley noted that males aged between 18 and 25 are the most violent group in Australia today, "but people [do] not live in fear of every young man".

That Feneley drew on the views of Paul Morgan is significant. SANE Australia is a mental health charity aimed at helping Australians affected by mental illness, both personally and through family, to lead a better life. A significant focus of their campaigning is the reduction of stigma. By including Morgan's expertise and insight, Feneley helped to balance and moderate the obviously horrific crime and its associations with mental illness. Feneley used Morgan's expertise most significantly when he placed emphasis on some of the structural factors involved in the murder:

Mr Morgan said ... there was a "very small by significant" correlation between schizophrenia and an increased risk of violence. "But that is concentrated in people who are generally younger males, who may have a propensity to violence anyway ... who are not getting treatment, and especially if they are mixed up in drugs and alcohol". Anthony Waterlow has a history of drug and alcohol abuse, and violence.

An article written by three authors, David Barrett, Rhett Watson, and Gemma Jones, published in *The Daily Telegraph* on 14 November 2009, explained that Anthony Waterlow was a "loner" who lived in "a lonely world". Barrett, Watson, and Jones explored some of the broader issues involved in the crime, looking beyond Waterlow's battle with mental illness. They documented a history of physical violence by Waterlow against his family that was compounded and exacerbated by his refusal to take anti-psychotic medication. They explained that as a young man he was officially diagnosed with paranoid schizophrenia, "but friends say he refused to take medication ... [and] bursts of violence against family members as the delusions gripped him eventually led to court-ordered apprehension violence orders". His sister, Chloe, who he would later kill after murdering his father, "had already made it known to others that she feared for the safety of her family" and that he had "once attacked her in a hotel". The three journalists documented more cases of violence:

In 2007 he twice appeared in court. Once for bashing friend and prominent jewelery designer Bridie Lander. He also tried to smash down two doors of neighbours in an Elizabeth Bay block of flats ... Even those who have previously been victims of Anthony's violence are loathe to blame him. Instead, there is a feeling that, like too many of the mentally ill, he fell through the cracks.

The purpose of this article, as it was in Feneley's piece, was to explore some of the broader social circumstances involved in the murders committed by Anthony Waterlow. The explanatory narrative so often reinforced in articles explored in this chapter was also tempered, with more attention given by Barrett, Watson, and Jones to Waterlow's history of violence, and reluctance to take anti-psychotic medication. This drew emphasis away from a simple cause-effect explanation between mental illness and violence. Anthony Waterlow was instead portrayed as someone who suffered greatly, and perhaps was as much a victim of this story as the deceased family members he killed. The three journalists consolidated this view when they concluded that he had fallen "through the cracks" of the mental health system.

SOLUTIONS, RECOMMENDATIONS

As was the case in accounts of fathers, mothers, and progeny, nearly all cases involved murder, and journalists used mental illness more frequently than any other explanatory device to account for how and why these crimes took place. Further research and scrutiny of media reporting guidelines is required on the reporting of violence, separate to further research on fair and accurate reporting related to mental health, so that journalists do not inadvertently cause harm and increase stigmatizing attitudes and discriminatory practices toward people experiencing mental health issues.

CONCLUSION

This chapter was divided into three sections based on the perpetrators of acts of violence that took place in the family setting. Categories were fathers, of which there were 24 articles dedicated to the stories of eleven separate men; mothers, where 22 articles reported on the stories of 24 mothers who harmed their children; and finally, progeny, where a total of 58 articles presented 17 cases of sons or daughter who killed, or planned to kill, one or both of their parents. The argument that unites these three sections is that in cases where violence occurred in the family setting, whether the perpetrator was a father, a mother, or their sons and/or daughters, Australian journalists used mental illness to explain how and why these crimes took place. But the analysis presented in this chapter has shown that the explanatory mental health narrative, while used in the vast majority of newspaper reports on family violence, was not employed uniformly across all three categories. This analysis offers support for an argument presented in chapter one of this text relating to the construction of mental health reporting for publication in newspapers. The analysis presented in this chapter yielded three additional findings that were common across all three categories. The first was the tendency for journalists to portray abhorrent murders as reflective of broader social problems, the second was the use of additional examples of violence as a means for sensationalizing news stories, and the third was the restrictions placed on journalists by sub-judice law and the effect these constraints had on the construction of news stories.

REFERENCES

American Psychiatric Association. (2013). *Diagnostic and statistical manual of mental disorders* (5th ed.). Arlington, VA: American Psychiatric Association.

Erickson, R. J. (2005). Why emotion work matters: Sex, gender, and the division of household labor. *Journal of Marriage and the Family*, *67*(2), 337–351. doi:10.1111/j.0022-2445.2005.00120.x

Garner, H. (2014). *This house of grief*. Melbourne: Text Publishing.

Hochschild, A. R. (1979). Emotion work, feeling rules, and social structure. *American Journal of Sociology*, *85*(3), 551–575. doi:10.1086/227049

Hunter Institute of Mental Health. (2014). *Reporting suicide and mental illness: A Mindframe resource for media professionals*. Newcastle, Australia: Hunter Institute of Mental Health.

Levinger, G. (1964). Task and social behaviour in marriage. *Sociometry*, *27*(4), 433–448. doi:10.2307/2785657

Pearson, M., & Polden, M. (2011). *The journalist's guide to media law*. NSW: Allen & Unwin.

Showalter, E. (1987). *The female malady: Women, madness and English culture, 1830-1980*. London: Virago.

Stone, K. (n.d.). What the new DSM-V says about post-partum depression and psychosis. *Post-partum Progress*. Retrieved from: http://www.postpartumprogress.com/what-the-new-dsm-v-says-about-post-partum-depression-psychosis

Uribe, R., & Gunter, B. (2007). Are "sensational" news stories more likely to trigger viewers' emotions than non-sensational news stories? *European Journal of Communication*, *22*(2), 207–228. doi:10.1177/0267323107076770

Voumard, S. (2016). *The media and the massacre: port arthur 1996-2016*. Melbourne: Transit Lounge Publishing.

Wondemaghen, M. (2013). Depressed but not legally mentally impaired. *International Journal of Law and Psychiatry*, *37*(2), 160–167. doi:10.1016/j.ijlp.2013.11.010 PMID:24268825

Chapter 9
Access to Evidence-Based Services for Individuals With Borderline Personality Disorder

Peter King
RMIT University, Australia

Jennifer Martin
Swinburne University, Australia

ABSTRACT

This chapter outlines the key features of the diagnosis of borderline personality disorder. This is a diagnosis that has attracted significant levels of stigma and has generally been viewed as difficult to treat. This has resulted in often inadequate service responses for people experiencing high levels of distress. Increased understanding is facilitated by exploring precipitating factors leading to this diagnosis, including invalidating and often traumatizing environments. Available evidence from Australian and international literature is considered, with main treatments identified to inform improved treatment outcomes. The need for attention to biological, psychological factors is highlighted and in particular acknowledgment of the high prevalence of trauma, particularly childhood sexual assault, amongst the mostly women who are given this diagnosis.

INTRODUCTION

Borderline Personality Disorder is thought to be one of the more difficult psychiatric diagnoses to treat. Individuals with a diagnosis of BPD experience feelings of immense emotional distress and feature extremes in an attempt to regulate emotions. An individual diagnosed with BPD can face difficulty in returning to an emotional baseline when aroused. Individuals feel judged or abandoned which makes effective coping during the ups and downs of life seem distant and unattainable. Chronic suicidality, self-injurious behaviours, risk taking, misdiagnosis, chaotic relationships and intense emotional responses add to the complexity of what becomes part of the daily life for an individual diagnosed with BPD. Added to the complex presentation is the conjecture within the mental health profession as to, how and where

DOI: 10.4018/978-1-5225-7402-6.ch009

individuals with BPD can be best supported to overcome this often-debilitating condition? This chapter presents the available evidence on issues of accessibility and effective treatments for BPD. It opens with an introduction to BPD that includes what BPD is considered to be in terms of diagnosis and symptoms. This is followed by background information relating to the origins of this diagnosis and contemporary diagnostic techniques and requirements as identified in the two main diagnostic manuals used in mental health services in Australia today, the Diagnostic and Statistical Manual of Psychiatry by the American Psychiatric Association (DSM-V) and the International Classification of Diseases (ICD-10-AM) by the World Health Organisation. The reported incidence of BPD – both globally and within Australia is looked at followed by consideration of precipitating factors, invalidating environments, trauma, social factors, and theories related to BPD. The focus of the second half of this chapter is on treatment responses.

BACKGROUND

What Is Borderline Personality Disorder?

Borderline personality disorder (BPD) can be defined as a mental health disorder impacting the feelings and thoughts of an individual and how the individual perceives others. These thoughts and feelings typically cause functional problems during everyday life (Biskin, 2015). BPD is seen as a complex psychiatric condition with several key characteristics including: (1) unstable mood changes that typically shift at different times; (2) impulsive behaviours and; (3) self-harm (commonly physical) or suicidal behaviours. More often, these characteristics occur during stressful situations and exceed what is considered to be normative type behaviour, causing significant distress to the individual. In addition, individuals diagnosed with BPD typically have relationships that are characterized by chaos and instability, caused by behaviours commonly mediated through feelings of abandonment and rejection that may be either real or imagined (Chanen, McCutcheon, Jovev, Jackson, & McGorry, 2007). Thus, overall, individuals diagnosed with BPD commonly have a pattern of instability, not only in mood fluctuations, but also in interpersonal relationships.

BPD symptoms are numerous. However, overall symptoms revolve around feelings of self-worth and value, relations to others, and behaviours (Zimmerman, Chelminski, & Young, 2008). The most common features include:

1. Fear of abandonment, causing the individual to resort to extreme measures to avoid abandonment or rejection;
2. A consistent pattern of intense, yet unstable, relationships, where the individual's partner is, at first idolized, and then believed to be cruel;
3. Changes in self-identity and self-image, commonly including goal and value changes;
4. Incidences of stress-related paranoia and a lack of contact with reality, which can last anywhere from a few minutes to a few hours;
5. Incidences of impulsive and/or risky behaviour, which may result in emotional, physical, or mental harm;
6. Incidences of suicidal and/or self-harm threats and/or behaviour;
7. Intense mood swings which can range from happiness, irritability, shame, and/or anxiety and can last for a few hours or a few days;

8. Continuous feelings of emptiness; and
9. Incidences of inappropriate and intense anger (Sajadi, Arshadi, Zargar, Mehrabizade Honarmand, & Haijari, 2015; Skodol, Gunderson, Pfohl, Widigier, Livesley, & Siever, 2002).

Given these features, individuals diagnosed with BPD are commonly thought to be overly sensitive (Zimmerman, Rothschild, & Chelminski, 2005).

BPD is believed to require sustained treatment for recovery (Livesley, Schroeder, Jackson, & Jang, 1994; Trull, Useda, Conforti, & Doan, 1997). Yet, BPD did not appear in the DSM manual until its third edition in 1980. During this time, the term "borderline" was used to refer to individuals displaying behaviours that could be classified somewhere between neurosis and psychosis. As time has passed, the definition of the term "borderline" has changed to reflect a series of symptoms found in unstable personality structures with the potential to negatively impact an individual's life. Areas of impact may include employment (such as loss or frequent change), education (such as poor completion levels), legal (due to conflicts and displays of anger), relationship (such as marriage and/or divorce), self-harm (such as cutting, burning and overdoes), abuse (such as being in abusive relationships), medical issues (such as unplanned pregnancies, physical altercations, and/or sexually transmitted diseases from unsafe actions, and, most significantly, suicide (Gunderson, Stout, McGlashan, Shea, Morey, Grilo… Skodol, 2011).

Diagnostic Classification

The diagnosis of BPD is classified in Australia using the criteria of the American Psychiatric Association's (APA) *Diagnostic and Statistical Manual of Mental Disorders, 5th edition, (DSM-V)* and/or the World Health Organization's, *International Statistical Classification of Diseases and Related Health Problems, 10th Revision, Australian modification (ICD-10-AM)*. Australian courts and private practitioners more readily refer to the DSM-V (301.83) whilst government funding is based on ICD-10-AM (F60.3). The majority of international research, including research mentioned in this chapter, is based on the DSM classification of BPD (American Psychiatric Association, 2013).

Although similar, there are differences between these DSM-V and ICD-10 diagnoses. Significantly, the ICD-10 and DSM-V are considered the same and applicable in an Australian court of law. The most important distinctions between them are: (1) the ICD-10-AM was produced by a global agency, with an Australian modification, whereas the DSM-V was produced by a national agency in the United States of America; (2) the ICD-10 focuses on reducing disease burdens related to mental disorders, whereas the DSM-V focuses on the mental illness aspect of classifications for psychiatrists; (3) the ICD-10 is approved by World Health Organisation (WHO) member countries, whereas the DSM-V is approved by the APA, and; (4) the ICD-10 is distributed broadly and with minimal costs, whereas the DSM-V accounts for a significant amount of the revenue for the American Psychiatric Association (American Psychological Association, 2009). Although there is little justification for maintaining both the DSM-V and ICD-10, it is noted that the DSM-V has a significant amount of additional information, which is not included in the ICD-10 (American Psychological Association, 2009).

Commonly, BPD symptoms manifest during adolescence or young adulthood (Guzder, Paris, Zelkowitz, & Feldman, 1999). However, diagnosis does not typically occur until the individual is an adult. BPD can be diagnosed through either the DSM-V (301.83) or the ICD 10 (F60.3). The diagnostic criteria for BPD under DSM-V include essential features, such as personality impairments in context of self and interpersonal, as well as pathological personality traits (DSM-V, 301.83). The specific criteria for a BPD diagnosis under the DSM-V include self-functioning impairments through identity and/or self-direction and interpersonal functioning impairments through empathy and/or intimacy. A BPD diagnosis under the DSM-V includes the pathological personality trait of negative affectivity, commonly characterised through emotional lability, anxiousness, separation insecurity, and depression (DSM-V, 301.83). Additionally, BPD diagnosis under DSM-V includes the pathological personality trait of disinhibition, commonly characterized by impulsivity and risk taking. Finally, a BPD diagnosis under DSM-V includes the pathological personality trait of antagonism, commonly characterized by hostility. The DSM-V diagnosis of BPD recognizes that these impairments affect personality functioning and personality trait expression (DSM-V, 301.83).

Under the ICD-10, BPD is classified as F60.31 – emotionally unstable personality disorder/borderline type (World Health Organization, 2015). According to the ICD-10, a specific personality disorder (such as BPD) is characterized through character and constitution and is considered to constitute a severe disturbance. This also includes the individual's behavioural tendencies and typically involves several personality areas (World Health Organization, 2015). Thus, BPD is characterised through behavioural tendencies that cause a significant amount of personal and social disruption (World Health Organization, 2015). Generally, under the ICD-10, a diagnosis of BPD can only occur if the symptoms are not caused by brain damage, disease or other medical conditions. An ICD-10 BPD diagnosis requires that an individual acts impulsively and does not consider the potential consequences of their behaviour. Further, an individual may be afflicted with affective instability, as well as unclear and/or disturbed beliefs, especially those related to personal image, aims/goals, and internal preferences (such as beliefs) (World Health Organization, 2015).

Precipitating Factors

There are different risk factors associated with BPD (Fromene, Guerin & Krieg, 2014). For example, risk factors are caused by hereditary predisposition, a stressful childhood, and/or personality (Siever & Koenigsberg, 2000; Zanarini, 1997, 2000).

Precipitating factors, or those features that increase the likelihood of BPD, include childhood abuse and/or neglect (Zanarini, 2000). However, there are other potential causes as well. For instance, some researchers believe that genetics influence the incidence of BPD, suggesting that personality disorders can be inherited from parents (Lieb, Zanarini, Schmahl, Linehan & Bohus, 2004). At the same time, researchers suggest that BPD can be associated with other mental health issues that are prevalent in family members. Some researchers believe that brain abnormalities influence the incidence of BPD, suggesting that there may be brain changes that affect emotional regulation, impulsivity, and aggression (Skodol, Gunderson, Pfohl, Widigier, Livesley, & Siever, 2002). Furthermore, it is believed that there are certain brain chemicals, such as serotonin, that affects mood, that may not be functioning correctly in individuals with BPD (Fromene & Guerin, 2014).

There are both legitimate and predetermined factors that precipitate the likelihood of BPD occurrence. For example, individuals with certain mood disorders (anxiety or depression) may have greater incidences of symptoms of BPD (Crowell, Beauchaine, & Linehan, 2009). According to the diathesis-stress model, the combination of stress and a genetic vulnerability may increase BPD development opportunities and likelihoods (Koerner & Linehan, 2000). This is because the underlying personality traits can be inherited from parents (Linehan et al., 1999, 1991). Thus, the diathesis-stress model shows that certain personality traits (impulsivity and emotional instability) coupled with ineffective stress management techniques can increase incidences of BPD (Linehan, 1993). This information leads to the implication that BPD is genetic (Crowell, Beauchaine, & Linehan, 2009; Distel, Willemsen, Ligthart, Derom, Martin, Neale, … Boomsma, 2010). Biological factors include irregular levels of serotonin, a neurotransmitter, commonly linked to depression, and also linked to BPD incidences (Koerner & Linehan, 2000; Lieb, Zanarini, Schmahl, Linehan, & Bohus, 2004). In other cases, researchers have found that the limbic system within the brain, commonly related to emotional response regulation, may impact the likelihood of BPD development (Crowell, Beauchaine, & Linehan, 2009; Distel, Willemsen, Ligthart, Derom, Martin, Neale, … Boomsma, 2010; Koerner & Linehan, 2000). Other significant possible causes include abuse (sexual, verbal, and emotional), separation/early loss of parent(s), and/or family chaos, especially during early childhood and the adolescence years (Lieb, Zanarini, Schmahl, Linehan, & Bohus, 2004).

Invalidating Environments

A common concept used in psychology is "invalidation" coined by Marsha Linehan (1993) through dialectical behaviour therapy, which encompasses more than disagreeing with another person's point of view. In terms of psychology, invalidation refers to communications by the attacker(s) that render the target's feelings, opinions, and emotions as being invalid (i.e. irrational, selfish, right, and/or wrong) (Allen, 2013; Crowe, 2004). When invalidation occurs, the invalidator ensures that it is known that the targets of emotions, viewpoints, and/or feelings have no impact and/or have no bearing at any time or in any way. In some cases, invalidation worsens to physical, verbal, or emotional abuse, and in rare cases murder. Predominantly, invalidation occurs in the form of verbal manipulations. These verbal manipulations are used to invalidate the victim subtly and in a confusing manner (Gunderson, 2006; Skodol, Gunderson, Pfohl, Widigier, Livesley, & Siever, 2002).

An invalidating environment does not necessarily mean that someone is abused and/or neglected. Invalidation commonly occurs through a blatant disregard of an individual's feelings (such as ignoring, ridiculing, denying, and/or judging) (Gunderson, 2006; Koerner & Linehan, 2000). Furthermore, the invalidator commonly emphasizes that the individual's feelings are wrong without attempting to understand these feelings (Fromene, Guerin, & Krieg, 2014; Krieg, 2009). Those who grow up and live in these invalidating environments eventually believe they do not matter as individuals, much less that their beliefs, thoughts, feelings, and/or actions matter to the invalidator. This significantly impacts their abilities to recognize, label, and trust their emotions, commonly leading to substance abuse or self-harm in efforts to remain in control (Lieb, Zanarini, Schmahl, Linehan, & Bohus, 2004; Linehan, Armstrong, Suarez, Allmon, & Heard, 1999; Linehan, Schmidt, Dimeff, Craft, Kanter, & Comtois, 1991). Thus, BPD is commonly characterized as the inability to regulate emotion and/or emotional sensitivity triggered through living in an invalidating environment (Crowell, Beauchaine, & Linehan, 2009; Distel, Willemsen, Ligthart, Derom, Martin, Neale, …Boomsma, 2010).

Trauma and Social Context

Through numerous studies, it is evident that there are many disorders, including BPD, that are caused by precipitating factors, such as early traumatic events that are instilled in the individual's personality organization (Baird, 2008; Van der Kolk, 1987, 1988). This has led to correlations between BPD and childhood trauma (Perry, Herman, Van der Kolk, & Hoke, 1990; Schore, 1994). One study found that 81% of those diagnosed with BPD presented with major childhood trauma (Baird, 2008). Childhood abuse situations will be re-enacted repeatedly until the victim is able to clarify and validate the feelings of injustice and fears of retribution (Van der Kolk, 1987, 1988).

There are striking similarities between the clinical descriptions of BPD and post-traumatic stress disorder (PTSD) (Clarkin, Hull, & Hurt, 1993). This is especially true when there is a history of repeated trauma over time (Baird, 2008; Clarkin, Hull, & Hurt, 1993). Common overlaps are affect regulation disturbances, which include symptoms and/or traits such as increased aggression and startle response, hypervigilance, increased incidences of depression and dysphoria, lack of impulse control (such as increased risk-taking), self-harm (including self-mutilation and substance/alcohol abuse/dependency), disassociation, paranoia, ideation, and intrusive memories (Perry, Herman, Van der Kolk, & Hoke, 1990; Schore, 1994). Yet, there is one significant difference in the descriptive characteristics between BPD and PTSD in that BPD requires no trauma in the history of the person (Baird, 2008; Clarkin, Hull, & Hurt, 1993). This is despite an undeniable link existing between childhood sexual abuse and BPD (Baird, 2008). Since many abuse survivors with BPD do not meet post-traumatic stress disorder criteria, it is postulated that BPD may be likened to a complicated post-traumatic syndrome (Herman, 1997; Perry, Herman, Van der Kolk, & Hoke, 1990). Therefore, it is necessary to allow for validation and integration of the trauma in order to achieve successful treatment (Van der Kolk, 1987, 1988).

Some researchers argue BPD occurs as a result of chronic terror during childhood, specifically during the early developmental period (Burns & Martin, 2014; Herman, 1997). As a result, it is expected that childhood terror is imposed on adult situations, providing a key factor in the development of BPD (Waudby, & Trull, 2002; Perry, Herman, Van der Kolk, & Hoke, 1990). Therefore, the pathology related to BPD is considered a failure in the early development period that allows for the ability of children to self-soothe an activity commonly associated with evocative memories (Baird, 2008; Perry, Herman, Van der Kolk, & Hoke, 1990). Self-soothing capacities refer to memories that are comforting that occurred with caregivers (Baird, 2008; Burns & Martin, 2014). It has become evident that childhood trauma is a significant preceptor in the development of BPD and affects treatment (Herman, 1997). In fact, other conclusions have been drawn, suggesting that if the childhood trauma is not addressed during psychotherapy, the trauma will continue to be re-enacted by the person (Nickell, Waudby, & Trull, 2002; Perry, Herman, Van der Kolk, & Hoke, 1990).

Not only do these individuals suffer from BPD, they also develop other mental health disorders and are commonly susceptible to alcohol and/or substance abuse (Gunderson, 2006). Furthermore, there are also societal and cultural factors contributing to variations in BPD prevalence. For example, development of BPD can be attributed to unstable familial situations, economic factors (such as job loss/change/income fluctuations), or trauma (Baird, 2008; Gunderson, 2006). Numerous other factors influence the development of BPD, such as inconsistent, inadequate and abusive parenting, which can potentially cause those that are biologically predisposed to BPD to have increased risks of developing the disorder (Leichsenring, Leibing, Kruse, New, & Leweke, 2011). Yet, there is no one cause that increases the risk of BPD development (Baird, 2008; Gunderson, 2006). Furthermore, it has been determined that although a genetic predisposition is necessary, environmental factors may increase the risk of developing BPD (Skodol, Gunderson, Pfohl, Widigier, Livesley, & Siever, 2002; Van der Kolk, 1988).

BIOSOCIAL THEORY

Research shows that BPD is a severe behavioural disorder as well as a perplexing one (Crowell, Beauchaine, & Linehan, 2009). The primary features of BPD are shown to be the inability to regulate emotion, increased impulsivity, identity disturbances, lack of sustainable interpersonal relationships, and self-harm behaviours (including suicide) (Crowe, 2004; Lieb, Zanarini, Schmahl, Linehan, & Bohus, 2004; Perry, Herman, Van der Kolk, & Hoke, 1990). These are explained to include additional difficulties, especially emotional and financial, on a host of people, including friends, family, and society in general (Perry, Herman, Van der Kolk, & Hoke, 1990). The biosocial theory of BPD, established in 1993, has resulted in one of the most delineated etiological models in relation to borderline pathology (Cavazzi & Becerra, 2014; Gill & Warburton, 2014). According to Linehan (1993), BPD centres around emotional dysregulation. Furthermore, it emerges due to biological vulnerabilities and environmental influences, proving that dysfunction is a significant factor in BPD (Arens, Grabe, Spitzer, & Barnow, 2011; Crowell, Beauchaine, & Linehan, 2009).

Original propositions stated that BPD developed through invalidating environments, commonly characterised by the intolerance of emotional expression. This is especially true in consideration of emotions that are not associated with observable events (Arens, Grabe, Spitzer, & Barnow, 2011; Fonseca-Pedrero, Paino, Lemos-Giraldez, Sierra-Baigrie, Gonzalez, Bobes, & Muniz, 2011). In invalidating environments, it is taught that emotions are not to be outwardly displayed, coped with internally and without parental support, as well as being unwarranted. This causes deficiencies in relation to the understanding, recognition, and regulation of emotions. This leads to variations between emotional inhibition and lability (Crowell, Beauchaine, & Linehan, 2009; Linehan, 1993).

Originally, the biosocial theory considered early emotional development separate to impulsivity (Linehan, 1993). Later research showed emotion can be influenced by impulsivity (Gratz & Roemer, 2004). Additionally, further research showed that approximately 40 to 90% of those diagnosed with BPD engage in self-harm or attempt suicide (Gill & Warburton, 2014; Koerner & Linehan, 2000). At the same time, it has been found that BPD development is likely to occur due to a combination of biological vulnerability predisposition and environmental risk factors (American Psychiatric Association, 2004; Arens, Grabe, Spitzer, & Barnow, 2011). Thus, invalidating environments are severely damaging to impulsive and emotionally sensitive children, further influenced by inconsistent punishments and anger escalation (Crowell, Beauchaine, & Linehan, 2009; Laporte & Guttman, 1996).

There are numerous controversies in relation to BPD. For example, researchers are indecisive as to whether or not BPD refers to transient psychotic state incidents or stable sets of personality traits (Arens, Grabe, Spitzer, & Barnow, 2011; Crowell, Beauchaine, & Linehan, 2009). According to the biosocial model one of the first borderline pathology traits to emerge is poor impulse control (Gratz & Roemer, 2004, 2008). As a result, this trait may be the one major difference that accounts for biological vulnerabilities that can be attributed to BPD and other related disorders (Koerner & Linehan, 2000; Laporte & Guttman, 1996). Emotional lability is also significant with this arising from environmental and individual characteristics that include: biological vulnerabilities in relation to environmental risks; opportunities for emotional dysregulation and behavioural dyscontrol (Lieb, Zanarini, Schmahl, Linehan, & Bohus, 2004; Linehan, Armstrong, Suarez, Allmon, & Heard, 1999; Linehan, Schmidt, Dimeff, Craft, Kanter, & Comtois, 1991; Linehan, 1993). These factors are believed to contribute to disruptive cognitive and social outcomes that may be heightened by emotional coping strategies that are found to be maladaptive (Laporte & Guttman, 1996).

TREATMENT RESPONSES TO BORDERLINE PERSONALITY DISORDER

The complexity of a BPD presentation lends itself to much confusion and conjecture within the mental health profession. There are a number of mitigating circumstances that add to the complexity of treating an individual with a BPD presentation. Mental health professionals are, at times, confused by a lack of formal policy and direction for an evidence informed approach to the therapeutic treatment of individuals with a diagnosis of BPD. Health professionals often find themselves struggling to comprehend the chronicity of an individual's thought pattern and risk. This confusion adds to the anxiety of all stakeholders and perceived lack of an adequate response for individuals with a diagnosis of BPD.

All too common does the conjecture around treatment, seriousness of suicide risk and perceived failure of individuals with a diagnosis of BPD to appear committed to treatment, result in judgments by mental health professionals and society in general. A number of studies cited in McGrath and Dowling (2012) examine these concerns by exploring the attitudes of nurses towards service consumers with BPD. These studies report the perception of individuals with BPD as being difficult, manipulative, demanding, destructive, or attention seeking. Judgments like those described by McGrath and Dowling (2012) contribute to the complexity of treatment needs for BPD thus resulting in an exacerbation of BPD features. Feelings of invalidation, judgment and abandonment then become the focus of the person and progression towards effective outcomes seems near impossible to both the consumer and mental health professional providing treatment.

Psychological interventions to have shown improvement, in individuals with BPD, include: Cognitive Behavioural Therapy, Metallization-Based Treatment (Bateman & Fonagy, 2010), Cognitive Analytic Therapy, Group Therapy, Schema-Focused Therapy, Dialectical Behaviour Therapy (Linehan, Armstrong, Suarez, Allmon, & Heard, 1999; Van den Bosch, 2005) and psychotherapies (De Maat, De Jonghe, Schoevers & Dekker, 2009). All treatment is focused on the recognition of emotional/behavioural difficulties, as well as emotional/behavioural regulation and management (Brown, Henriques, Xie, Hollander, & Beck, 2005; Linehan, Armstrong, Suarez, Allmon, & Heard, 1999; Lynch, Morse, Mendelson, & Robins, 2003). The remainder of this chapter examines guidelines for treatments from the United States, the United Kingdom, Australia and the main features of treatments proven to be effective.

United States Guidelines

All western developed countries have similar, if not the same, treatment options (Beatson & Rao, 2014; Fromene & Guerin, 2014). Under the United States guidelines, BPD is considered to be an extremely serious mental illness. Moreover, it is characterized by unstable emotions, behaviours, and relationships. BPD was first listed in in the DSM III, commonly used to diagnose mental illnesses by psychiatrists and psychologists. However, there are commonly incidences of co-existing disorders that accompany BPD, such as anxiety, depression, self-harm, suicidal behaviours, and substance/alcohol abuse (Crowell, Beauchaine, & Linehan, 2009; Gill & Warburton, 2014). At the same time, research showed that dialectical behaviour therapy was beneficial in that it reduced suicide attempts in women by 50%, showing greater promise for treatment options beyond psychotherapy (Gill & Warburton, 2014; Olenchek, 2008; Safer, Telch, & Agras, 2011). Dialectical behaviour therapy was also important because emergency room and inpatient services were not needed as much because dialectical behaviour therapy focused on the retention of individuals with BPD in therapy. However, despite treatment successes, there have been incidences of

BPD under- or misdiagnoses, easily reduced by inquiring about symptoms and personal/familial medical history (Koons, Robins, Tweed, Lynch, Gonzalez, Morsh, ... Bastian, 2001; Safer, Telch, & Agras, 2011).

At the same time, it was argued by researchers that BPD was one of the most difficult mental health disorders to treat (Crowell et al., 2009; Gill & Warburton, 2014). However, it has been shown that BPD can be treated, allowing individuals with BPD to have improved quality of life (Koerner & Linehan, 2000; Koons, Robins, Tweed, Lynch, Gonzalez, Morsh, ... Bastian, 2001). One of the most effective treatments is considered to be psychotherapy (Linehan, Armstrong, Suarez, Allmon, & Heard, 1999; Lynch, Morse, Mendelson, & Robins, 2003). It is also noted that medication is also used in certain situations in order to manage specific symptoms (Olenchek, 2008; Safer, Telch, & Agras, 2011). Researchers agree that when the same individual is under the care of multiple professionals, all professionals must work to develop a cohesive treatment plan (Skodol, Gunderson, Pfohl, Widigier, Livesley, & Siever, 2002; Van der Kolk, 1987, 1988). United States therapists typically turn to psychotherapy as a first option for those with BPD. Although it is shown that psychotherapy is effective towards some symptoms, it cannot necessarily treat all symptoms associated with BPD (Domes, Winter, Schnell, Voha, Fast, & Herpertz, 2006). Other treatment options include cognitive behavioural therapy, schema-focused therapy, group therapy, and medications (Gill & Warburton, 2014).

The Federal Food and Drug Administration has not approved any medications for BPD treatment. Moreover, few studies show the effectiveness or necessitation of medication for treating BPD. Despite this, there are many people diagnosed with BPD on medications in conjunction with therapy. It has been seen that medication does not cure BPD (Koons, Robins, Tweed, Lynch, Gonzalez, Morsh, ... Bastian, 2001); however, it does help with symptom management, such as anxiety, depression, and/or aggression (Crowell, Beauchaine, & Linehan, 2009). Alternative treatment options exist as well. It is suggested that especially for women, Omega-3 fatty acids may be beneficial in treating BPD. Omega-3 fatty acids may be comparable to mood stabilizers, yet with fewer side effects (Lynch, Morse, Mendelson, & Robins, 2003). At the same time, evidence shows that proper treatment commonly results in clients exhibiting fewer or less severe symptoms (Koerner & Linehan, 2000; Koons, Robins, Tweed, Lynch, Gonzalez, Morsh, ... Bastian, 2001).

Australian Guidelines

Australian mental health policy and practice focuses on recovery aimed at living well using a strengths approach. Australian guidelines offer systems training for emotional predictability and problem solving, cognitive analytic therapy, schema-focused psychotherapy, transference-focused psychotherapy, cognitive-behavioural therapy, interpersonal psychotherapy, mentalization-based therapy, and dialectical behaviour therapy (Australian Government, 2011; Fromene, Guerin & Krieg, 2014). At the same time, Australian researchers suggest that psychiatric management is equally effective to dialectical behaviour therapy in consideration of symptom severity, distress, and depression (Fromene & Guerin, 2014; Fromene, Guerin & Krieg, 2014). It has also been suggested that effective clinical care is equally effective to cognitive analytic therapy for those between 14 and 18 years of age in the improvement of psychopathology (Beatson & Rao, 2014). Other effective therapy types include conversational and supportive psychotherapy, and a therapeutic community approach (Australian Government, 2011; Beatson & Rao, 2014; Fromene & Guerin, 2014).

The most effective therapies adopt a theoretical approach that is both explicit and integrated and is followed in full by the treatment team (Australian Government, 2011; Beatson & Rao, 2014). The approach is discussed in its entirety with the individual diagnosed with BPD and is supervised by a trained therapist, who also receives support and supervision by other members of the treatment team (Fromene & Guerin, 2014). It is important for the supervising therapist to consider the emotions of the individual and remain focused on assisting the individual to create change in behaviours, thoughts, and actions (Fromene, Guerin, & Krieg, 2014; Wetzelaer, Farrell, Evers, Jacob, Lee, Brand, ... Arntz, 2014). It is also important for treatment considerations to include the availability of treatment, as well as the preference of the individual. The individual's psychiatric symptom severity must be considered in the assessment of a treatment method, as well as how impaired the psycho-social functioning is.

Most importantly, the treatment team must consider how willing the individual is to participate in therapy, as well as the motivations for engaging in therapy, the ability of the person to maintain appropriate therapeutic boundaries, and professional support availability (Australian Government, 2011; Beatson & Rao, 2014). As such, those diagnosed with BPD need to receive structured therapies designed for BPD treatment and supervised by at least one trained and qualified professional (Bendit, 2014; Fromene & Guerin, 2014; Fromene, Guerin, & Krieg, 2014). Furthermore, it is important to take the needs of the individual into account when developing session frequency, including at least one per week in most situations (Meaney-Tavares & Hasking, 2013; Wetzelaer, Farrell, Evers, Jacob, Lee, Brand, ... Arntz, 2014; Winsper, Marwaha, Lereya, Thompson, Eyden, & Singh, 2015).

United Kingdom Guidelines

The United Kingdom focuses on person-centred care. It is believed that treatment is most effective if it considers the needs and preferences of the individual. Thus, within the United Kingdom, emphasis is placed on allowing those with BPD to make informed decisions regarding care and/or treatment after receiving all information regarding options from professionals (Rogers & Dunne, 2013). When providing treatment for individuals diagnosed with BPD, good communication is emphasized between the individual and the professional. It is also important to support the verbal communication with written communication, designed to meet the needs of the person. At the same time, the United Kingdom emphasizes implementation priorities. These include service access for all people, autonomy and choice, the opportunity to develop a relationship with the treatment provider based on optimism and trust, proper assessment, developing an effective care plan and management for the treatment ending and transition support (Rogers & Dunne, 2013).

Psychological treatment obtained for BPD in the United Kingdom focuses on the use of a theoretical approach, designed both explicitly and through integration, by the treatment team and therapist. This approach is detailed to the individual receiving treatment. It, most importantly, provides for structured care and includes provisions for therapist supervision (Harvey, Black, & Blum, 2010). Psychotherapy must last at least 3 months. At the same time, treatment should not be limited to BPD or related symptoms/behaviours, such as self-harm, emotional instability, risk-taking behaviour, and/or transient psychotic symptoms (Rogers & Dunne, 2013). Thus, it is expected that BPD treatment in the United Kingdom encompass the entire person, not the disorder only.

EVIDENCE-BASED PRACTICE

The Australian Psychological Society Ltd (2010), the largest of all non-medical representative organisations for health professionals in Australia, state that the delivery of "...evidence-based psychological interventions by appropriately trained mental health professionals is seen as best practice..." (p. 1) when delivering therapeutic interventions. The concept of evidence-based practice refers to a mental health professional's capacity to draw upon the empirical research, of a particular intervention, and integrate the core concepts into their decision making and to deliver an informed therapeutic approach (Webber, 2011). Evidence-based approaches and interventions identified for individuals with a diagnosis of BPD treatment include: cognitive analytic therapy, cognitive behaviour therapy, transference-focused therapy, dialectical behaviour therapy and mentalization-based therapy. Despite these possibilities and treatment options, there are differing factors that affect recovery and symptom improvement time (Domes, Winter, Schnell, Voha, Fast, & Herpertz, 2006). As a result, individuals diagnosed with BPD would do well to maintain their patience and support network (Safer, Telch, & Agras, 2011).

Cognitive Analytic Therapy

Cognitive analytic therapy is an interpersonal therapy that repeats patterns found in relationships, while also providing integration based on various theoretical perspectives. These perspectives may include cognitive and analytic concepts in consideration of self (Australian Psychological Society Ltd, 2010; Lawn & McMahon, 2015; Ryle & Kerr, 2002). Cognitive analytic therapy features the assumption that individuals with BPD have developed characteristic reciprocal roles, reflecting their early formative experiences. These roles typically focus on their primary caregivers. However, it is recognized that, optimally, individuals with BPD internalize the different healthy and adaptive roles that allow them to evaluate other people's behaviour and respond appropriately (Ryle & Kerr, 2002; Stoffers, Völlm, Rücker, Timmer, Huband, & Lieb, 2012).

During cognitive analytic therapy, individuals diagnosed with BPD learn how to enact both portions of a reciprocal role. It is possible that the individual enacts either the adult or the child. In this context, an individual abused as a child may present as an abused victim, yet show ways that they are abusive towards others (potentially including the therapist). In this scenario, the reciprocal role can be illustrated as being disrespectful towards others and/or self (Australian Psychological Society Ltd, 2010; Lawn & McMahon, 2015). This scenario shows that on one hand, there is too much pain attached, prohibiting the individual from being able to experience that role, causing the individual to position themselves in the opposite role of the abuser (Ryle & Kerr, 2002; Stoffers, Völlm, Rücker, Timmer, Huband, & Lieb, 2012).

As a result, cognitive analytic therapy concerns itself with internalized reciprocal roles which influence interpersonal relations and self-management. It is assumed through cognitive analytic therapy that these roles create "templates" that show implications regarding the expectations of the individuals, including feelings and behaviours that are characterized in relationships. Therefore, these templates project pressures placed by the individual with BPD on others, expecting them to behave predictably. The reciprocal roles show how the individual expects the other person to act towards them. This can be considered an abusive to abused role, commonly associated with feelings of anger and worthlessness (Lawn & McMahon, 2015; Ryle & Kerr, 2002; Stoffers, Völlm, Rücker, Timmer, Huband, & Lieb, 2012).

Thus, the reciprocal role commonly involves a parent and child, whereupon the parent provides negative behaviours towards the child, and the child relives the experiences of childhood. Through cognitive analytic therapy, this reciprocal role is transformed to reflect positive behaviours from the parent towards the child and feelings of security in the child (Australian Psychological Society Ltd, 2010; Crowe, 2004).

It is important to be aware that cognitive analytic therapy focuses on empathic validation of the internalized experience of the individual diagnosed with BPD. At the same time, cognitive analytic therapy does not always assume that the recollection of the experience is accurate (Australian Psychological Society Ltd, 2010; Lawn & McMahon, 2015). Therefore, cognitive analytic therapy utilizes procedures related to reciprocal roles that focus on sequences of mental and behavioural processes. These processes are commonly associated with affect from awareness and guides the action (such as feeling safe), yet lead to procedures of self-defeat, such as seeking constant reassurance (Ryle & Kerr, 2002; Stoffers, Völlm, Rücker, Timmer, Huband, & Lieb, 2012).

Cognitive Behaviour Therapy

Cognitive behaviour therapy differs from cognitive analytic therapy. Cognitive behaviour therapy is known as a talking therapy focusing on the effect of thoughts, beliefs, and attitudes on feelings and behaviour. A secondary goal is to teach coping skills individuals diagnosed with BPD can use to deal with different problems (Lawn & McMahon, 2015; Norrie, Davidson, Tata, & Gumley, 2013). Cognitive behaviour therapy utilizes a combination of cognitive and behaviour therapy. Thus, cognitive behaviour therapy is based on the assumption that thoughts regarding particular situations can affect feelings and behaviour. Cognitive behaviour therapy focuses on stopping the cycle of negative thinking and is considered to be relatively flexible in order to adapt to the unique needs of the individual (Australian Psychological Society Ltd, 2010; Lawn & McMahon, 2015). Thus, current evidence as to the effects of cognitive behaviour therapy suggests that it can effectively treat problems with anger, anxiety, and panic attacks. At the same time, cognitive behaviour therapy is reputed to be able to treat mood disorders, such as BPD or depression (Norrie, Davidson, Tata, & Gumley, 2013). This treatment is useful for those with substance/alcohol abuse issues, eating disorders, obsessive-compulsive disorders, phobias, sexual/relationship problems, or sleep problems (Ryle & Kerr, 2002; Stoffers, Völlm, Rücker, Timmer, Huband, & Lieb, 2012). In fact, in some situations, cognitive behaviour therapy has been shown to be as equally effective as medication for certain conditions, such as depression and anxiety disorders. However, cognitive behaviour therapy is designed to be a short-term treatment (Australian Psychological Society Ltd, 2010; Lawn & McMahon, 2015).

One course of cognitive behaviour therapy may encompass twelve sessions spread out over twelve weeks, resulting in one per week. Cognitive behaviour therapy sessions may be delivered in various ways: individually, in a group, self-help books, and/or computer programmes (Ryle & Kerr, 2002; Stoffers, Völlm, Rücker, Timmer, Huband, & Lieb, 2012). Therefore, the focal point of cognitive behaviour therapy sessions is to explore problems for individuals to work on and the related goals, plan how problems can be addressed appropriately, and explore feelings, thoughts, and/or behaviours. Ultimately, the goal of cognitive behaviour therapy is to teach the individual diagnosed with BPD coping skills for different situations (Lawn & McMahon, 2015; Norrie, Davidson, Tata, & Gumley, 2013). Furthermore, cognitive behaviour therapy tends to favour equality and an environment without judgement as the individual and therapist work together (Australian Psychological Society Ltd, 2010; Lawn & McMahon, 2015).

This suggests that the therapist needs to seek and consider the views and reactions of the individual. This can allow the therapist to develop the progression of therapy programs. Through collaboration, the individual is actively involved in therapeutic goal-setting (Ryle & Kerr, 2002; Stoffers, Völlm, Rücker, Timmer, Huband, & Lieb, 2012).

Transference Focused Therapy

Another therapy used for those diagnosed with BPD is transference focused therapy. This type of therapy focuses on contemporary psychoanalytic therapy. Psychoanalytic therapy is believed to be effective because this type of thinking is believed to enhance understanding and treatment of personality disorders (Arntz, Stupar-Rutenfrans, Bloo, van Dyck, & Spinhoven, 2015). The treatment of these personality disorders, and specifically BPD, through the use of transference focused therapy includes different modifications of the technique to meet individual needs (Australian Psychological Society Ltd, 2010; Stern & Yeomans, 2015). Transference focused therapy emphasizes that symptoms, including behavioural manifestations, can be explained by internal mental or emotional factors. It is believed that these factors cannot commonly be seen visibly (Arntz, Stupar-Rutenfrans, Bloo, van Dyck, & Spinhoven, 2015). Therefore, transference focused therapy emphasizes that attention must be paid to these factors and is considered essential to treatment through psychotherapy. In fact, some of these factors may influence the treatment process and psychotherapy goals. Thus, problematic behaviours and symptoms previously found to be unclear, may become clear through the analysis of the experiences (Australian Psychological Society Ltd, 2010; Stern & Yeomans, 2015).

Transference focused therapy has, as a result, been shown to be efficient in the treatment of BPD symptoms. Research shows that other treatments focus on the reduction of symptoms. This is commonly done through the emphasis and use of coaching and guidance through therapy, which teaches individuals how to control their behaviours (Australian Psychological Society Ltd, 2010; Stern & Yeomans, 2015). However, transference focused therapy uses different actions. Transference focused therapy places a tremendous amount of emphasis on the assessment and evaluation of the individual, as well as the establishment of a treatment contract (useful because it determines what conditions must be met by either party and are mutually agreed upon as the basic therapeutic framework).

However, transference focused therapy places an even higher emphasis on assisting individuals in understanding shifts between personal experiences and the experiences associated with other people (Arntz, Stupar-Rutenfrans, Bloo, van Dyck, & Spinhoven, 2015; Australian Psychological Society Ltd, 2010; Stern & Yeomans, 2015). These types of shifts (or splits) are shown within different experiences, both past and present, can exist in different scenarios, such as in places of employment, socially with peers and friends, with family, and within the treatment relationship. Therefore, transference focused therapy is divided into two major phases. The first phase is important because it establishes the treatment structure, including setting limits on the destructiveness of the person (Arntz, Stupar-Rutenfrans, Bloo, van Dyck, & Spinhoven, 2015; Australian Psychological Society Ltd, 2010; Stern & Yeomans, 2015). The second phase emphasizes the exploration of the individual's mind and identity. However, there is an obvious overlap between the phases in order to account for initial observations and explorations. Finally, transference focused therapy may have continuous limit-setting occur between the therapist, treatment team, and individual (Arntz, Stupar-Rutenfrans, Bloo, van Dyck, & Spinhoven, 2015; Australian Psychological Society Ltd, 2010; Stern & Yeomans, 2015).

Dialectical Behaviour Therapy

Considered the "Gold Standard" of treatments for individuals diagnosed with BPD, with over 30 randomised clinical trials (Safer, Telch, & Agras, 2011) vouching for its efficacy, dialectical behaviour therapy was developed through the efforts of American psychologist Marsha Linehan. Dialectical behaviour therapy is underpinned by a behavioural therapy approach (Fromene & Guerin, 2014; Jackson & Burgess, 2000). However, Linehan adapted cognitive behavioural therapy in order to meet the needs of individuals diagnosed with BPD or those individuals that experience intense emotions (Koerner & Linehan, 2000; Koons, Robins, Tweed, Lynch, Gonzalez, Morsh, ...Bastian, 2001). Specifically, dialectical behaviour therapy is useful for those that have repeated chaos enduing features, such as self-harm, attempted suicide, alcohol/substance abuse, bulimia/anorexia, and relationships that are unstable (Linehan, 2000; Linehan, Armstrong, Suarez, Allmon, & Heard, 1999; Olenchek, 2008).

Due to the efforts of researchers to improve dialectical behaviour therapy and the success of the treatment in individuals diagnosed with BPD, the treatment is recognized as being the most effective psychological treatment for those with BPD. The goal of dialectical behaviour therapy is to change an individual's behaviour that is considered to be unhelpful (Koerner & Linehan, 2000; Lieb, Zanarini, Schmahl, Linehan, & Bohus, 2004). However, dialectical behaviour therapy differs from cognitive behaviour therapy because the entire person is accepted, rather than just positive traits. Furthermore, there is an increased importance on the relationship between the individual and therapist when engaged in dialectical behaviour therapy. The purpose for this is to utilize this relationship as a continuous motivation tactic for the individual, encouraging change (Australian Psychological Society Ltd, 2010; Linehan, Wilks, & Chelsey, 2015). The goals of dialectical behaviour therapy revolve around learning to manage and control difficult emotions. This is done by allowing the individual to experience these emotions, which will then teach them to recognize and accept them for what they are, rather than have inappropriate reactions and behave in unfitting ways (Australian Psychological Society Ltd, 2010; Koerner & Linehan, 2000; Lieb, Zanarini, Schmahl, Linehan, & Bohus, 2004; Linehan, Wilks, & Chelsey, 2015). Therefore, the overarching goal of dialectical behaviour therapy is to find a balance between self-acceptance and change.

There are four major elements that encompass standard dialectical behaviour therapy: (1) individual therapy; (2) group skills training; (3) phone coaching and; (4) consultation groups for therapists. These combined elements allow the greatest opportunities for change within the individual diagnosed with BPD. Research shows that the group skills training used in dialectical behaviour therapy is important because it teaches individuals appropriate behavioural skills (Australian Psychological Society Ltd, 2010; Koerner & Linehan, 2000; Linehan, Wilks, & Chelsey, 2015). Two educators teach skills and the individuals in the group practice the newly-taught skills in everyday life situations, both in groups and individually (Australian Psychological Society Ltd, 2010; Koerner & Linehan, 2000). In most cases, groups meet for two and a half hours per week for approximately 24 weeks. However, this curriculum is commonly repeated at least once to obtain group skills training availability for an entire year. In other cases, subsets of skills are taught in order to meet the needs of particular individuals with differing circumstances (Lieb, Zanarini, Schmahl, Linehan, & Bohus, 2004; Linehan, Wilks, & Chelsey, 2015).

At the same time, the individual therapy element of dialectical behaviour therapy is used to enhance client motivation. Individual therapy also allows individuals the opportunity to apply the skills learnt in group therapy in relation to challenges that are specific to their lives (Australian Psychological Society Ltd, 2010; Koerner & Linehan, 2000). Standard dialectical behaviour therapy models have individual and group therapy running concurrently. Crisis coaching is commonly conducted over the phone and provides assistance in effective skill use when faced with difficult situations in everyday life. The goal of crisis coaching is to allow individuals support in between therapy sessions (Lieb, Zanarini, Schmahl, Linehan, & Bohus, 2004; Linehan, Wilks, & Chelsey, 2015). The purpose of consultation opportunities between the treatment team is to provide support to therapists when treating individuals. BPD is commonly considered to be severe, complex, and requires a considerable amount of time to treat. Therefore, through consultations, the treatment team is kept motivated and adherent in order to provide effective treatment to individuals. The treatment teams meet weekly or fortnightly and are composed of those professionals that work with individual clients, as well as those engaged in group skills training (Koerner & Linehan, 2000; Linehan, Wilks, & Chelsey, 2015).

There are four behavioural skill sets taught in dialectical behaviour therapy: (1) mindfulness; (2) distress tolerance; (3) interpersonal effectiveness and; (4) emotional regulation. The first skill set – mindfulness – is designed to teach the individual how to be present and fully aware in a given moment. The second skill set – distress tolerance – is designed to teach the individual how to be tolerant of pain while enduring difficult situations, instead of trying to change it. The third skill set – interpersonal effectiveness – is designed to teach the individual ways to ask for what is desired and how to decline requests, yet maintain existing relationships and self-respect. The fourth and final skill set – emotional regulation – is designed to teach the individual ways to change emotions that the individual wishes to change (Koerner & Linehan, 2000; Lieb, Zanarini, Schmahl, Linehan, & Bohus, 2004; Linehan, Wilks, & Chelsey, 2015). Current research shows that the skills training obtained in dialectical behaviour therapy constitutes an effective intervention that may address a wide array of needs of certain individuals in different settings (Koerner & Linehan, 2000; Lieb, Zanarini, Schmahl, Linehan, & Bohus, 2004; Linehan, Wilks, & Chelsey, 2015).

Research and past experience shows that individuals obtaining dialectical behaviour therapy are faced with multiple issues that require treatment. Therefore, dialectical behaviour therapy is developed from a hierarchy of treatment targets (Australian Psychological Society Ltd, 2010; Koerner & Linehan, 2000). This hierarchy is useful for the therapist to ascertain what order treatment should occur and is based on priority. The first priority is to resolve life-threatening behaviours, including suicidal and self-injury behaviours. The second priority is to resolve therapy-interfering behaviours, including behaviours that will interfere with the provision of effective treatment. These behaviours are not limited to the individual, but can be conducted by the therapist and includes actions, such as late attendance for sessions, cancelling sessions, and/or not working together to meet treatment objectives (Lieb, Zanarini, Schmahl, Linehan, & Bohus, 2004; Linehan, Wilks, & Chelsey, 2015). The third priority is to resolve behaviours that interfere with quality of life. These may include crises related to housing, employment, and/or financial, as well as problems with personal relations with friends/family/significant other and co-existing mental disorders. The fourth priority is to resolve skills deficiencies through acquisition. To resolve this priority, new skills (behaviours) are taught in order to eliminate ineffective and/or inappropriate behaviours in order to assist individuals in reaching their goals (Lieb, Zanarini, Schmahl, Linehan, & Bohus, 2004; Linehan, Wilks, & Chelsey, 2015).

There are four stages to dialectical behaviour therapy. These stages are defined by behaviour severity. However, therapists commit themselves to working with individuals to meet goals at each stage in the therapeutic process. The overall goal of dialectical behaviour therapy is to teach the individual the skills necessary to have a life that is considered to be worth living. The first stage accepts that the individual is miserable and participates in behaviours that are "out of control". Thus, during the first stage, the individual is commonly engaging in self-destructive behaviours (Koerner & Linehan, 2000; Lieb, Zanarini,

Schmahl, Linehan, & Bohus, 2004). Since individuals are commonly volatile during this stage, the primary goal is to achieve behavioural control. During the second stage, the individual may feel desperate and suffer due to previous traumatic and invalidating experiences. However, the individual's behaviour is under control and there is an inhibited emotional experience. As a result, the goal of the second stage is to assist the individual to experience full emotions, allowing for post-traumatic stress disorder issues to be treated (Australian Psychological Society Ltd, 2010; Linehan, Wilks, & Chelsey, 2015). The third stage involves assisting the individual in learning how to live. This is done through assisting to define life-long goals, establish and build self-respect, which will assist the individual in achieving a life of peace and happiness. The final stage of dialectical behaviour therapy involves assisting the individual in determining a spiritual existence in life and establishing a deeper meaning to life. This stage is not for all individuals but is beneficial for those that need to feel connected on a deeper level. This stage is designed to assist the individual in learning how to transition from feeling incomplete to a life of happiness (Australian Psychological Society Ltd, 2010; Lieb, Zanarini, Schmahl, Linehan, & Bohus, 2004).

Mentalization Based Therapy

Mentalization based therapy is a psycho-dynamically-oriented psychotherapy designed to assist individuals diagnosed with BPD. The focus of this type of therapy is to assist individuals to learn how to separate and differentiate personal thoughts and feelings from those of other people. Mentalization refers to the ability of people to understand behaviours and feelings, as well as the association with specific mental states, in both self and others (Australian Psychological Society Ltd, 2010; Bateman & Fonagy, 2010). Contemporary thought suggests that individuals diagnosed with BPD do not have the same capacity as others for mentalization. At the same time, mentalization is found in traditional therapy, yet does not have the primary focus that it has in mentalization based therapy. Mentalization is utilized in a safe, supportive setting during therapy. However, as the approach is psychodynamic, it is not as directive as other therapies, such as cognitive behaviour therapy and/or dialectical behaviour therapy. Commonly, mentalization based therapy focuses on learning/practicing skills in social relationships, as well as independently with the therapist (Australian Psychological Society Ltd, 2010; Bateman & Fonagy, 2010).

Medication

Psychiatric medications refer to any pharmacological compound prescribed to treat mental health disorders or to aid in symptom reduction. The most common types of psychiatric medications include antidepressants and mood stabilizers (Brown, 2001; Jackson & Burgess, 2000; Krieg, 2009). Treatment guidelines (Australian Government, 2011) and research suggest that psychiatric medications do not provide an overall improvement to individuals with a diagnosis of BPD. Although there is no evidence that psychiatric medication improves BPD overall, some improvements are noted when using psychiatric medication to treat particular features of BPD rather than the full spectrum of symptoms. In times of extreme distress or trauma memory recall from somatic markers, individuals with a diagnosis of BPD may experience psychotic like features including disassociation and perceptual disturbances such as "voices". Other times an individual with emotion modulation difficulties, such as extremes in emotional expression, may require the prescription of a mood stabiliser. Depressed mood is another common feature for individuals with a diagnosis of BPD; at times of prolonged mood decline antidepressants have been found to be useful in the short term.

CONCLUSION

Borderline personality disorder is a diagnosis that is commonly misunderstood with high levels of stigma attached to it due to the challenging behaviours often experienced that may interfere with the therapeutic relationship. The fact that there is not a medication to successfully treat BPD is a main distinguishing feature from other psychiatric diagnoses that generally respond to a combination of medical, psychological and social interventions. This chapter has shown the frequent association between trauma and BPD, and in particular childhood sexual abuse, noting however that trauma does not need to be present to be given this diagnosis. A number of proven successful interventions are presented in this chapter that share a number of common features challenging the misconception that BPD cannot be treated. Further research, to be published elsewhere, has been conducted by the author in his doctoral thesis, entitled *Effective Interventions for Working With Individuals with Borderline Personality Disorder* (King, 2017). This includes Australian mental health practitioners' views on what are the most effective treatments for BPD, most suitable locations for treatment and the most appropriate professionals to best respond.

REFERENCES

Allen, D. M. (2013). Invalidation in Families: What Are The Hidden Aspects? *Psychology Today.* Retrieved from: https://www.psychologytoday.com/us/blog/matterpersonality/201309/invalidation-in-families-what-are-the-hidden-aspects

American Psychiatric Association. (2004). *Practice guidelines for the treatment of psychiatric disorders.* Washington, DC: APA.

American Psychiatric Association. (2013). *Diagnostic and statistical manual of mental disorders* (5th ed.). Arlington, VA: American Psychiatric Publishing.

American Psychological Association. (2009). ICD vs. DSM. *Monitor on Psychology, 40*(9), 65.

Arens, E. A., Grabe, H. J., Spitzer, C., & Barnow, S. (2011). Testing the biosocial model of borderline personality disorder: Results of a prospective 5-year longitudinal study. *Personality and Mental Health, 5*(1), 29–42. doi:10.1002/pmh.143

Arntz, A., Stupar-Rutenfrans, S., Bloo, J., van Dyck, R., & Spinhoven, P. (2015). Prediction of treatment discontinuation and recovery from Borderline Personality Disorder: Results from an RCT comparing Schema Therapy and Transference Focused Psychotherapy. *Behaviour Research and Therapy, 74*, 60–71. doi:10.1016/j.brat.2015.09.002 PMID:26432172

Australian Government. (2011). *Clinical Practice Guideline for the Management of Borderline Personality Disorder (BPD).* Canberra, ACT: National MedicalResearch Council.

Australian Psychological Society Ltd. (2010). *Evidence-based Psychological Interventions in the Treatment of Mental Disorders: A Literature Review.* Melbourne: Australian Psychologcal Society.

Baird, L. (2008). Childhood Trauma in the Etiology of Borderline Personality Disorder: Theoretical Considerations and Therapeutic Interventions. *Hakomi Forum, 19*(20-21), 31-42.

Bateman, A., & Fonagy, P. (2010). Mentalization-based treatment for borderline personality disorder. *World Psychiatry; Official Journal of the World Psychiatric Association (WPA)*, *9*(1), 11–15. doi:10.1002/j.2051-5545.2010.tb00255.x PMID:20148147

Beatson, J., & Rao, S. (2014). Psychotherapy for borderline personality disorder. *Australasian Psychology*, *22*(6), 529–532. doi:10.1177/1039856214555531 PMID:25319122

Bendit, N. (2014). Reputation and science: Examining the effectiveness of DBT in the treatment of borderline personality disorder. *Australasian Psychology*, *22*(2), 144–148. doi:10.1177/1039856213510959 PMID:24191293

Biskin, R. S. (2015). The Lifetime Course of Borderline Personality Disorder. *Canadian Journal of Psychiatry*, *60*(7), 303–308. doi:10.1177/070674371506000702 PMID:26175388

Brown, G. K., Ten Have, T., Henriques, G. R., Xie, S. X., Hollander, J. E., & Beck, A. T. (2005). Cognitive therapy for the prevention of suicide attempts: A randomized controlled trial. *Journal of the American Medical Association*, *294*(5), 563–570. doi:10.1001/jama.294.5.563 PMID:16077050

Brown, R. (2001). Australian Indigenous mental health. *The Australian and New Zealand Journal of Mental Health Nursing*, *10*(10), 33–41. doi:10.1046/j.1440-0979.2001.00189.x PMID:11421971

Burns, E., & Martin, A. J. (2014). ADHD and Adaptability: The Roles of Cognitive, Behavioural, and Emotional Regulation. *Australian Journal of Guidance & Counselling*, *24*(2), 227–242. doi:10.1017/jgc.2014.17

Cavazzi, T., & Becerra, R. (2014). Psychophysiological Research of Borderline Personality Disorder: Review and Implications for Biosocial Theory. *Europe's Journal of Psychology*, *10*(1), 185–203. doi:10.5964/ejop.v10i1.677

Chanen, A., McCutcheon, L., Jovev, M., Jackson, H., & McGorry, P. (2007). Prevention and early intervention for Borderline Personality Disorder. *The Medical Journal of Australia*, *187*(7), 18–21. PMID:17908019

Clarkin, J. F., Hull, J. W., & Hurt, S. W. (1993). Factor structure of borderline personality disorder criteria. *Journal of Personality Disorders*, *7*(2), 137–143. doi:10.1521/pedi.1993.7.2.137

Crowe, M. (2004). Never good enough–part 1: Shame or Borderline Personality Disorder? *Journal of Psychiatric and Mental Health Nursing*, *11*(11), 327–334. doi:10.1111/j.1365-2850.2004.00732.x PMID:15149381

Crowell, S. E., Beauchaine, T. P., & Linehan, M. M. (2009). A Biosocial Developmental Model of Borderline Personality: Elaborating and Extending Linehan's Theory. *PMC*, *135*(3), 495–510. PMID:19379027

Distel, M. A., Willemsen, G., Ligthart, L., Derom, C. A., Martin, N. G., Neale, M. C., ... Boomsma, D. I. (2010). Genetic covariance structure of the four main features of borderline personality disorder. *Journal of Personality Disorders*, *24*(4), 427–444. doi:10.1521/pedi.2010.24.4.427 PMID:20695804

Domes, G., Winter, B., Schnell, K., Voha, K., Fast, K., & Herpertz, S. C. (2006). The influence of emotions on inhibitory functioning in Borderline Personality Disorder. *Psychological Medicine*, *36*(08), 1163–1172. doi:10.1017/S0033291706007756 PMID:16700964

Fonseca-Pedrero, E., Paino, M., Lemos-Giraldez, S., Sierra-Baigrie, S., Gonzalez, M. P., Bobes, J., & Muniz, J. (2011). Borderline personality traits in nonclinical young adults. *Journal of Personality Disorders*, *25*(4), 542–556. doi:10.1521/pedi.2011.25.4.542 PMID:21838568

Fromene, R., & Guerin, B. (2014). Talking with Australian Indigenous Clients with a Borderline Personality Disorder Diagnosis: Finding the Context behind the Label. *The Psychological Record*, *64*(3), 569–579. doi:10.100740732-014-0058-3

Fromene, R., Guerin, B., & Krieg, A. (2014). Australian Indigenous Clients with a Borderline Personality Disorder Diagnosis: A Contextual Review of the Literature. *The Psychological Record*, *64*(3), 599.

Gill, D., & Warburton, W. (2014). An Investigation of the Biosocial Model of Borderline Personality Disorder. *Journal of Clinical Psychology*, *70*(9), 866–873. doi:10.1002/jclp.22074 PMID:24585693

Gratz, K. L., & Roemer, L. (2004). Multidimensional assessment of emotion regulation and dysregulation: Development, factor structure, and initial validation of the Difficulties in Emotion Regulation Scale. *Journal of Psychopathology and Behavioral Assessment*, *26*(1), 41–54. doi:10.1023/B:JOBA.0000007455.08539.94

Gratz, K. L., & Roemer, L. (2008). The relationship between emotion dysregulation and deliberate self-harm among female undergraduate students at an urban commuter university. *Cognitive Behaviour Therapy*, *37*(1), 14–25. doi:10.1080/16506070701819524 PMID:18365795

Gunderson, J. G. (2006). *A BPD Brief: An introduction to Borderline Personality Disorder*. New York: Borderline Personality Disorder Resource Center.

Gunderson, J. G., Stout, R. L., McGlashan, T. H., Shea, M. T., Morey, L. C., Grilo, C. M., ... Skodol, A. E. (2011). Ten-year course of borderline personality disorder: Psychopathology and function from the Collaborative Longitudinal Personality Disorders study. *Archives of General Psychiatry*, *68*(8), 827–837. doi:10.1001/archgenpsychiatry.2011.37 PMID:21464343

Guzder, J., Paris, J., Zelkowitz, P., & Feldman, R. (1999). Psychological risk factors for borderline pathology in school-age children. *Journal of the American Academy of Child and Adolescent Psychiatry*, *38*(2), 205–212. doi:10.1097/00004583-199902000-00021 PMID:9951221

Harvey, R., Black, D. W., & Blum, N. (2010). Systems Training for Emotional Predictability and Problem Solving (STEPPS) in the United Kingdom: A Preliminary Report. *Journal of Contemporary Psychotherapy*, *40*(4), 225–232. doi:10.100710879-010-9150-4

Herman, J. L. (1997). *Trauma and Recovery*. New York: Basic Books.

Jackson, H., & Burgess, P. M. (2000). Personality Disorders in the Community: A report from the Australian National Survey of Mental Health and Wellbeing. *Social Psychiatry and Psychiatric Epidemiology*, *12*(53), 1–8. PMID:11213842

King, P. (2017). *Effective interventions for working with individuals with borderline personality disorder* (Unpublished PhD thesis). RMIT University, Melbourne, Australia.

Koerner, K., & Linehan, M. (2000). Research on dialectical behavior therapy for patients with borderline personality disorder. *The Psychiatric Clinics of North America*, *23*(1), 151–167. doi:10.1016/S0193-953X(05)70149-0 PMID:10729937

Koons, C. R., Robins, C. J., Tweed, J. L., Lynch, T. R., Gonzalez, A. M., Morsh, J. Q., ... Bastian, L. A. (2001). Efficacy of dialectical behavior therapy in women veterans with borderline personality disorder. *Behavior Therapy*, *32*(2), 371–390. doi:10.1016/S0005-7894(01)80009-5

Krieg, A. (2009). The experience of collective trauma in Australian Indigenous communities. *Australasian Psychology*, *17*(1_suppl), 28–32. doi:10.1080/10398560902948621 PMID:19579102

Laporte, L., & Guttman, H. (1996). Traumatic childhood experiences as risk factors for borderline and other personality disorders. *Journal of Personality Disorders*, *10*(3), 247–259. doi:10.1521/pedi.1996.10.3.247

Lawn, S., & McMahon, J. (2015). Experiences of care by Australians with a diagnosis of borderline personality disorder. *Journal of Psychiatric and Mental Health Nursing*, *22*(7), 510–521. doi:10.1111/jpm.12226 PMID:26122817

Leichsenring, F., Leibing, E., Kruse, J., New, A. S., & Leweke, F. (2011). Borderline personality disorder. *Lancet*, *377*(9759), 74–84. doi:10.1016/S0140-6736(10)61422-5 PMID:21195251

Lieb, K., Zanarini, M. C., Schmahl, C., Linehan, M. M., & Bohus, M. (2004). Borderline personality disorder. *Lancet*, *364*(9432), 453–461. doi:10.1016/S0140-6736(04)16770-6 PMID:15288745

Linehan, M. (1993). *Cognitive–behavioral treatment of borderline personality disorder*. New York: Guilford Press.

Linehan, M. M. (2000). The empirical basis of Dialectical Behavior Therapy: Development of new treatments versus evaluation of existing treatments. *Clinical Psychology: Science and Practice*, *7*(1), 113–119. doi:10.1093/clipsy.7.1.113

Linehan, M. M., Armstrong, H. E., Suarez, A., Allmon, D., & Heard, H. L. (1991). Cognitive- behavioral treatment of chronically parasuicidal borderline patients. *Annals of General Psychiatry*, *48*(12), 1060–1064. doi:10.1001/archpsyc.1991.01810360024003 PMID:1845222

Linehan, M. M., Schmidt, H., Dimeff, L. A., Craft, J. C., Kanter, J., & Comtois, K. A. (1999). Dialectical behavior therapy for patients with borderline personality disorder and drug dependence. *The American Journal on Addictions*, *8*(4), 279–292. doi:10.1080/105504999305686 PMID:10598211

Linehan, M. M., Wilks, M., & Chelsey, R. (2015). The Course and Evolution of Dialectical Behavior Therapy. *American Journal of Psychotherapy*, *69*(2), 97–110. doi:10.1176/appi.psychotherapy.2015.69.2.97 PMID:26160617

Livesley, W. J., Schroeder, M. L., Jackson, D. N., & Jang, K. L. (1994). Categorical Distinctions in the Study of Personality Disorder—Implications for Classification. *Journal of Abnormal Psychology*, *103*(1), 6–17. doi:10.1037/0021-843X.103.1.6 PMID:8040482

Lynch, T. R., Morse, J. Q., Mendelson, T., & Robins, C. J. (2003). A randomized trial of dialectical behavior therapy for depressed older adults: Post-treatment and six month follow- up. *The American Journal of Geriatric Psychiatry*, *11*(1), 33–45. doi:10.1097/00019442-200301000-00006 PMID:12527538

Meaney-Tavares, R., & Hasking, P. (2013). Coping and Regulating Emotions: A Pilot Study of a Modified Dialectical Behavior Therapy Group Delivered in a College Counseling Service. *Journal of American College Health*, *61*(5), 303–309. doi:10.1080/07448481.2013.791827 PMID:23768227

Nickell, A. D., Waudby, C. J., & Trull, T. J. (2002). Attachment, parental bonding and borderline personality disorder features in young adults. *Journal of Personality Disorders*, *16*(2), 148–159. doi:10.1521/pedi.16.2.148.22544 PMID:12004491

Norrie, J., Davidson, K., Tata, P., & Gumley, A. (2013). Influence of therapist competence and quantity of cognitive behavioural therapy on suicidal behaviour and inpatient hospitalisation in a randomised controlled trial in borderline personality disorder: Further analyses of treatment effects in the BOSCOT st. *Psychology and Psychotherapy: Theory, Research and Practice*, *86*(3), 280–293. doi:10.1111/papt.12004 PMID:23420622

Olenchek, C. (2008). Dialectical Behavior Therapy — Treating Borderline Personality Disorder. *Socialwork Today*, *8*(6), 22.

Perry, J. C., Herman, J. L., Van der Kolk, B. A., & Hoke, L. (1990). Psychotherapy and psychological trauma in borderline personality disorder. *Psychiatric Annals*, *26*(1), 33–43. doi:10.3928/0048-5713-19900101-08

Rogers, B., & Dunne, E. (2013). A Qualitative Study on the Use of the Care Programme Approach with Individuals with Borderline Personality Disorder. *Journal of Psychosocial Nursing and Mental Health Services*, *51*(10), 38–45. doi:10.3928/02793695-20130628-03 PMID:23855437

Ryle, A., & Kerr, I. B. (2002). *Introducing Cognitive Analytic Therapy. Principles and Practices*. Retrieved from http://www.ucl.ac.uk/clinical-psychology/competency-maps/pd- framework/Specific psychological interventions/Cognitive Analytic Therapy for webpage.pdf

Safer, D. L., Telch, C. F., & Agras, W. S. (2011). Dialectical behavior therapy for bulimia nervosa. *The American Journal of Psychiatry*, *158*(4), 632–634. doi:10.1176/appi.ajp.158.4.632 PMID:11282700

Sajadi, S. F., Arshadi, N., Zargar, Y., Mehrabizade Honarmand, M., & Haijari, Z. (2015). Borderline Personality Features in Students: The Predicting Role of Schema, Emotion Regulation, Dissociative Experience and Suicidal Ideation. *International Journal of High Risk Behaviors & Addiction*, *4*(2). doi:10.5812/ijhrba.20021v2 PMID:26401490

Schore, A. N. (1994). *Affect regulation and the origin of the self: The neurobiology of emotional development*. Hillsdale, NJ: Lawrence Erlbaum and Associates.

Siever, L. J., & Koenigsberg, H. W. (2000). *The frustrating no-mans-land of borderline personality disorder. Cerebrum*. New York: The Dana Forum on Brain Science.

Skodol, A. E., Gunderson, J. G., Pfohl, B., Widigier, T. A., Livesley, W. J., & Siever, L. J. (2002). The borderline diagnosis I: Psychopathology, comorbidity, and personality structure. *Biological Psychiatry*, *51*(12), 936–960. doi:10.1016/S0006-3223(02)01324-0 PMID:12062877

Stern, B., & Yeomans, F. (2015). *Transference-Focused Psychotherapy (TFP)*. New York: The Center for Transference-Focused Psychotherapy.

Stoffers, J. M., Völlm, B. A., Rücker, G., Timmer, A., Huband, N., & Lieb, K. (2012). Psychological therapies for people with borderline personality disorder. *The Cochrane Database Of Systematic Reviews*, (8).

Trull, T. J., Useda, J. D., Conforti, K., & Doan, B.-T. (1997). Borderline Personality Disorder Features in Nonclinical Young Adults: 2. Two Year Outcome. *Journal of Abnormal Psychology*, *106*(2), 307–314. doi:10.1037/0021-843X.106.2.307 PMID:9131850

Van der Kolk, B. A. (1987). *Psychological trauma*. Washington, DC: American Psychiatric Press.

Van der Kolk, B. A. (1988). Trauma spectrum: The interaction of biological and social events in the genesis of the trauma response. *Journal of Traumatic Stress*, *1*(3), 273–290. doi:10.1002/jts.2490010302

Wetzelaer, P., Farrell, J., Evers, S. M., Jacob, G. A., Lee, C. W., Brand, O., ... Arntz, A. (2014). Design of an international multicentre RCT on group schema therapy for borderline personality disorder. *BMC Psychiatry*, *18*(14), 319. doi:10.118612888-014-0319-3 PMID:25407009

Winsper, C., Marwaha, S., Lereya, S. T., Thompson, A., Eyden, J., & Singh, S. P. (2015). Clinical and psychosocial outcomes of borderline personality disorder in childhood and adolescence: A systematic review. *Psychological Medicine*, *45*(11), 2237–2251. doi:10.1017/S0033291715000318 PMID:25800970

World Health Organization. (2015). *The ICD-10 Classification of Mental and Behavioural Disorders*. Retrieved from http://www.who.int/classifications/icd/en/bluebook.pdf

Zanarini, M. C. (2000). Childhood experiences associated with the development of borderline personality disorder. *The Psychiatric Clinics of North America*, *23*(1), 89–101. doi:10.1016/S0193-953X(05)70145-3 PMID:10729933

Zanarini, M. C., & Frankenburg, F. R. (1997). Pathways to the development of borderline personality disorder. *Journal of Personality Disorders*, *11*(1), 93–104. doi:10.1521/pedi.1997.11.1.93 PMID:9113824

Zimmerman, M., Chelminski, I., & Young, D. (2008). The frequency of personality disorders in psychiatric patients. *The Psychiatric Clinics of North America*, *31*(3), 405–420. doi:10.1016/j.psc.2008.03.015 PMID:18638643

Zimmerman, M., Rothschild, L., & Chelminski, I. (2005). The prevalence of DSM-IV personality disorders in psychiatric outpatients. *The American Journal of Psychiatry*, *162*(10), 1911–1918. doi:10.1176/appi.ajp.162.10.1911 PMID:16199838

Chapter 10
Working With Lesbian, Gay, Bisexual, and Transgender People in Care Relationships

Gabriel Aleksandrs
Carers Victoria, Australia

ABSTRACT

This chapter details some key considerations for health and human services professionals working with lesbian, gay, bisexual, and transgender (LGBT) people in care relationships. Reflecting on the impacts of stigma and discrimination as well as the social, cultural, and political contexts of LGBT communities and carers, this chapter will explore some of ways these factors (as well as heterosexist and cis-genderist assumptions about families and partners) impact the identification, support, and recognition of LGBT people in care relationships. Finally, this chapter will recommend strategies to reduce poor mental health and wellbeing outcomes among people in care relationships where one or all people involved are LGBT, and explore some key actions that may assist health and human services better support and include LGBT people in care relationships.

INTRODUCTION

Research on the physical and mental health of lesbian, gay, bisexual and transgender (LGBT) populations has identified that LGBT people face unique hardships and obstacles to wellbeing. These can include experiences of physical and mental abuse, persecution or economic disadvantage, and can occur within a range of public life domains such as employment, education, criminal-justice law and relationship recognition. These hardships can be directly linked to negative discriminatory societal responses to diversity of sexual orientation, gender identity or expression and include exclusion or discrimination in personal spheres, such as within significant interpersonal relationships (Rosenstraich, 2013; Moleiro & Pinto, 2015).

For LGBT people in care relationships, intersections might arise between these hardships and the experience of providing or receiving informal support to or from another person. This can result from

DOI: 10.4018/978-1-5225-7402-6.ch010

direct stressors, dynamics of the care relationship itself, or circumstances arising within a person's family or community, economic or socio-political context.

This chapter specifically refers to two sub-cohorts of "carers". One cohort is L, G, B, and/or T people who support a person/s with a chronic illness, disability, mental illness, substance abuse issues or who have aged-related needs. The other sub-cohort are non-LGBT people who care for L, G, B and/or T person/s who (due to one of these same circumstances) require support. Other terms include "people in care relationships" and "LGBT people in care relationships", these refer to carers as above, but also to LGBT people receiving care.

BACKGROUND

Access to Health and Human Services

Literature on LGBT people's use of health and human services acknowledges the impact of stigma attached to non-heterosexual orientations and transgender identities is often a determining feature of the difficulties people experience in accessing them (Johnson, Mimiaga & Bradford, 2008). Emergent research on the experiences of LGBT people seeking or using health and human services (inclusive of carer supports) has recognised a variety of potential barriers to, and gaps in, appropriate service provision as well as fear of self-disclosure among LGBT service users (Albuquerque, de Lima Garcia, da Silva Quirino, Alves, Belém, dos Santos Figueiredo,... & de Abreu, 2016; Coon, 2007).

Many services designed for community and individual wellbeing, safety or capacity building (such as housing, policing, justice, legal, education and employment services) are perceived as unreliable or untrustworthy by LGBT people. LGBT populations have reported inequitable assistance and discriminatory practices in these sectors and highlighted many providers are simply inappropriate or ill-prepared to meet LGBT client needs (Aldridge & Somerville, 2014; Campo & Taylor, 2015; Rossman, Salamanca & Macapagal, 2017).

Circumstances surrounding LGBT communities suggest the need for tailored health and human services, which target the unique challenges and risks they face (Burwick, Gates, Baumgartner & Friend, 2014; Coon, 2007). LGBT people experience sizeable disparities in health and wellbeing outcomes compared to non-LGBT people. Among these are poorer mental health, greater suicide and self-harm risk, increased risks to sexual health, chronic illness, high rates of substance misuse as well as a higher likelihood of being a victim to bullying, violence and harassment (McKay, 2011; Scott, Pringle & Lumsdaine, 2004; Whitehead, Shaver & Stephensen, 2015).

Experiences of discrimination, stigma and harassment on the basis of sexual orientation and gender identity is recognised as a key determinant of health and connected to poorer mental health outcomes among LGBT people (Rutherford, McIntyre, Daley & Ross, 2012). Research on LGBT mental health has identified links between discrimination and levels of depression, suicidal ideation and anxiety (Rosenstreich, 2013; Leonard, Pitts, Mitchell, Lyons, Smith, Patel,... & Barrett, 2012).

Furthermore, while research on comparative health risks and outcomes between the distinct subgroups under the LGBT umbrella remains innovative, significant disparities and differences between each cohort are noted in available data (LGBTI Health Alliance, 2016; Whitehead, Shaver, & Stephenson, 2016). Where there is overlap between cohorts, for example gay transgender men, these risks may be magnified.

Wellbeing of Carers

LGBT people in care relationships are subject to these and other health disparities. Research on the health and wellbeing of carers (and former carers) has identified higher rates of psychological distress and self-reported poorer physical health than people who do not provide care (Schofield, Bloch, Herman, Murphy, Nankervis, & Singh, 1998).

Negative outcomes are not only due to caring, but also attributed to indirect, secondary stressors: a lack of support outside the care relationship and daily life concerns such as poor health, can both impact carers lives (Stalker, 2003). However, it is important to note carers are regularly exposed to stressors and distressing events at a significantly high rate, which increase the risk of common mental disorders (Stansfeld, Smuk, Onwumere, Clark, Pike, McManus, ... & Bebbington, 2014) as well as physical injury (Brown & Mully, 1997; Tong, Haig, Nelson, Yamakawa, Kandala, & Shin, 2003) and illness (Schofield, Bloch, Herman, Murphy, Nankervis, & Singh, 1998).

Indirect impacts on carers (such as limited time, stretched resources or insufficient energy to achieve desired goals in priority life areas) may negatively impact their social life, increase isolation, or create clashes between care relationships and employment. This can subsequently impact intimate partnerships and other family or friend relationships (Oyebode, 2003). Such indirect impacts are an important consideration for policymakers and service providers aiming to mediate health and psychological strains on carers (Stansfeld, Smuk, Onwumere, Clark, Pike, McManus, ... & Bebbington, 2014).

Amplified disadvantage can occur among LGBT carers, where direct or indirect stressors related to care responsibilities combine with anxieties due to L, G, B and/or T discrimination. The experience of real or perceived discrimination can also influence a person's wellbeing. Anxieties regarding the cultural safety of a service provider can be a barrier to using carer or related services, which may otherwise sustain the quality of their relationships. For example, an LGBT carer who is concerned about reactions towards them at a carer support group may choose not to access this form of support, which is known to otherwise alleviate social isolation for others who feel welcome. Also, LGBT people supported in care relationships may experience barriers to accessing services and community due to stigma or discrimination experienced as an LGBT person, as well as due to a disability, mental or chronic illness or their age-related care needs.

Inclusion Criteria

Finally, in some literature, 'LGBTI' is used in an effort to include intersex people and recognise their contributions to LGBT communities. References to L, G, B and T people in this chapter are made with acknowledgment some LGBT people are intersex. However, not all intersex people are LGBT (OII Australia, 2012). Therefore, 'LGBTI' is considered insufficient and inappropriate to refer to intersex experiences here.

While there is overlap with LGBT experiences for some intersex people, major differences between intersex, sexuality and transgender issues remain. These include the nature of acts of violence and discrimination used against intersex people, such as non-consensual medical surgeries. Additionally, there are differences between sexual and gender identity issues and those related to intersex body experiences (Androgen Insensitivity Support Syndrome Support Group Australia (AISSGA), Intersex Trust Aotearoa New Zealand (ITANZ) Organisation Intersex International Australia (OIIAU), Black E., Bond K., (AISSGA), Briffa, T., (OIIAU/AISSGA), Carpenter M., (OIIAU/Intersex Day Project, Cody C., (OIIAU),

David, A., (OIIAU)… BEECHAC, Yovanovic, 2017, pp. 2-4). Conflation of intersex and LGBT issues is problematic in the context of health and discrimination experiences. Therefore, 'intersex' is excluded from the acronym throughout this chapter except where the literature referenced includes it. Inappropriate inclusion of 'intersex' in 'LGBTI' frames illustrates while the acronym may seem convenient, it is not inevitably matched by shared experiences among the communities it refers to.

Interaction Between Carers and Services

Fredriksen-Goldsen and Hooyman (2007) note that although studies identify poor physical and mental health outcomes among carers, there is less exploration on whether or how health or human services can address them, particularly in relation to traditionally marginalised groups. It has also been identified that primary and frequent carers can experience lower life satisfaction than people who care less often (Borg & Hallberg, 2006).

Despite this, health, welfare and government services are often inadequate to address these issues and people with care responsibilities risk not having their needs or concerns addressed alongside those they support. Literature on care relationships cite carers and caring family members who felt overlooked, inadequately informed by professionals (Theed, Eccles & Simpson, 2017), excluded from care teams and care planning, and who had their skills or knowledge downplayed (Williams, 2007; 2012).

An online survey conducted in 2017 questioned 3,516 unpaid carers aged 18-75 across Australia, France, Germany, Italy, Spain, the UK and the US. It found 28 per cent of carer respondents felt their role was unrecognized by their healthcare system, and approximately 43 per cent of surveyed carers living in suburban areas did not feel supported at all by social/welfare services. This survey also found 54 per cent of respondents did not have time to book or attend their own medical appointments, while about 42 per cent put the health of the person they are caring for above their own (Embracing Carers, 2017).

In addition, literature on carers identifies that care relationships can be hidden within a range of contexts, while particular cohorts of carers are even less likely to be identified (Knowles, Combs, Kirk, Griffiths, Patel, & Sanders, 2016). Carer isolation may also increase in countries and contexts where client centered or consumer directed models of care and self-management approaches for people are increasing (Knowles, Combs, Kirk, Griffiths, Patel, & Sanders, 2016; Ottmann, Laragy & Haddon, 2009). If gaps for carer inclusion are not addressed within these service approaches, a risk of damage to the quality of care relationships and new stresses within them remain (Ottmann, Laragy, & Haddon, 2009).

Likewise, ambiguity of relationships between formal service providers and carers has been well documented. Twigg and Atkin (as cited in Rogers & Barnes, 2003, p. 121) identified four policy and service provider approaches to carers, which describe how carers fall either within or beyond health and human services system concerns or responses:

1. The first was *carers as a resource*. This model primarily saw carers as a broad spectrum of people with no distinction between friends, neighbours or primary carers, who could provide support to a service user. These carers are viewed to function in the background to formal service provision and only considered when they are struggling;
2. The second is *carers as co-workers,* where carers are seen as working with formal service providers who may negotiate with carers to delineate between informal and formal care. While the main focus of this model is still the client, carers are considered more central than in the resource model. Despite conflicts of interest being recognised in the 'co-worker' model, these are usually dismissed

in the belief carers want to perform the role. Enabling this is seen as the best way for services to build a relationship with the carer;

3. The third model is the *carers as a co-client*, which concentrates on people who are primary carers with considerable responsibilities. It includes the likelihood of co-existing carer needs, which may need to be met alongside a client. This approach recognises carer needs may conflict with those of the service user's, and that prioritising of need can ignite tensions which need consideration;
4. Finally, there is the *superseded carers* model, which frequently guides service provider interactions with carers supporting people with intellectual disabilities, physical disabilities or mental ill health. Service providers do not sustain care relationships in this instance but rather attempt to remove the need for them. This is done by focussing on the service user and increasing their independence or through interventions, which aim to reduce or remove dependence on a carer.

Throughout this chapter, readers are encouraged to consider how bias towards particular family structures, or discrimination against particular service users, may influence work with LGBT people in care relationships. Readers should seek to identify circumstances where carers might be vulnerable to being considered a resource, a co-worker, a co- client or superseded, or where attitudes to LGBT people receiving care may influence how staff respond to the care relationship and caregiver.

Forms of Discrimination and Stigma Towards LGBT People

Barriers to services, discriminatory treatment and unsuitable supports jeopardize the wellbeing of LGBT people and accrue substantial human and economic cost (Banks 2003). The high societal and economic value of care relationships, combined with their regularity across society (CANCA, 2017), underlies the importance of both mainstream and targeted LGBT services being capable to respond to them appropriately.

A key to providing useful responses to LGBT client or carer needs is recognising homophobia, heterosexism, bi-phobia, transphobia and their impacts. Homophobia typically refers to fears and hatred of lesbians or gay men based on their desires and sexual practices, which can lead to discriminatory behaviour, physical violence or verbal abuse (Leonard, Marshall, Hillier, Mitchell & Ward, 2010).

Heterosexism is related to homophobia insomuch as it refers to assumptions and beliefs that all people are, or at least should be, heterosexual (Leonard, 2002). Heterosexist perspectives perpetuate discrimination against LGBT people through implication that non-heterosexual sexualities are harmful, abnormal and a risk to societal wellbeing (Leonard, 2002; Rosenstreich, 2013; Smith & Ingran, 2004). However, heterosexism is not expressed only by direct hatred for LGBT people, but also through unconscious or deliberate omission of LGBT needs and perspectives. Regardless of its presentation, heterosexism results in heterosexual behaviors, identity or norms, being privileged over those of sexual minorities who are consequently discredited.

For LGBT people in care relationships heterosexist views and assumptions about family, intimate partnerships, parenting and communities among health and human services staff are an additional hurdle (Willis, Ward & Fish, 2011). Heterosexist (and cis-sexist) assumptions by service staff can reduce awareness and identification of LGBT service users and their care relationships (Willis, Ward, & Fish, 2011). This can obscure LGBT status, inhibit self-expression and client help seeking around particular needs (Irwin, 2007).

Homophobia can also extend to bisexuals who are in same gender relationships and may be experienced alongside bi-phobia. Bi-phobia is similarly based on an aversion to sexual desires or practices; however, fear and hatred of bisexual people can also result from mono-sexist beliefs. In other words, the view that only 'single-gender sexual orientations' (heterosexuality and homosexuality) are legitimate (Ross, Dobinson & Eady 2010, p. 496). Mono-sexist views are not limited to heterosexual populations and can be held by gay or lesbian people, thus impacting the safety and inclusion of bisexual people in gay, or shared "LGBT" environments (McLean, 2008).

Likewise, transphobia is defined as an irrational hatred towards individuals who do not conform to societal gender expectations. Enabled by cultural ideologies of heterosexist views of masculine and feminine expression (Rosenstreich, 2013), transphobic views reinforce gender non-conformity between sex and gender as an objectionable characteristic. Transphobia correlates with cis-genderism, which refers to the view conformity between assigned sex at birth and gender identity is normal or natural; or alternatively the view that people whose gender identity is incongruent with the sex they were assigned at birth are odd or threatening (Leonard, Lyons, & Bariola, 2015, cited in Blumer, Ansara & Watson, 2013; Preciado, 2013).

As the focus of transphobia is on gender identity and expression, transgender people of any sexual orientation are vulnerable to experiencing it. Similar to biphobia, it is not only heterosexual people who may be transphobic. Literature on transgender and gender diverse experiences identifies transphobia and cis-genderist interactions among lesbians, gays, and bisexuals (Nadal, Whitman, Davis, Erazo & Davidoff, 2016, p. 499; Cashore & Tuason, 2008, pp. 388–390).

MULTIPLE MARGINALITIES AND INTERSECTION OF LIVED EXPERIENCES

Terminology and Identity

LGBT communities are overlapping, yet separate groups whose experiences of sexual orientation, gender expression and identity are shaped by a range of intersectional lived experiences. It is essential service providers understand how discrimination related to sexual and gender identity or expression may intersect with non-LGBT related marginalities.

Central to the provision of care relationship support is whether people identify with the term "carer" or not. This may depend on a range of individual and relationship characteristics. For example, care relationships may be concealed due to stigma associated with mental illness disability, or a chronic illness (Koschorke, Padmavati, Kumar, Cohen, Weiss, Chatterjee, ... & Balaji, 2017). Carers may hide a care relationship out of respect for another person's decision to not disclose their condition or disability (Kittikorn, Street & Blackford 2006).

Furthermore, despite carer or "caregiver" being a reasonably established term in many health and human service settings, there is fluidity in the way people identify with it. Indeed, there has been contestation regarding the usefulness of this term and arguments it is divisive (Molyneaux, Butchard, Simpson & Murray, 2010). Similarly, its relevance to Aboriginal and culturally diverse communities has been questioned (Hill, Cass, Newton & Valentine, 2012), while disability researchers have challenged carer language dichotomies which focus on dependency or imply loss of autonomy (Stalker 2003).

Perceptions of the term carer orientate around supportive tasks, which originate from preluding affiliations, friendships or familial circumstances. However, distinguishing care relationships from other patterns of care in families and society, or interdependent characteristics of personal, gender and family relationships is difficult (Rogers & Barnes, 2003).

LGBT communities by their nature challenge more traditional definitions of gender and family models, while their relationships may exist within private or selective spheres where they feel safe to express them (Fish, 2006). Nonetheless, caregiving can implement and ascribe value to a range of relationships or social bonds that LGBT people may be part of (Williams, 2012). These include intimate partnerships and "family of choice" – including ex-partners or non-LGBT allies/supporters/friends (Barrett, Whyte, Comfort, Lyons & Crameri, 2015; Kia, 2012; Muraco & Fredricksen Goldsen, 2014). They may also be parent-child relationships (Parslow & Hegarty, 2013; Washington, McElroy, Albright, Oliver, Lewis, Meadows, & Elliott, 2015) or relationships between biological family members, such as siblings (Coon, 2007).

Whether responsibilities are named "caring" or not, people in care relationships require assistance, preferably before the toll on their physical and mental health becomes unsustainable. This does not mean replacing all informal supports – but rather working collectively with carers and service users to remove or mitigate damaging stress factors; and supporting relationships which help them thrive.

As care relationships express a variety of bonds, the health and wellbeing of people in care relationships can be improved when they are able to express themselves in ways independent of the need for support or the ability to provide it. When optimally supported and functioning well, care relationships should enhance emotional and physical independence, confidence, and the autonomy of all parties. Care relationships must also tap into community resources and capacity.

Higher rates of poor mental and physical health and disability among LGBT people suggests many have an increased likelihood of requiring informal care from a friend, partner of family member over their life course or knowing a person who does. With this in mind it is also worth noting that care relationships can be reciprocal and interdependent where two or more people exchange distinct types of support for one another, or the same type of support at various times (Greenberg, 1995; Stalker, 2003). The dichotomy between service user and carer is not always clear-cut. Reciprocity has been identified as a protective factor against carer stress and it is important for services to recognise and support this aspect of care relationships (del-Pino-Casado, Frías-Osuna & Palomino-Moral, 2011).

Disability, Illness and Stigma

Discrimination, stigma and systemic inequality directed at people with disabilities, chronic or mental illness, or because of care responsibilities, can add pressures to everyday life. This can create impediments to care relationships being visible, positive or advantageous.

For example, LGBT people with a disability have cited ableism within LGBT communities as an issue (Harley, Nowak, Gassaway & Savage, 2002; Jowett & Peel, 2009), as well as being desexualized in the eyes of the public and service providers (McCann, Lee & Brown, 2016). Assumptions about what make bodies "normal", attractive, capable of intimacy and sexual function can obscure LGBT identities among people with disabilities (Chappell, 2015).

People in care relationships may also face poor disability access to LGBT community venues and events, which would otherwise provide a sense of belonging. Alternatively, they may experience social stigma related to a disability or mental illness. Exclusion like this can increase distress among LGBT people who are already at heightened risk of experiencing poor mental health. Discrimination in multiple spaces, such as disabled communities and LGBT communities for example, may be especially stressful if a person is struggling to accept their sexual orientation or gender identity, or feels alone due to homophobia in wider society or among disability networks.

Ageism

Ageism, too, can further marginalise people in care relationships. Ward (2000) notes that ageism can be a violation of human and civil rights by categorising and discriminating against people based on age. This deprives older people of autonomy, choice and can force dependent status on them. Ward highlights ageist views that perceive growing older as undesirable and enables community disassociation from ageing. Ageism is not limited to the general public and can also be institutionalised within professional healthcare practices, which has implications for care relationships. For example, a doctor may assume a person is incapable of providing support because of their age and ignore their observations about a patient.

Ageism can also impact LGBT people in unique ways. For instance, a social worker may assume an elderly man is heterosexual and living with a 'friend' simply because he has a grandchild. Rather than imagining the possibility the man may have formed a gay relationship later in life, the social worker's perceptions reflect tendencies in the field of gerontology to overlook the diversity of gay and lesbian ageing (Price, 2012). Haghiri-Vijeh (2013) notes cases of LGBT people who were excluded from end of life decision-making processes while their partners were in care. Experiences of ageism within LGBT communities and negative perceptions of ageing among gay men have also been raised (Tinney, Dow, Maude, Purchase, Whyte, & Barrett, 2015).

Gender

Lesbian, bisexual and transgender women can experience intersections of marginalisation due to gender related discrimination within public spheres and their families. For instance, research has identified gay men and lesbians are more likely to undertake parent care than heterosexuals (Glaesser & Patel, 2016). However, community expectations – or the carer's own expectations – of traditional gender roles (Reczek & Umberson, 2016) alongside assumptions lesbian or bisexual daughters were "single" may increase the likelihood they would be assumed to care for parents in comparison to their male counterparts (Parslow & Hegarty, 2013). It is not unlikely transgender women may also experience expectations of "nurturing" or "caring" behaviour upon transition and expression of their gender identity.

Race, Religion and Culture

Assumptions about race, religion or culture can also compromise health and human services provision and have flow on effects for the wellbeing of ethnically and faith diverse LGBT people seeking supports. Pallotta-Chiarolli and Rajkhowa (2017) note that being LGBT within a minority ethnic or faith community means navigating, negotiating and living between varied and multiple conventions, expectations and social codes regarding gender, sexuality and ethnicity. Young same sex attracted and gender diverse refugee and asylum seekers, for example, can experience significant ongoing stress and fear about the impacts of being out, and also the impacts of this upon their families due to shame and humiliation (Canales & Leonard, 2016).

Assumptions LGBT people do not exist within minority faith or ethnic communities can be prevalent within the communities themselves or originate beyond them. The perception, inclusion and influence of LGBT people is problematic in global, post-colonial countries and contexts where histories of colonialism, racism and segregation cross with contemporary, "Western" ideas of sexuality and gender identity.

Colonization of gender and sexualities can result in erasure of identities such as race, ethnicity, nationalism, class and gender and subsequently extend invisibility of LGBT sub-cohorts such as lesbian women, even in physical and cultural spaces that aim to disrupt hetero-normativity (Reygan, 2016). Similarly, the oppression of local diverse sexualities and genders may stem from views that see being L, G, B and/or T is a symptom of secular or decadent moralities of urban white culture (Pallotta-Chiarolli & Rajkhowa, 2017). Racism may also be experienced within LGBT communities (Walters & Old Person Jr, 2014).

Furthermore, cultural norms vary in relation to stigma and meanings attached to health conditions or disabilities, which can influence people's interaction with health and human services or their likelihood to provide care. Some research has identified a sense of "duty" among some ethnic and religious groups, yet human services do not always respond in culturally sensitive ways (Greenwood, Habibi, Smith & Manthorpe, 2015). It has been noted that social work literature, for instance, remains wanting for tools or guidelines to address the intersection of multiple marginalities, identities and experiences of LGBT people of colour (Walters & Old Person Jr, 2014). Without guidance, staff run the risk of responding poorly or focusing on a carer's ethnicity and assumed cultural preferences over their needs specific to their lived experience of gender or sexuality.

Case Study: Jin

Jin supports her mother who has severe arthritis, chronic depression and anxiety. Since the death of Jin's father, her mother has struggled at home alone, so Jin spends two hours daily travelling to and from her mother's house to assist with meals, personal care and transport to medical appointments. Jin also provides financial support to her mother, which is placing strain on Jin's relationship.

Jin is in a lesbian relationship of three years. Her partner is not "out" to her Chinese family, who hope she will marry a Chinese man. Jin's partner's family think her and Jin are just friends as they are studying at university together. Jin's partner is covering more of their household bills.

Jin's mother began phoning her late at night. During these calls, she swings between sobbing about her husband's death and becoming abusive, telling Jin she is a 'disgusting lesbian'. Being awakened late during the night and the stress of these calls is making Jin depressed, as is an increase in arguments with her partner.

Jin's mother was recently admitted to hospital due to a severe depressive episode. However, when she was discharged the duty social worker saw no need to refer her to extra supports because Jin's mother said via an interpreter she had a dutiful daughter and it was the 'traditional Chinese way' for the community to look after its own.

Refugee Experience

LGBT refugee or migration experiences can also influence help seeking of LGBT people (Canales & Leonard, 2016). Past discrimination by service providers can deter LGBT people from accessing health and human services or self- disclosure. Likewise, distrust towards service providers can exist among refugee LGBT people who experienced persecution, violence and threats in their countries of origin (Reading & Ruben, 2011). There are high rates of post-traumatic stress and trauma among refugee populations (Reading & Ruben, 2011). Reluctance to use services can be particularly detrimental in populations who collectively cope with high rates of trauma as ripple effects spread through whole communities.

Even in countries where LGBT people have significant legal protections, they face more vulnerability than cis-gendered heterosexual populations to poor health. Substantial evidence indicates LGBT persons experience significant health inequalities and poorer outcomes than heterosexual persons worldwide (World Health Organization, 2013).

Mental Health System Experiences and Mental Health Outcomes for LGBT People

Cognizance of high rates of mental ill health among LGBT people is vital when working with those who are in care relationships, whether they are caregivers or receiving care. Risks to mental health, combined with threats to wellbeing associated with the direct or indirect stressors of caregiving, create a potential for crisis flashpoints in care relationships, which require monitoring and mitigation.

Research has identified LGBT people's experiences of discrimination can extend to their use of mental health services (Croghan, Moone & Olson, 2014; Kidd, Veltman, Gately, Chan & Cohen, 2011; Rutherford, McIntyre, Daley, & Ross, 2012). This includes an unhelpful legacy of stigmatising clinical theories and diagnosis ascribed to LGBT people, which was at the heart of many psychiatric institutions and practices (Drescher, 2015; Whitehead, Shaver, & Stephenson, 2016).

For a large part of modern gay, lesbian, bisexual and transgender history, LGBT people have been categorised by psychiatric pathological views that associate non-heterosexual attractions or transgender identities with disease, developmentally disruptive external factors (such as sexual abuse, or "excessive mothering") and other kinds of psychological inferiority (Drescher, 2015). This coincided with a range of heterosexist views, perpetuated within health, scientific and psychiatric circles at different times and which have served to exclude LGBT people. For example, some of these views labeled LGBT people as biologically inferior or suggested they have hormonal disorders, while others presented LGBT people as genetically inferior, emotionally inept or morally dangerous (Fish, 2006).

Moleiro and Pinto (2015) note although the American Psychiatric Association removed homosexuality from the Diagnostic and Statistical Manual in 1973, formal pathologisation of homosexuality did not cease with this change. The DSM-II contained the diagnosis of 'sexual orientation disturbance', which was then replaced by 'ego dystonic homosexuality' in the DSM-III, by 1980. Both these diagnoses continued to legitimise sexual "conversion" therapies among people with homosexual attraction who were distressed by or sought to change their orientation. Furthermore, the World Health Organization's International Classification of Diseases (ICD-10) did not remove homosexuality until 1992 and still contains a diagnosis similar to 'ego-dystonic homosexuality' which is due to be modified in the next revision (Moleiro & Pinto, 2015, pp. 2-3).

Likewise, the World Health Organization is moving towards declassifying transgender identity as a mental disorder in the ICD-10 by no longer classifying "Transsexualism" under the category of "Mental health and disorders". It is proposed, instead to be classified as "Gender incongruence of adolescence and adulthood" under the category "Conditions related to sexual health" (Thomas, Pega, Khosla, Verster, Hana, & Say, 2017). 'Gender identity disorder' was only recently removed from the DSM and debate persists among transgender people as to whether it should remain at all. As Moleiro and Pinto (2015) note, many believe inclusion of transgender identity within diagnostic tools plays a significant role in perpetuating and rationalizing prejudice toward transgender people.

Transgender populations face unique obstacles accessing mental health care. Some include poor access to sensitive and capable professionals; difficulty finding information about gender dysphoria, hormone therapies or surgeries; inadequate access to safe prescription and supervision of hormone therapy; and poor affordability and availability of surgeries (Lo & Horton, 2016).

These obstacles impact core domains gender affirmation traverses, such as the social (e.g. name, pronoun), psychological (e.g. internal, felt self), medical (e.g. hormone therapy, surgeries, or body modification), and legal, such as official gender markers or legal name change (Reisner, Poteat, Keatley, Cabral, Mothopeng, Dunham,... & Baral, 2016). Achieving gender affirmation will also depend on a person's context (e.g. country and region), issues of economics or poverty, and the criminalisation of sexual and gender minorities.

This can cause mental distress and slow down outcomes transgender people highly anticipate. It can also increase the risk of violence and discrimination as they go through visible physical changes or when mismatching legal identification reveals transgender identity. Seeking mental health support to cope with such circumstances can be difficult. The complexities of accessing treatments to transition have added to the perception of service providers as "gatekeepers" among transgender and gender diverse people (Cruz, 2014).

For example, the World Professional Association for Transgender Care (WPATH) Standards of Care stipulates that mental health professionals are the first point of contact for transgender people seeking affirmation of their gender. Referral for hormone therapy or surgery requires a mental health professional's assessment of a person's eligibility, suitability and readiness, with lower genital surgery often requiring two mental health professional referrals. In addition, the use of DSM-5 is embedded in the Standards of Care to assess whether distress is not accounted for by another diagnosis (Schulz, 2018). This may result in reluctance among transgender people to disclose poor mental health where this may jeopardize medical transition or result in a perception of impaired decision-making capacity.

Health and human service staff should avoid assumptions that client distress is related to gender identity or sexuality, rather than a range of issues in other life domains. Discerning stressors and avoiding conflation of LGBT status with mental illness is crucial when supporting a care relationship where the mental distress of a transgender person is an issue.

Case Study: Emma

'Emma' is a transgender woman who lives with bi-polar 2 and PTSD. She has managed on a low dose of medication and meditation classes for three years. Over recent months her panic attacks increased after she was harassed by a group of men on a train who tried to rip off her dress. Emma's long-term bisexual partner Alice supported Emma to report the incident to police and assisted Emma to resume

regular counseling. When Alice suggested Emma review her medication, Emma said she was fearful her symptoms would result in her psychiatrist refusing her female hormone prescriptions and gender reassignment surgery. Alice fully supports Emma's gender transition, but knows that the last time Emma increased her medication during a relapse of severe symptoms it helped.

Alice is experiencing insomnia, she cries often and worries about Emma. On occasion, she has left work early to meet and comfort Emma and ensure she does not self-harm. Recently she took Emma to hospital during a panic attack where she couldn't breathe. Emma did not present as a woman at emergency because she was afraid of how staff would react. Emma requested strict confidentiality from Alice about her symptoms getting worse and hides them from her GP. Despite these issues Emma and Alice remain excited about Emma's transition and Emma only has three more psychiatrist appointments over four months before she will be approved for hormone therapy.

SOLUTIONS AND RECOMMENDATIONS

Proposed solutions to improve LGBT access to health and human services include: addressing discrimination against LGBT people globally and within broader society, (Carroll & Mendos, 2017); legislative protections; improved service delivery standards and LGBT inclusive guidelines (Daley & MacDonnell, 2011); staff training on LGBT community needs (Irwin, 2007); de-stigmatisation/de-pathologisation of LGBT people (Lim, Brown & Jones, 2013); and the development of models of health and community care that increase both safety and relevance of services for LGBT consumers (Barrett, Turner & Leonard, 2013).

Consider Issues Surrounding 'Families of Choice'

Some carer support agencies and programs recognise the likelihood of LGBT people seeking "families of choice" due to possible or actual rejection by family of origin as a result of their sexual orientation or gender identity. Indeed, available research indicates a high value ascribed to friends as potential caregivers among LGBT people (Croghan, Moone & Olson 2014; Fredriksen-Goldsen, Kim, Muraco & Mincer, 2009).

It has been suggested that care circles initiated by partners, friends and community allies were a development among LGBT communities during the AIDS crisis when friends and partners were heavily impacted (Glaesser & Patel 2016; Shiu, Muraco, & Fredriksen-Goldsen, 2016). It is no surprise the protective nature of care relationships with friends and partners may be appealing or favoured, especially if formal services and family or community of origin, are seen as unsafe or inappropriate (Fredriksen-Goldsen, Kim, Muraco, & Mincer, 2009). It is not just the provision of care, which is valued. Family of choice can be a source of refuge for LGBT people who are caregivers and support them in their role as a carer enabling them to carry on during times of stress (Butler 2017; Dykewomon, 2017; Price, 2011).

However, friend and family of choice care remains under-researched (Shiu, Muraco, & Fredriksen-Goldsen, 2016). Furthermore 'families of choice' should not be assumed just because a person is L, G, B and/or T. This presumes circumstances, community connections and personal capacity capable of close and well-resourced relationships, which are supportive in family-like ways. This may not be the case.

In addition, some people may not have access to deeply reciprocal relationships with others who are physically able to meet their care needs (Hash & Nettling, 2009). Where illness carries tremendous stigma, such as in severe mental illness, people may find close relationships difficult to maintain. Some LGBT people may also be reliant on or supporting a person they are not "out" to or is homophobic (Barrett & Crameri, 2015) thus isolating them from other communities. Improved clarity of the relationship between care giving and families of choice, particularly among marginalised extended communities, is required. This will better inform targeted, helpful health and human service interventions, and aid the development of strengths-based approaches that reflect the full range of relationships LGBT people are in, and the extent to which these relationships are supportive to service users.

Relationship Recognition

It should be noted too, family of choice might be reluctantly used or a substitute term for people who would like more legitimacy afforded to their relationships or those of their loved ones. Legal recognition for LGBT people is inconsistently granted from country to country. Not all people wish to marry and some LGBT people may indeed prefer to accentuate less conventional relationships or see families of choice as a form of political resistance to conventional relationships overseen by the State (Price, 2011). Legal relationship recognition has been highlighted in many global LGBT human rights campaigns; likewise, many LGBT relationship recognition campaigns have focused on human rights, equality and the practical barriers insufficient legal recognition of partner relationships can create.

Beyond the legalities, common societal views of what constitutes families (including among non-LGBT people) can vary significantly and change over time, as can the visibility or acknowledgement of LGBT family structures. For example, Mizielińska and Stasińska (2017) cite shifts in Poland during public and political debates regarding two civil union bills proposed by SLD (the Democratic Left Alliance party) in 2011.Their research identified changes within Polish public discourse on LGBT families over the last decades from very conservative and traditional definitions of family in the early 2000s to more open definitions by 2010–2011. They note media debate shaped the public conversation on civil unions by contextualizing same-sex unions within wider-ranging changes in the way families function. They also found many voices in the public sphere regardless of whether they were for or against same-sex unions acknowledged the existence of LGBT parents.

Legislation does not always accommodate changing social views however, and as Mizielińska and Stasińska (2017) note 'family is a construct that suits a specific vision of society and its politics. It is nothing fixed and permanent' (p. 1812). It is therefore not surprising the rights afforded to LGBT people and the social recognition of their relationships are vulnerable to political and social volatilities.

The civil union's bills in Poland would have enabled tax benefits, widow pensions, the right to inheritance and social insurance to married gay and lesbian couples (however it excluded rights to adoption). Nevertheless, the civil partnership act or recognition of same-sex families did not prevail in Poland (Mizielińska & Stasińska, 2017), which no doubt had significant repercussions for some Polish LGBT people in care relationships.

Similarly, other issues have been identified for LGBT people in care relationships living in the United States. These include: being ineligible for government and workplace family benefits and leave; and high levels of discrimination in employment and housing, including public housing and long-term care housing (Fredriksen-Goldsen, Kim, Muraco, & Mincer, 2009). Again, progress addressing these issues remains dependent on political climates, which, at least currently for LGBT Americans, appears fickle.

Service providers ignoring or misunderstanding legal protections, and rejecting LGBT carers as powers of attorney (Croghan et. al 2014), partners (Valenti & Katz, 2014) or beneficiaries (Czaja, Sabbag, Lee, Schulz, Lang, Vlahovic,... & Thurston, 2016) has also been raised. There has been some success in achieving recognition of child guardianship via second parent adoption and recognition for non-biological parents in some countries such as the United States (Knauer, 2016) and Australia, where law is increasingly including and recognising gay and lesbian couples and their children (Sifris, 2014). However, where lesbian and gay parents cannot adopt (including transgender people in lesbian or gay relationships) remains an issue. From this perspective families of choice may not seem compensatory for people who would rather alter the legal expression of their closest relationships if they had the opportunity.

LGBT people in care relationships can experience discrimination and may face the indignity of requests to "prove" their relationship to service providers in countries where they are not legally recognised. Conscious recognition of how care dynamics are impacted by legal or social inequities can improve the sensitivity of service responses to mental distress among consumers, carers and families who struggle to have their bonds recognised legally and socially.

Marriage equality is one measure, that can influence access to income support programs — either by increasing or decreasing access — or by altering the household income or composition considered to determine eligibility for programs (Burwick, Gates, Baumgartner, & Friend, 2014). However, the right to marry needs to be matched with the principle that all marriages are equal; alongside non-discrimination laws on the basis of sexual orientation and gender identity which cover all life domains. This would better meet the needs of LGBT people across the range of care relationships discussed in this chapter. Despite the complexities of families of choice as a broad concept, they nonetheless remain a source of support for many service users and carers, and require recognition by service providers.

RECOMMENDATIONS AND TIPS FOR PRACTICE

There are many affirmative actions that health and human services can take in response to LGBT people in care relationships to help mitigate the impacts of discrimination and care relationship stress.

Address Heteronormative and Cis-Gendered Service Delivery

As touched on earlier in this chapter there are a growing number of affirmative practice guides available to assist health and human services develop inclusive practices for LGBT service users. Many of these provide a starting point and go some way in reducing discriminatory heteronormative and cis-gendered practices. In some countries, sector accreditation and minimum standards in LGBT inclusive service provision, such as the Rainbow Tick in Australia (Gay and Lesbian Health Victoria, n.d.), have been designed for the community, health and human services sectors as well as service benchmarking initiatives like the Health Equality Index by the Human Rights Campaign Foundation.

Work in this area also includes guidelines on the primary care of LGB health consumers in a range of countries including the US, Australia, UK, Canada and Ireland (McNair, 2010) and social work guides for best practice working with LGB people in Ireland (IASW, 2011). Guides associated with these standards can assist with the adoption of LGBT inclusive policies and practices. Similarly, literature initiatives addressing hetero and cis-normative practices have provided overviews of best practice. Examples of practical actions within these standards, guides and available literature include things like:

- Use open gender neutral/appropriate language and terminology with service users when referring to relationships and gender identity (Irish Association of Social Workers, 2011; The Joint Commission, 2011);
- Design service forms which capture sexual and gender diversity or amend government mandated templates and documentation to ensure they are LGBT inclusive (Barrett & Crameri, 2015);
- Understand legal service provider obligations and anti-discrimination laws which, protect LGBT people and the range of jurisdictions in which they apply (The Joint Commission, 2011);
- Create a welcoming environment, e.g. display posters affirming LGBT communities, use images of LGBT people in service materials (Friedrickson-Goldsen & Hooyman, 2007), display rainbow, bisexual and transgender flags (Barrett & Crameri, 2015) ensure LGBT specific service brochures are available;
- Build mutually beneficial partnerships between LGBT community groups and health and human service providers to collaborate and pool resources with the goal to create effective care pathways and supports for LGBT people in care relationships (Coon, 2007);
- Train staff to ask questions regarding sexual and gender identity appropriately at service gateways (LGBTI Health Alliance, 2013) and challenge their assumptions about sexuality and gender (Barrett & Crameri, 2015);
- Be clear to service users and carers that all genders and sexualities are respected and considered equal (Barrett & Crameri, 2015);
- Incorporate affirmative recruitment policies, ensure equitable treatment and inclusion of LGBT staff (The Joint Commission, 2011).

The complex issues surrounding the development of carer and consumer experience and outcome measurement instruments, evaluations and assessments exceed this chapter's discussion. Suffice to say these are common tools in health, mental health and other human services settings that vary in application and domains of measurement, and are often tailored to services provided.

Furthermore, reliable measurement of service user and caregiver experience and outcomes at various points of the service journey over time is useful. Quality service validation and outcome measurement tools can increase knowledge of how carer or consumer concerns change, decrease or escalate over time. Ideally these instruments and tools can build service capacity to identify changes at various stages of care relationships and during different interventions (e.g. when a person is admitted, treated or discharged from a program/service). Service experience and outcome measurement instruments that capture LGBT data are required to detect causes of positive and negative outcomes for LGBT people in care relationships in a range of circumstances and service contexts.

However, measuring LGBT service experience requires ascertaining not only who LGBT people are, but also any capacity to record and report on this data. Data collection can be influenced by circumstances such as whether people are "out" about their sexuality (LGBTI Health Alliance, 2013; Valenti & Katz, 2014) or in a heterosexual relationship at the time but are bisexual, for example. Counting transgender people can be complex if they are not "perceived" as trans, are assumed to be cis-gendered or they identify as either 'male' or 'female' only. Transgender people may also provide different responses to queries regarding their gender at various stages of their journey, or identify in ways that are inconsistent with a range of legal documentation services may refer to (LGBTI Health Alliance, 2013).

These issues require consideration and consultation with LGBT communities, organisations, specialist service providers, activists and community groups (where possible) to design relevant, respectful data collection and measurement tools and decide how the information will be collected, by who, and under what circumstances.

Be Person Centered and Relationship Aware in LGBT Service Delivery

Outcomes for services wanting to improve LGBT consumer and carer inclusion depend largely on whether they understand an L, G, B and/or T person's lived experience, choices and views from a holistic perspective. This includes but is not limited to consideration of:

- The variability of desire among LGBT people to use an 'LGBT specific' service;
- How connected service users feel (or want to be) to LGBT communities;
- The separate and overlapping nature of gender and sexuality;
- Whether multiple identities are significant to a person and whether an order is attached to them (e.g. their ethnicity, religion, identity as a carer, gender identity, experience as a person with a disability);
- Pre-existing relationships the service user is party to (whether these are in the LGBT community or not), the importance and purpose ascribed to them and ways these are defined.

Ascertaining the priority of concerns for LGBT people and their allies in care relationships requires open in-depth inquiry and discernment to ensure quality support and referral. This is particularly the case in mental health or carer counseling settings where distress may be expressed in raw forms at crisis points. For example, poor mental health or increased anxiety among LGBT (or ally) carers could be due to any one or a combination of factors such as:

- A lack of support for their care role;
- Care relationship conflicts, or conflict external to the care relationship;
- Heightened concerns about the person they support (e.g. risk the person will self-harm or a sudden change in physical health);
- Discrimination against either themselves or the person they support;
- General poor health and human service system responses;
- A lack of service recognition of expertise within the care relationship or poor service recognition pre-existing support strategies;
- Significant care responsibilities being required over a prolonged period;
- Whether the carer provides support to more than one person.

Understand Service User Family Roles and Dynamics From LGBT Perspectives to Inform Work With LGBT People in Care Relationships

While LGBT consumer guides are useful, addressing care relationship needs is also required. Family-focused and integrated service approaches to supporting care relationships must reflect the range of relationships LGBT people are in, and consider the unique strains LGBT people are vulnerable to experiencing within their families and communities of origin (Fricdrickson-Goldsen & Hooyman, 2007).

For example, information about sexual orientation and/or gender identity needs to be handled appropriately in family and care relationship contexts. Staff working with LGBT people in care relationships should ensure the status of their consent to disclose sexual or gender identity is clear. Health and human service staff need to explicitly clarify how information is recorded as well as how or where it is used and who with (LGBTI Health Alliance, 2013). This can avoid negative or damaging impacts of unwelcome disclosures, which may harm the foundations of a care relationship or reduce support to people who are party to them or lead to trauma or mental illness for the carer. Available literature on LGBT care relationships and caregiving also identify some useful actions and strategies, which include but are not limited to the following strategies:

- Identify carer and carer peer support groups that welcome LGBT people or develop LGBT support groups (Barrett & Crameri, 2015; Coon, 2007);
- Support consumer and carer peer groups and peer workers to improve LGBT literacy and awareness (Barrett & Crameri 2015);
- Develop or adopt policies ensuring equal visitation and the right for service users to identify a support person (or persons) of their choice (The Joint Commission, 2011);
- Provide professional development and training on the needs of those in care relationships (Schofield, Bloch, Herman, Murphy, Nankervis, & Singh, 1998) – this could include carer identification, referral, supports, carer advocacy and advanced planning with carers;
- Understand the law and ethics context which form a backdrop to all aspects of caring (Ross, 2003) and ensure this informs service practices with care dyads. Understand how this context intersects with laws impacting the rights afforded to LGBT people;
- Incorporate language, processes, procedures and practices that include and conceptualise family in a broad sense (Price, 2011) and which recognise LGBT parent arrangements and partnerships.

Consider Your Service's Approach and Tools

Systematic identification of carers at risk of poor mental health is a priority and it is a breach of care if the significant numbers of carers who meet the criteria for psychological distress are not offered support. In reference to palliative care, Hudson (2013) notes the challenge workers experience in supporting carers implies potential merit in recognising carers as "care recipients" to justify much needed time, resources and interventions where appropriate.

Screening consumers at health, disability, youth, aged, and mental health service gateways to ascertain if they have a carer partially addresses identification of carers. Additional clarification whether consumers provide care to another person would also be of assistance. This can enable prompt referral to interventions for people in care relationships and improve service provision for carers experiencing distress or poor health, whether it is related to their care role or not. In mental health settings screening for care responsibilities combined with competent data collection could aid understanding of the mental health impacts of care relationships, the mental needs of carers, which services carers use and how useful they find them.

Care responsibilities can be established without using the term "carer" and this may increase the likelihood of identification of care relationships. Asking questions of service users around their day-to-day life is helpful, such as 'are there people who rely on you to help with things?' or 'are there people you rely on to help you regularly or from time to time?' Regardless of whether service data collection fields refer to the existence of carers, face-to-face inquiry should reflect everyday lives and relationships. A list of thoughtful standardized intake instruments can be a useful prompt, particularly if they have been developed in consultation with communities a service is targeting.

Work and Plan Mutually, Particularly Where the Care Relationship Is at Risk

Where people in care relationships have negotiated issues of emergency planning, and a service user has made choices and decided to access supports in identified circumstances with the assistance of their carer, it is important that health and human services staff honor these choices. New care plans and support strategies for people in care relationships should include all parties and provide space for the carer to manage their health or self-care alongside the service user's needs.

Empowering LGBT people to clarify wishes is vital, especially where care responsibilities may not be as readily assumed as it would of "spouses" or biological families. This is particularly the case, if additional legal or practical steps are required to ensure the rights of primary carers, family members or partners are recognised. Identification of consumer preferences for nominated persons, guardians and medical powers of attorney is as important as identifying 'a carer'.

Connect With LGBT Organisations to Raise LGBT Literacy

Social isolation among LGBT people and their allies in care relationships can also be addressed through increasing awareness and recognition of care relationships within LGBT communities. This can include highlighting community access issues and barriers people in care relationships may face due to disability, mental or chronic illness, or age-related needs. LGBT people working in health and human services may be well positioned to play a unique role bridging the knowledge gap between services (including carer supports) and their own communities. Peer supports are an important source of social interaction and education (Broady & Aggar, 2017). LGBT consumer and carer peer leaders could increase care relationship literacy in LGBT communities. Peer carer and consumer reference groups, committees and organisations should reach out and encourage participation of LGBT people via LGBT community networks and at LGBT events.

Limitations

It has been noted that broader political, economic and social settings in which human services are positioned, including national and global contexts, also contribute to the possibilities and limitations of their interventions (Johnson, Mimiaga, & Bradford, 2008). Likewise, it is essential to concede this chapter's deliberations are limited by the research and literature they are based on. These are primarily from countries and settings where social welfare, health and human services, and social safety nets are available in adequate capacity to warrant discussion within social science and related professions. Conclusions are shaped by the views, experiences and perceptions of those who contributed to this literature as well as the chapter's author.

Another central limitation of this chapter is the emergent nature of literature on LGBT carers. Social work research specifically on LGBT people who provide regular informal support, or on LGBT social support systems, remains limited (Orel & Coon, 2016, p. 41; Willis, Ward & Fish, 2011, p. 1306). In addition, knowledge about LGBT people in care relationships is framed by persisting questions regarding the lived experiences of LGBT people which from a global view can be vastly different from one nation-state to the next.

However, there is no reason why existing knowledge (for example on carers, LGBT communities, health and wellbeing, disability, ageing, cultural and religious diversity and physical and mental illnesses) cannot be combined and contrasted to collectively inform health and human service professionals enough to further inquiry and initiate some service adjustments.

CONCLUSION

As a general social policy category, caregiving has undergone significant study and research. This is particularly the case in countries where de-institutionalisation has resulted in a greater policy focus on independent community living. However, a defining feature of this research is a lack of mature critical perspectives and an emphasis on dichotomies of carer vs service user rather than the relationship between them (Lloyd, 2003). In addition, research on caregiving generally focuses on biological family and marital relationships (Shiu, Muraco, & Fredriksen-Goldsen, 2016). Expansion of existing literature on carer relationship perspectives that focus beyond cis-gendered family frames would be useful.

Ending global inequalities among LGBT people, including human rights abuses against them, their families and communities, is an urgent and complex task. LGBT people in care relationships also must deal with the impacts of inequality and discrimination, which in turn may increase the likelihood of LGBT people being in a care relationship.

Workers in health and human services need to examine service systems and practices that perpetuate discrimination and health inequalities against LGBT people. For example, it is noted that the medical paradigm has been a causal power contributor to social isolation and exclusion of LGBT people, and prevented them from being recognised in family units. Countries that are anti-LGBT continue to treat people from these communities with shock therapy, medications and surgical procedures to alter "abnormality" in an attempt to treat and cure. Furthermore, health service provider assumptions and discrimination toward LGBT people may persist if underlying beliefs and attitudes shaped by medical, religious and cultural values are not addressed (Haghiri-Vijeh, 2013).

Unique circumstances of stigma and discrimination experienced by LGBT people, especially human rights abuses within mental health and human services settings, require proactive consideration by workers when planning supports for LGBT people (and their allies) providing or receiving care. Cultural safety for LGBT consumers and carers is particularly important when mental health interventions are required.

Reducing deficits in health and human service provision for LGBT people will address many barriers they may face in seeking validation of their relationships. However, service providers also need to voice resistance to discrimination against LGBT people and advocate for improvements to the rights granted them wherever possible to establish an environment for best practice with LGBT cohorts.

In addition, health and human service providers should ensure inclusion, recognition and support of care relationships is embedded in the design, implementation, review and evaluation of services. Professional practices should recognise the interdependent reciprocal qualities of care relationships and the intersection of LGBT, cultural, or disabled identities; as well as the social, economic, cultural and political context of LGBT service users and carers (Coon, 2007). Given the regularity of care relationships and the significant contribution they provide communities, it is essential that supports reach hidden carer cohorts like LGBT people. This can enable more sustainable, healthy, safer, connected and productive communities and reduce the financial and human costs of long-term care.

FUTURE RESEARCH

Research on caring in the LGBT community is in the initial stages of development, while existing empirical studies on caregiving and LGBT people are qualitative in methodology. Subsequently there is little quantitatively verified information on LGBT caregiving, including the demands on LGBT caregivers, supports to LGBT people in care relationships and the psychological impacts of care. Fredriksen-Goldsen and Hooyman (2007) note a lack of theoretical grounding to LGBT caregiving research and suggest life course and longitudinal approaches might provide more in-depth knowledge. This includes information on: whether people within diverse communities have similar or different life courses; the impact of specific risk or protective factors over different life stages; generational experiences of being in a care relationship; and the influence of family context and structure (Fredriksen-Goldsen & Hooyman, 2007).

Willis et al. (2011) also note LGBT carers are often spoken about as a single social identity, with bisexual and transgender issues being subsumed into gay and lesbian research and practice. Failure to distinguish between sexual orientation and gender assumes the same needs for both and has resulted in data not being separately analysed in research. A lack of available research evidence on transgender and bisexual carers is subsequently noted. Research on differing kinds of care practices within transgender communities is identified as an issue that should generate questions for future social work inquiry.

Available research on LGBT carers identifies that LGBT carers have poorer health and wellbeing outcomes than non-LGBT carers (Shiu, Muraco, & Fredriksen-Goldsen, 2016). This reflects broader health inequalities among LGBT populations. While issues for LGBT people and their allies in care relationships raised in this chapter are not universal, they may influence intervention outcomes and the choice of particular approaches. Health and human service providers need to examine how discrimination and stigma; and views, assumptions and societal or political treatment of LGBT people, may affect work with, or support for, the health and wellbeing of LGBT people in care relationships.

REFERENCES

Albuquerque, G. A., de Lima Garcia, C., da Silva Quirino, G., Alves, M. J. H., Belém, J. M., dos Santos Figueiredo, F. W., ... de Abreu, L. C. (2016). Access to health services by lesbian, gay, bisexual, and transgender persons: Systematic literature review. *BMC International Health and Human Rights*, *16*(1), 2. doi:10.118612914-015-0072-9 PMID:26769484

Aldridge, D., & Somerville, C. (2014). *Your Services Your Say: LGBT people's experiences of public services in Scotland*. Stonewall.

Australia, O. I. I. (2012). *Intersex for allies*. Melbourne: OII Australia. Retrieved from https://oii.org.au/21336/intersex-for-allies

Banks, C., Muhajarine, N., Waygood, K., Duczek, L., & Hellquist, G. (2003). *The cost of homophobia: Literature review on the human impact of homophobia in Canada*. Gay & Lesbian Health Services of Saskatoon.

Barrett, C., & Crameri, P. (2015). *An extra degree of difficulty. An evidence based guide to the experiences and needs of older LGBTI carers and the carers of older LGBTI people. Australian Research Centre in Sex, Health and Society*. Melbourne, Australia: La Trobe University.

Barrett, C., Turner, L., & Leonard, L. (2013). *Beyond a rainbow sticker. A report on How^2 create a gay, lesbian, bisexual, transgender and intersex (GLBTI) inclusive service 2012-2013*. Melbourne: Gay and Lesbian Health Victoria.

Barrett, C., Whyte, C., Comfort, J., Lyons, A., & Crameri, P. (2015). Social connection, relationships and older lesbian and gay people. *Sexual and Relationship Therapy*, *30*(1), 131–142. doi:10.1080/14681994.2014.963983 PMID:25544830

Borg, C., & Hallberg, I. R. (2006). Life satisfaction among informal caregivers in comparison with non-caregivers. *Scandinavian Journal of Caring Sciences*, *20*(4), 427–438. doi:10.1111/j.1471-6712.2006.00424.x PMID:17116152

Broady, T., & Aggar, C. (2017). Carer interventions: An overview of service effectiveness. *Journal of the Australasian Rehabilitation Nurses Association*, *20*(2), 5.

Brown, A. R., & Mulley, G. P. (1997). Injuries sustained by caregivers of disabled elderly people. *Age and Ageing*, *26*(1), 21–23. doi:10.1093/ageing/26.1.21 PMID:9143433

Burwick, A., Gates, G., Baumgartner, S., & Friend, D. (2014). *Human Services for Low-Income and At-Risk LGBT Populations: The Knowledge Base and Research Needs. Project Brief. OPRE Report Number 2014-84*. Washington, DC: Office of Planning, Research and Evaluation, Administration for Children and Families, U.S. Department of Health and Human Services.

Butler, S. S. (2017). Older lesbians receiving home care: Formal and informal dimensions of caregiving. *Journal of Women & Aging*, 1–20. PMID:28632089

Campo, M., & Tayton, S. (2015). *Intimate partner violence in lesbian, gay, bisexual, trans, intersex and queer communities*. Retrieved from https://aifs.gov.au/cfca/publications/intimate-partner-violence-lgbtiq-communities

Carroll, A., & Mendos, L. R. (2017). *State-Sponsored Homophobia 2017: A World Survey of Sexual Orientation Laws: Criminalisation, Protection and Recognition*. Retrieved from https://ilga.org/downloads/2017/ILGA_State_Sponsored_Homophobia_2017_WEB.pdf

Cayleff, S. (2008). Feeding the hand that bit you: Lesbian daughters at mid-life negotiating parental caretaking. *Journal of Lesbian Studies*, *12*(2-3), 237–254. doi:10.1080/10894160802161398 PMID:19042735

Chappell, P. (2015). Queering the social emergence of disabled sexual identities: Linking queer theory with disability studies in the South African context. *Agenda (Durban, South Africa)*, *29*(1), 54–62.

Coon, D. W. (2007). Exploring interventions for LGBT caregivers: Issues and examples. *Journal of Gay & Lesbian Social Services, 18*(3-4), 109–128. doi:10.1300/J041v18n03_07

Croghan, C. F., Moone, R. P., & Olson, A. M. (2014). Friends, family, and caregiving among midlife and older lesbian, gay, bisexual, and transgender adults. *Journal of Homosexuality, 61*(1), 79–102. doi:10.1080/00918369.2013.835238 PMID:24313254

Cruz, T. M. (2014). Assessing access to care for transgender and gender nonconforming people: A consideration of diversity in combating discrimination. *Social Science & Medicine, 110*, 65–73. doi:10.1016/j.socscimed.2014.03.032 PMID:24727533

Czaja, S. J., Sabbag, S., Lee, C. C., Schulz, R., Lang, S., Vlahovic, T., ... Thurston, C. (2016). Concerns about aging and caregiving among middle-aged and older lesbian and gay adults. *Aging & Mental Health, 20*(11), 1107–1118. doi:10.1080/13607863.2015.1072795 PMID:26247917

Daley, A. E., & MacDonnell, J. A. (2011). Gender, sexuality and the discursive representation of access and equity in health services literature: Implications for LGBT communities. *International Journal for Equity in Health, 10*(1), 40. doi:10.1186/1475-9276-10-40 PMID:21957894

Darlington Statement: Joint consensus statement from the intersex community retreat in Darlington, March 2017. (2017). Working Paper. Sydney, NSW: QUT.

del-Pino-Casado, R., Frías-Osuna, A., & Palomino-Moral, P. A. (2011). Subjective burden and cultural motives for caregiving in informal caregivers of older people. *Journal of Nursing Scholarship, 43*(3), 282–291. PMID:21884374

Drescher, J. (2015). Out of DSM: Depathologizing homosexuality. *Behavioral Science, 5*(4), 565–575. doi:10.3390/bs5040565 PMID:26690228

Drescher, J. (2015). Queer diagnoses revisited: The past and future of homosexuality and gender diagnoses in DSM and ICD. *International Review of Psychiatry (Abingdon, England), 27*(5), 386–395. doi:10.3109/09540261.2015.1053847 PMID:26242413

Dykewomon, E. (2017). The caregiver and her friends. *Journal of Lesbian Studies*, 1–8. PMID:28339346

Embracing Carers. (2017). *Embracing the Critical Role of Caregivers Around the World.* Darmstadt, Germany: Merck GKaA.

Fish, J. (2006). *Heterosexism in health and social care*. Springer. doi:10.1057/9780230800731

Fredriksen-Goldsen, K. I., & Hooyman, N. R. (2007). Caregiving research, services, and policies in historically marginalized communities: Where do we go from here? *Journal of Gay & Lesbian Social Services, 18*(3-4), 129–145. doi:10.1300/J041v18n03_08

Fredriksen-Goldsen, K. I., Kim, H. J., Muraco, A., & Mincer, S. (2009). Chronically ill midlife and older lesbians, gay men, and bisexuals and their informal caregivers: The impact of the social context. *Sexuality Research and Social Policy Journal of NSRC, 6*(4), 52–64. doi:10.1525rsp.2009.6.4.52 PMID:20436796

Gay and Lesbian Health Victoria. (n.d.). *LGBTI Inclusive Practice*. Retrieved from https://www.glhv.org.au/lgbti-inclusive-practice

Glaesser, R. S., & Patel, B. R. (2016). Psychological Trauma and LGBT Caregivers: A Conceptual Framework to Guide Practice. *Journal of Evidence-Informed Social Work, 13*(5), 458–468. doi:10.1080/23761407.2016.1166825 PMID:27119978

Greenberg, J. S. (1995). The Other Side of Caring: Adult Children with Mental Illness as Supports to Their-Mothers in Later Life. *Social Work, 40*(3), 414–423. PMID:7761928

Greenwood, N., Habibi, R., Smith, R., & Manthorpe, J. (2015). Barriers to access and minority ethnic carers' satisfaction with social care services in the community: A systematic review of qualitative and quantitative literature. *Health & Social Care in the Community, 23*(1), 64–78. doi:10.1111/hsc.12116 PMID:25135207

Haghiri-Vijeh, R. (2013). The Importance of Including the Needs of the LGBTIQ Community in the Millennium Development Goals and Education of Healthcare Professionals. *Journal of Global Citizenship & Equity Education, 3*(1), 68.

Harley, D. A., Nowak, T. M., Gassaway, L. J., & Savage, T. A. (2002). Lesbian, gay, bisexual, and transgender college students with disabilities: A look at multiple cultural minorities. *Psychology in the Schools, 39*(5), 525–538. doi:10.1002/pits.10052

Hash, K. M., & Netting, F. E. (2009). It takes a community: Older lesbians meeting social and care needs. *Journal of Gay & Lesbian Social Services, 21*(4), 326–342. doi:10.1080/10538720802497910

Hill, T., Cass, B., Newton, B., & Valentine, K. (2012). *Indigenous carers.* Social Policy Research Paper No. 45.

Hudson, P. (2013). Improving support for family carers: Key implications for research, policy and practice. *Palliative Medicine, 27*(7), 581–582. doi:10.1177/0269216313488855 PMID:23780618

Irish Association of Social Workers (IASW). (2011). *Lesbian, Gay & Bisexual People: A Guide to Good Practice for Social Workers.* Retrieved from https://www.iasw.ie/download/4/5f24c87f-8792-4df1-a8d6-294bdbe6e851.PDF

Irlam, C. B. (2012). *LGBTI Data: developing an evidence-informed environment for LGBTI health policy.* Sydney: National LGBTI Health Alliance.

Irwin, L. (2007). Homophobia and heterosexism: Implications for nursing and nursing practice. *The Australian Journal of Advanced Nursing, 25*(1), 70.

Johnson, C. V., Mimiaga, M. J., & Bradford, J. (2008). Health care issues among lesbian, gay, bisexual, transgender and intersex (LGBTI) populations in the United States: Introduction. *Journal of Homosexuality, 54*(3), 213–224. doi:10.1080/00918360801982025 PMID:18825859

Jowett, A., & Peel, E. (2009). Chronic illness in non-heterosexual contexts: An online survey of experiences. *Feminism & Psychology, 19*(4), 454–474. doi:10.1177/0959353509342770

Kia, H. (2012). "I'm part of this family": How five care-giving partners of gay men story their experiences. *Journal of Gay & Lesbian Social Services, 24*(2), 140–157. doi:10.1080/10538720.2012.669369

Kidd, S. A., Veltman, A., Gately, C., Chan, K. J., & Cohen, J. N. (2011). Lesbian, gay, and transgender persons with severe mental illness: Negotiating wellness in the context of multiple sources of stigma. *American Journal of Psychiatric Rehabilitation*, *14*(1), 13–39. doi:10.1080/15487768.2011.546277

Kittikorn, N., Street, A. F., & Blackford, J. (2006). Managing shame and stigma: Case studies of female carers of people with AIDS in Southern Thailand. *Qualitative Health Research*, *16*(9), 1286–1301. doi:10.1177/1049732306293992 PMID:17038758

Knauer, N. J. (2016). lgbt older adults, chosen family, and caregiving. *The Journal of Law and Religion*, *31*(2), 150–168. doi:10.1017/jlr.2016.23

Knowles, S., Combs, R., Kirk, S., Griffiths, M., Patel, N., & Sanders, C. (2016). Hidden caring, hidden carers? Exploring the experience of carers for people with long-term conditions. *Health & Social Care in the Community*, *24*(2), 203–213. doi:10.1111/hsc.12207 PMID:25706665

Koschorke, M., Padmavati, R., Kumar, S., Cohen, A., Weiss, H. A., Chatterjee, S., ... Balaji, M. (2017). Experiences of stigma and discrimination faced by family caregivers of people with schizophrenia in India. *Social Science & Medicine*, *178*, 66–77. doi:10.1016/j.socscimed.2017.01.061 PMID:28213300

Leonard, W. (2002). *What's the difference? Health issues of major concern to gay lesbian bisexual transgender and intersex (GLBTI) Victorians. Ministerial Advisory Committee on Gay and Lesbian Health (MACGLH)*. Melbourne: Department of Human Services.

Leonard, W., Lyons, A., & Bariola, E. (2015). *A Closer Look at Private Lives 2*. Retrieved from https://www.glhv.org.au/sites/default/files/Closer_Look_Private_Lives2.pdf

Leonard, W., Marshall, D., Hillier, L., Mitchell, A., & Ward, R. (2010). *Beyond homophobia: meeting the needs of same sex attracted and gender questioning (SSAGQ) young people in Victoria. A policy blueprint* (Doctoral dissertation). William Buckland Foundation.

Leonard, W., Pitts, M., Mitchell, A., Lyons, A., Smith, A., Patel, S., & Barrett, A. (2012). *Private Lives 2: The second national survey of the health and wellbeing of gay, lesbian, bisexual and transgender (GLBT)*. Australians.

Lim, F. A., Brown, D. V. Jr, & Jones, H. (2013). Lesbian, gay, bisexual, and transgender health: Fundamentals for nursing education. *The Journal of Nursing Education*, *52*(4), 198–203. doi:10.3928/01484834-20130311-02 PMID:23471873

Lloyd, L. (2003). Caring Relationships: Looking Beyond Welfare Categories of Carers' and Service Users'. *Research Highlights in Social Work*, 37-55.

Lo, S., & Horton, R. (2016). Transgender health: An opportunity for global health equity. *Lancet*, *388*(10042), 316–318. doi:10.1016/S0140-6736(16)30675-4 PMID:27323923

McCann, E., Lee, R., & Brown, M. (2016). The experiences and support needs of people with intellectual disabilities who identify as LGBT: A review of the literature. *Research in Developmental Disabilities*, *57*, 39–53. doi:10.1016/j.ridd.2016.06.013 PMID:27372882

McKay, B. (2011). Lesbian, gay, bisexual, and transgender health issues, disparities, and information resources. *Medical Reference Services Quarterly*, *30*(4), 393–401. doi:10.1080/02763869.2011.608971 PMID:22040245

McLean, K. (2008). Inside, outside, nowhere: Bisexual men and women in the gay and lesbian community. *Journal of Bisexuality*, *8*(1-2), 63–80. doi:10.1080/15299710802143174

McNair, R. P., & Hegarty, K. (2010). Guidelines for the primary care of lesbian, gay, and bisexual people: A systematic review. *Annals of Family Medicine*, *8*(6), 533–541. doi:10.1370/afm.1173 PMID:21060124

Mejia-Canales, D., & Leonard, W. (2016). *Something for them.* Retrieved from https://www.glhv.org.au/sites/default/files/2016-09/somethingforthcm.pdf

Mizielińska, J., & Stasińska, A. (2017). "There Is Nothing Like a Family": Discourses on Families of Choice in Poland. *Journal of Homosexuality*, *64*(13), 1793–1815. doi:10.1080/00918369.2016.1267460 PMID:27918870

Moleiro, C., & Pinto, N. (2015). Sexual orientation and gender identity: Review of concepts, controversies and their relation to psychopathology classification systems. *Frontiers in Psychology*, *6*, 1511. doi:10.3389/fpsyg.2015.01511 PMID:26483748

Molyneaux, V., Butchard, S., Simpson, J., & Murray, C. (2011). Reconsidering the term 'carer': A critique of the universal adoption of the term 'carer'. *Ageing and Society*, *31*(3), 422–437. doi:10.1017/S0144686X10001066

Muraco, A., & Fredriksen-Goldsen, K. I. (2014). The highs and lows of caregiving for chronically ill lesbian, gay, and bisexual elders. *Journal of Gerontological Social Work*, *57*(2-4), 251–272. doi:10.1080/01634372.2013.860652 PMID:24224896

Nadal, K. L., Whitman, C. N., Davis, L. S., Erazo, T., & Davidoff, K. C. (2016). Microaggressions toward lesbian, gay, bisexual, transgender, queer, and genderqueer people: A review of the literature. *Journal of Sex Research*, *53*(4-5), 488–508. doi:10.1080/00224499.2016.1142495 PMID:26966779

National LGBTI Health Alliance. (2016). *The Statistics at a Glance: The Mental Health of Lesbian, Gay, Bisexual, Transgender and Intersex People in Australia.* Retrieved 28th August, 2017 from http://lgbtihealth.org.au/statistics/

Orel, N. A., & Coon, D. W. (2016). The Challenges of Change: How Can We Meet the Care Needs of the Ever-Evolving LGBT Family? *Generations (San Francisco, Calif.)*, *40*(2), 41–45.

Ottmann, G., Laragy, C., & Haddon, M. (2009). Experiences of disability consumer-directed care users in Australia: Results from a longitudinal qualitative study. *Health & Social Care in the Community*, *17*(5), 466–475. doi:10.1111/j.1365-2524.2009.00851.x PMID:19689678

Oyebode, J. (2003). Assessment of carers' psychological needs. *Advances in Psychiatric Treatment*, *9*(1), 45–53. doi:10.1192/apt.9.1.45

Pallotta-Chiarolli, M., & Rajkhowa, A. (2017). Systemic Invisibilities, Institutional Culpabilities and Multicultural-Multifaith LGBTIQ Resistances. *Journal of Intercultural Studies (Melbourne, Vic.)*, *38*(4), 429–442. doi:10.1080/07256868.2017.1341013

Parslow, O., & Hegarty, P. (2013). Who cares? UK lesbian caregivers in a heterosexual world. *Women's Studies International Forum*, *40*, 78–86. doi:10.1016/j.wsif.2013.03.003

Price, E. (2011). Caring for mum and dad: Lesbian women negotiating family and navigating care. *British Journal of Social Work*, *41*(7), 1288–1303. doi:10.1093/bjsw/bcr015

Price, E. (2012). Gay and lesbian carers: Ageing in the shadow of dementia. *Ageing and Society*, *32*(3), 516–532. doi:10.1017/S0144686X11000560

Reading, R., & Rubin, L. R. (2011). Advocacy and empowerment: Group therapy for LGBT asylum seekers. *Traumatology*, *17*(2), 86–98. doi:10.1177/1534765610395622

Reczek, C., & Umberson, D. (2016). Greedy spouse, needy parent: The marital dynamics of gay, lesbian, and heterosexual intergenerational caregivers. *Journal of Marriage and the Family*, *78*(4), 957–974. doi:10.1111/jomf.12318 PMID:27672229

Reisner, S. L., Poteat, T., Keatley, J., Cabral, M., Mothopeng, T., Dunham, E., ... Baral, S. D. (2016). Global health burden and needs of transgender populations: A review. *Lancet*, *388*(10042), 412–436. doi:10.1016/S0140-6736(16)00684-X PMID:27323919

Reygan, F. (2016). Black lesbian (non) representation in 'gay'media in Cape Town: Constructing a globalized white, male, affluent, gay consumer. *African Identities*, *14*(1), 85–98. doi:10.1080/14725843.2015.1100105

Rogers, H., & Barnes, M. (2003). Caring voices: Carers' participation in policy and practice. *Research Highlights in Social Work*, 117-136.

Rosenstreich, G. (2011). LGBTI people mental health and suicide. *National LGBTI Health Alliance*, 1-12.

Rosenstreich, G. (2013). *LGBTI People Mental Health and Suicide* (2nd ed.). Sydney: National LGBTI Health Alliance.

Ross, L. E., Dobinson, C., & Eady, A. (2010). Perceived determinants of mental health for bisexual people: A qualitative examination. *American Journal of Public Health*, *100*(3), 496–502. doi:10.2105/AJPH.2008.156307 PMID:20075326

Ross, M. (2003). The legal framework of caring. *Research Highlights in Social Work*, 177-194.

Rossman, K., Salamanca, P., & Macapagal, K. (2017). A qualitative study examining young adults' experiences of disclosure and non-disclosure of LGBTQ identity to healthcare providers. *Journal of Homosexuality*. (accepted for publication)

Rutherford, K., McIntyre, J., Daley, A., & Ross, L. E. (2012). Development of expertise in mental health service provision for lesbian, gay, bisexual and transgender communities. *Medical Education*, *46*(9), 903–913. doi:10.1111/j.1365-2923.2012.04272.x PMID:22891911

Schofield, H., Bloch, S., Herman, H., Murphy, B., Nankervis, J., & Singh, B. (1998). *Family Caregivers: Disability, Illness and Ageing*. St Leonards, N.S.W: Allen & Unwin in association with the Victorian Health Promotion Foundation (VicHealth).

Schulz, S. L. (2018). The Informed Consent Model of Transgender Care: An Alternative to the Diagnosis of Gender Dysphoria. *Journal of Humanistic Psychology*, *58*(1), 72–92. doi:10.1177/0022167817745217

Scott, S. D., Pringle, A., & Lumsdaine, C. (2004). *Sexual Exclusion–Homophobia and health inequalities: a review*. London: Health First.

Shiu, C., Muraco, A., & Fredriksen-Goldsen, K. (2016). Invisible care: Friend and partner care among older lesbian, gay, bisexual, and transgender (LGBT) adults. *Journal of the Society for Social Work and Research*, *7*(3), 527–546. doi:10.1086/687325 PMID:28367277

Sifris, A. (2014). *Gay and lesbian parenting: The legislative response.* Retrieved from https://aifs.gov.au/publications/families-policy-and-law/10-gay-and-lesbian-parenting-legislative-response

Smith, N. G., & Ingram, K. M. (2004). Workplace Heterosexism and Adjustment Among Lesbian, Gay, and Bisexual Individuals: The Role of Unsupportive Social Interactions. *Journal of Counseling Psychology*, *51*(1), 57–67. doi:10.1037/0022-0167.51.1.57

Stalker, K. (2003). Chapter One. In G. Grant & P. Ramcharan (Eds.), *Reconceptualising Work with 'carers': New Directions for Policy and Practice*. Jessica Kingsley Publishers.

Stansfeld, S., Smuk, M., Onwumere, J., Clark, C., Pike, C., McManus, S., ... Bebbington, P. (2014). Stressors and common mental disorder in informal carers–An analysis of the English Adult Psychiatric Morbidity Survey 2007. *Social Science & Medicine*, *120*, 190–198. doi:10.1016/j.socscimed.2014.09.025 PMID:25259657

The Joint Commission. (2011). *Advancing effective communication, cultural competence, and patient- and family-centered care for the lesbian, gay, bisexual, and transgender (LGBT) community: A field guide*. Retrieved from https://www.jointcommission.org/lgbt/

Theed, R., Eccles, F., & Simpson, J. (2017). Experiences of caring for a family member with Parkinson's disease: A meta-synthesis. *Aging & Mental Health*, *21*(10), 1007–1016. doi:10.1080/13607863.2016.1247414 PMID:27802771

Thomas, R., Pega, F., Khosla, R., Verster, A., Hana, T., & Say, L. (2017). Ensuring an inclusive global health agenda for transgender people. *Bulletin of the World Health Organization*, *95*(2), 154–156. doi:10.2471/BLT.16.183913 PMID:28250518

Tinney, J., Dow, B., Maude, P., Purchase, R., Whyte, C., & Barrett, C. (2015). Mental health issues and discrimination among older LGBTI people. *International Psychogeriatrics*, *27*(9), 1411–1416. doi:10.1017/S1041610214002671 PMID:26223452

Tong, H. C., Haig, A. J., Nelson, V. S., Yamakawa, K. S. J., Kandala, G., & Shin, K. Y. (2003). Low back pain in adult female caregivers of children with physical disabilities. *Archives of Pediatrics & Adolescent Medicine*, *157*(11), 1128–1133. doi:10.1001/archpedi.157.11.1128 PMID:14609905

Valenti, K., & Katz, A. (2014). Needs and perceptions of LGBTQ caregivers: The challenges of services and support. *Journal of Gay & Lesbian Social Services*, *26*(1), 70–90. doi:10.1080/10538720.2013.865575

Walters, K. L., & Old Person, R. L. (2008). Lesbians, gays, bisexuals, and transgender people of color: Reconciling divided selves and communities. *Social Work Practice with Lesbian, Gay, Bisexual, and Transgender people*, 41-68.

Ward, D. (2000). Ageism and the abuse of older people in health and social care. *British Journal of Nursing (Mark Allen Publishing)*, *9*(9), 560–563. doi:10.12968/bjon.2000.9.9.6292 PMID:11904891

Washington, K. T., McElroy, J., Albright, D., Oliver, D. P., Lewis, A., Meadows, S., & Elliott, S. (2015). Experiences of sexual and gender minorities caring for adults with non-AIDS-related chronic illnesses. *Social Work Research*, *39*(2), 71–81. doi:10.1093wrvu030

Whitehead, J., Shaver, J., & Stephenson, R. (2016). Outness, stigma, and primary health care utilization among rural LGBT populations. *PLoS One*, *11*(1), e0146139. doi:10.1371/journal.pone.0146139 PMID:26731405

Williams, C. (2007). "Permission to speak": A carer's experience. *Australian Health Review*, *31*(2), 167–171. doi:10.1071/AH070167 PMID:17470035

Williams, C. (2012). Chronic illness and informal carers: 'Non-persons' in the health system, neither carers, workers or citizens. *Health Sociology Review*, *21*(1), 58–68. doi:10.5172/hesr.2012.21.1.58

Willis, P., Ward, N., & Fish, J. (2011). Searching for LGBT carers: Mapping a research agenda in social work and social care. *British Journal of Social Work*, *41*(7), 1304–1320. doi:10.1093/bjsw/bcr114

World Health Organization. (2013). *Addressing the causes of disparities in health service access and utilization for lesbian, gay, bisexual and trans (LGBT) persons.* 52nd Directing Council. 65th Session of the Regional Committee. Concept Paper, 30.

Chapter 11
Mental Health Education and Literacy in Schools:
The Australian Experience

Matthew Dale
Mind Australia, Australia

ABSTRACT

This chapter will look at the current situation concerning youth mental health in Australia and provide information about youth mental health literacy, which was first coined by Jorm in 1997. A literature review of current Australian mental health promotion and education programs being offered in schools will be conducted as well as examples of some of the better-known ones that have been implemented internationally. The evolution of mental health education in Australian schools will be examined so as to provide a perspective of how some of the current programs came into being or existence. The main aim of this chapter will be to highlight the high prevalence of mental illness that exists amongst young people in Australia and how implementing mental health education in schools can be beneficial and helpful in improving their mental health and wellbeing. Mental health education in schools can help in breaking down the stigma surrounding mental illness. Another benefit is that young people will be able to identify mental health problems earlier amongst their peers and in themselves, which can lead to early help seeking, especially due to young people gaining a higher level of mental health literacy through mental health education programs.

INTRODUCTION

Australia has been active during the past 20 years in the development and implementation of Mental Health Policy and Mental Health Promotion. In the Fourth National Mental Health Plan 2009 - 2014 (Commonwealth of Australia, 2009), the Australian government in its wisdom and foresight choose to make Prevention and Early Intervention as its Priority Area 2. In the Summary of Actions (Commonwealth of Australia, 2009) in point one it noted that it would "work with schools, workplaces and communities to deliver programs to improve mental health literacy and enhance resilience" (p.32). Following on from

DOI: 10.4018/978-1-5225-7402-6.ch011

that it included as a further action to "implement targeted prevention and early intervention programs for children and their families through partnerships between mental health, maternal and child health services, schools and other related organisations" (p.32). One of the indicators for monitoring that this change had been made was to observe the "proportion of primary and secondary schools with mental health literacy components included in their curriculum" (p.32).

It is interesting to note that with all the best intentions of the Australian government to make Prevention and Early Intervention a mental health priority in the Fourth National Mental Health Plan that this was inexplicably missing from the Fifth National Mental Health Plan of 2017 - 2022. The Black Dog Institute in its *'Submission in response to the Draft 5th National Mental Health Plan'* (Back Dog, 2016) said that the plan was "silent on prevention and yet it is potentially a powerful solution to chronic mental illness and should be included as a key strategy" (p.10). It went on to add that "prevention programs are most effective when implemented early" and that they "strongly believed that school-based prevention is critical to reducing the overall burden of mental illness on the community" (p.10).

This chapter will look at the current situation that exists in Australian schools concerning youth mental health and the seriousness of this health problem. It will explore why mental health education in schools is so important and the benefits for implementing it into curriculum. It will also investigate why being mental health literate is significant in improving both peers and a young person's own mental health.

Before examining the various mental health promotion and education programs that currently exist in Australian schools, it will look at what has happened in Australian schools from a historical perspective, including initiatives such as MindMatters and KidsMatter. The Australian experience of mental health education in schools will also be compared to the international experience by examining what exists as well as what has worked and not been so successful overseas.

The chapter will also reflect on what are some of the problems and barriers that exist in implementing mental health education in Australian schools as well as the benefits of introducing it into the school curriculum and the future of mental health education in Australian schools.

YOUTH MENTAL HEALTH IN AUSTRALIA

There has been considerable research and study carried out about the onset of mental illnesses and mental health problems in people, not only in Australia but around the world. The evidence suggests that three in four mental health disorders emerge by the age of 24 and half by the age of 14 (Kessler, Berglund, Demler, Jin, Merikangas, & Walters, 2005; Sawyer, Arney, Baghurst, Clark, Graetz, & Kosky, 2000; McGorry, Purcell, Hickie, & Jorm, 2007). In 2013 - 2014, around a quarter of all young people aged 16-24 years in Australia had a mental disorder (approximately 26% or 671,000 young people). One in seven children and adolescents aged 4 - 17 years experienced a mental disorder in 2013 - 2014, which is equivalent to 14% or 560,00 young people. Depression impacts on the lives of 1 in 35 or 2.8% of young Australians aged 4-17. The statistics for anxiety are even greater where 1 in 10 adolescents aged 18 - 25 and 1 in 25 children aged 13 - 17 experience the condition. (Orygen Youth Health, 2008). Of concern was the fact that there was an increase of probable serious mental illness in the age group 15 - 19 from 18.7% in 2012 to 22.8% in 2016 (Mission Australia, 2016). Lawrence and colleagues (2015) commented that mental disorders were the leading cause of illness and disability for young people aged 10 to 19 years, ahead of any physical disease.

There is evidence to support that only about one-third of young people and adolescents with a mental disorder will actually seek help. Of that one-third only about 30% of young people will seek referrals for psychological therapy (McGorry, Purcell, Hickie, & Jorm, 2007; Rickwood, Deane, Wilson, & Ciarrochi, 2005). As can be seen from the previous statistics about youth mental health and mental illness, it is a serious health problem in Australia which something needs to be done about soon. Young people and adults responsible for looking after young people need to improve their mental health literacy so that young people who are presenting with early mental health problems can seek appropriate mental health treatment. Early intervention and prevention is crucial and mental health promotion and education programs in schools, as long as they are implemented properly, will go a long way to addressing some of these problems and concerns.

WHY IMPLEMENT MENTAL HEALTH EDUCATION IN SCHOOLS?

The importance and significance of implementing mental health education in schools, both locally here in Australia as well as overseas cannot be underestimated. Later in this chapter there will be a discussion about the benefits of doing so as well as some of the challenges and implications that present themselves to schools in trying to introduce mental health promotion to the curriculum. Within schools you are able to assemble a captive audience where they can be educated about important mental health and wellbeing information. This can be delivered and rolled out to large numbers of young people at the same time. In Australia, as in most countries, it is compulsory to attend school up until a certain age. In the state of Victoria it is currently 17. Barry and Jenkins (2007) highlighted just how important the emotional and social development of young people is during the time that they attend school and that it provides an excellent opportunity to create a positive environment where they can thrive.

Schools are able to create a sense of community and belonging which will help some young people who are either socially isolated or more at risk of developing mental illness than other students, to be able to maintain good mental health. The onset of mental illness is high in childhood and adolescence. It is well known from the evidence that 75% of all mental illnesses develop before the age of 24 so it makes sense to target this age group with effective, evidence-based mental health education programs so as to be more preventative than reactive, when a young person becomes unwell. By introducing Mental Health Education into schools, it will help to improve mental health outcomes for Australians by reducing the incidence or impact of risk factors while building up people's protective factors and thus help children and adolescents to access support early if difficulties do arise. Well-planned and thought out Mental Health Education programs can also have an impact on improving the mental health literacy of young people and students which in turn can lead to building stronger resilience during adverse times and help in breaking down the stigma that exists in relation to mental illness. The positive outcome of all of this would see young people accessing mental health services earlier. Good mental health in childhood also provides a solid foundation for managing the transition to adolescence and adulthood, engaging successfully in education and making a meaningful contribution to society (KidsMatter, Primary 2017). Working with children and young people is one potentially cost-effective way to address the impact of mental health difficulties in the community, both today and into the future. (Response Ability, 2012).

HISTORICAL CONTEXT OF MENTAL HEALTH EDUCATION IN AUSTRALIAN SCHOOLS

In 1996 the Australian government commissioned an audit to be conducted to look at Mental Health Education in Australian Secondary Schools. It was funded under the National Mental Health Community Awareness Program which was a National Mental Health Strategy initiative designed to reduce the stigma and discrimination experienced by people with a mental illness, their families and carers (Youth Research Centre and Centre for Social Health, 1996). A number of interesting findings from this audit helped guide the Australian government in the future direction of mental health education in Australian schools. It examined the National Curriculum at the time with regard to the school context of welfare while exploring the feasibility of implementing the World Health Organisation's 'Health Promoting Schools' policy.

The audit data focused on such things as what current policies on mental health and mental health education that there were, the perceptions and attitudes towards mental health in schools, particular classroom curriculum approaches, what welfare approaches were being used in schools and the involvement of community and other external agencies in school mental health education as well as what mental health education were available.

An important part of the audit report was to look at what current issues surrounded mental health education in schools as well as what the future direction of it might look like in Australian schools and what current education programs were already in operation. Issues included what actual coverage of mental health education was there in schools?; what professional development was being provided to teaching staff at schools in regards to mental health education?; how much involvement and support were external community and non-government agencies providing to schools?; where does mental health and mental illness education fit into the curriculum?; where can mental illness education be incorporated into existing programs and what medical interventions and suicide prevention programs are being conducted in secondary schools? Out of this audit the Australian government set up a mental health promotion initiative for secondary schools called MindMatters. The success of this would later produce the KidsMatter initiative for primary school students.

MindMatters

The original MindMatters pilot project began in November 1997 and lasted for about 18 months. The role out was delivered in 24 schools which included government and non-government schools. The pilot came about after an audit was completed in 1996, which examined what Mental Health Education there was in Australian secondary schools and if it was an appropriate setting for the promotion of mental health among young people. Upon completion of the evaluation of the MindMatters pilot it was decided to mass produce the resources and to disseminate these to schools with a secondary enrolment across Australia. This was carried out by Australian Principals Associations Professional Development Council and the Curriculum Corporation (Principals Australia Institute, 2017).

KidsMatter Primary

The Australian government saw the benefit of implementing a mental health education initiative such as MindMatters in secondary schools and realised that it might be even more important and beneficial to introduce a program that provided intervention for primary school aged children to deal with mental health problems earlier. Hence, KidsMatter Primary was introduced in 2006 and piloted in 101 schools over three years (2006 - 2009). This involved the Australian Psychological Society, the Australian Principals Associations Professional Development Council, beyondblue and the Australian Government Department of Health and Ageing (Principals Australia Institute, 2017).

The Gatehouse Project

The Gatehouse Project was a research project conducted in Victorian secondary schools between 1996 and 2001. Its aim was to promote the health and emotional wellbeing of young people by increasing connectedness and providing skills for managing life's ups and downs. Bond and colleagues (2002) referred to the Gatehouse Project as a school-based primary prevention program that offers a framework for building the capacity of school communities to address the emotional and mental health needs of students. A systematic process was used to create a whole school of change in regard to policies, programs, practices and structures. It was evaluated by using a randomised controlled trial. Findings found a reduction in the health risk behaviours of young people as well as system level changes within schools. The work of the Gatehouse Project is being further developed through the Adolescent Health and Social Environments Program (AHSEP), as well as there being national and international adaptations (Centre for Adolescent Health, 2017). An aim of the Gatehouse Project was to embed mental health promotion within the core business of school; that is to have connectedness to school and engagement with learning. The project used a variety of universal and targeted strategies at multiple levels to promote the emotional wellbeing of students combined with a whole school approach which would enhance and improve the social climate. It recognized that intervention was required for students who were more at risk due to the social environment that they came from (Bond, Butler, Glover, & Patton, 2002). The project identified three key priority areas for action; building a sense of security and trust; enhancing skills and opportunities for good communication; and building a sense of positive regard through valued participation in aspects of school life. The project emphasized the importance of healthy attachments or a sense of positive connection with teachers and peers (Bond, Butler, Glover, & Patton, 2002). The Gatehouse Project provided schools with a process of which to build on and develop new policies, programs and practices from an evidence-based platform. This included the establishment of an adolescent health team, reviews of programs, policies and practices, strategic planning to address risk and protective factors, training and implementation as well as monitoring and evaluation.

CURRENT MENTAL HEALTH EDUCATION PROGRAMS IN AUSTRALIAN SCHOOLS

MindMatters

MindMatters was originally developed by a team of academic researchers and health educational professionals. The 'whole of school' and holistic approach used by MindMatters was informed by the Health Promoting School concept and the Comprehensive School Mental Health Model, both of which were developed by the World Health Organisation (World Health Organisation Regional Office for Europe, 1994). Currently in Australia over 1,400 secondary schools are using MindMatters in some shape or form. Also, over 10,000 school staff and significant others have attended professional development sessions and in excess of 76,000 modules have been completed. Over 33,000 people are signed up to MindMatters. As can be seen from these figures its use is quite widespread. MindMatters is currently the key national mental health initiative for secondary schools in Australia (Principals Australia Institute, 2017). Principals Australia Institute (2017) defined it on it's website as the following, "It promotes mental health and wellbeing of students in secondary schools through a flexible framework that provides useful professional learning, resources and support. The resources enable staff to work with the school community to implement four components." The initiative is funded by the Australian Government Department of Health with beyondblue being designated as the lead contract for it while Principals Australia Institute staff help to deliver the program in each of the states. The MindMatters mental health framework is built around four key components. These include:

Component 1: Positive school community
Component 2: Student skills for resilience
Component 3: Parents and families
Component 4: Support for students experiencing mental health difficulties

Together these components provide a holistic and comprehensive view of student mental health and wellbeing within the wider school community. Each component is explored through a number of standalone online modules covering different topics. These modules include animation, video, interactive tools and downloadable resources and take around one hour to complete. Each module has a facilitator guide and can be explored individually or in a group. Special face-to-face events and experienced support from Principals Australia Institute project officers complement the online resources and help schools to implement what they have learnt (MindMatters, 2017). Central to the MindMatters philosophy is that of promotion, prevention and early intervention. It is about preventing the onset of early mental health problems through promoting positive mental health through a whole of school community approach and by providing students with the skills to improve relationships and build resilience. Staff are provided with professional guidance to help identify students who may be struggling with their mental health and knowledge on how to best support and help these students (MindMatters, 2017).

The attraction and advantage of MindMatters is that it is flexible in being to implement it into a school's curriculum so as to suit their own strategy / strategies and unique circumstances. Also the mental health resources has benefits not only for students but also staff and students' families. Sheehan and colleagues (2002) highlighted that "MindMatters can be distinguished from previous single-topic health education projects because it places mental health within the core educational business of schools rather than identifying it as a 'health topic'" (p. 113). They go on to say that "the professional development of teachers is fundamental to the success of the innovation". The main focus of MindMatters is on organisational structures, the social environment and the individual within this context.

KidsMatter and KidsMatter Early Childhood

After MindMatters was evaluated and the findings were disseminated, the Australian government saw the value and importance of developing a mental health education program for children of primary school age. It recognised that providing early intervention and prevention at an even earlier age than secondary school could make a difference in the mental health and wellbeing of children. KidsMatter is a national collaboration between the education and health sectors. It was jointly developed by beyondblue, Principals Australia Institute (PAI), Early Childhood Australia (ECA) and the Australian Psychological Society (APS), with funding from the Australian Government Department of Health and Ageing and beyondblue. (beyondblue 2016) KidsMatter Primary is a flexible, whole-school approach to improving children's mental health and wellbeing for primary schools. It can be tailored to schools' local needs.

Through KidsMatter Primary, schools undertake a two-to three-year cyclical process in which they plan and take action to be a positive community; one that is founded on respectful relationships and a sense of belonging and inclusion, and that promotes:

- Social and emotional learning (including evidence-based social and emotional learning programs);
- Working authentically with parents, carers and families;
- Support for students who may be experiencing mental health difficulties.

When schools take on KidsMatter, they build on the work that they are already doing in these areas (KidsMatter Primary, 2017). There are three parts that make up the KidsMatter framework. They are:

1. **Guiding Principles:** The beliefs that underpin KidsMatter;
2. **The Core Components:** The areas in which schools can most effectively concentrate their learning, planning and action;
3. **The Whole School Approach:** The essential elements for working together as a school community.

The four components that make up the KidsMatter / KidsMatter Early Childhood Framework are:

Component 1: Creating a sense of community.
Target Areas: A school community that promotes mental health and wellbeing and respectful relationships, belonging and inclusion.
Component 2: Developing children's social and emotional skills.
Target Areas: Effective social and emotional learning curriculum for all students and opportunities for students to practice and transfer their social and emotional skills.
Component 3: Working with parents and carers.
Target Areas: Collaborative working relationships with parents and carers, support for parenting and parent and carer support networks.
Component 4: Helping children who are experiencing mental health difficulties.

Target Areas: Understanding mental health difficulties and improving help-seeking and responding to students experiencing mental health difficulties (KidsMatter Primary, 2017).

KidsMatter recommended that schools should follow a 7-step implementation process related to focusing attention on the four components, as follows:

Step 1: Define the issues by writing a summary statement to describe the school's current situation related to each component.
Step 2: Set goals based on each summary statement.
Step 3: Identify any concerns in achieving the goals.
Step 4: Develop a broad range of options/strategies to address concerns and achieve goals.
Step 5: Evaluate the feasibility of each option/strategy.
Step 6: Formalise the component plan.
Step 7: Implement the plan and review (Askell-Williams, Lawson, & Slee, 2013).

beyondblue Mental Health Education Programs for Australian Schools

Australia's well known and respected depression and anxiety initiative, beyondblue, has produced several mental health education programs for primary and secondary schools as well as resources for universities and pre-schools. The better-known programs are KidsMatter and MindMatters which have already been previously spoken about. Other school mental health education programs include the following.

SenseAbility

The SenseAbility program has been designed and developed for secondary school students aged 12 - 18. SenseAbility is a strengths-based resilience program designed for those working with young Australians aged 12-18 years. It consists of a suite of modules developed to enhance and maintain emotional and psychological resilience. It was created with classroom delivery in mind, but the modules can easily be adapted to benefit young people in other structured environments such as TAFEs and youth organisations. The program is based on cognitive-behavioural principles, the evidence-based approach which says that our thoughts play a critical role in influencing feelings and consequent behaviour. SenseAbility consists of seven modules, a DVD and a CD with downloadable curriculum materials and resources. The seven modules include:

1. Essential skills
2. Sense of self-worth
3. Sense of control
4. Sense of belonging
5. Sense of purpose
6. Sense of future
7. Sense of humour (beyondblue, 2016)

The SenseAbility package has been designed to be delivered by teachers in the classroom and lesson plans have already been developed for teachers to use. It has been designed to fit in with the Australian curriculum framework which will make it easier for school leaders and staff to deliver and assess the SenseAbility program.

Secondary Schools Program (Years 8-10)

The Secondary Schools Program (beyondblue 2016) was developed specifically for the middle secondary years 8 - 10 which is a critical time both emotionally and socially in the lives of young people. It is a 30 session program that is intended to be delivered over three years, with students participating each year in 10 weekly classroom sessions of 30 - 45 minutes duration. The sequentially developed sessions are based on cognitive behavioural theories. The program is built around the development of six senses that act as protective factors against mental health problems:

1. Sense of self-worth
2. Sense of control
3. Sense of belonging
4. Sense of purpose
5. Sense of future
6. Sense of humour

Program delivery is based on principles of best-practice in effective teaching using a range of interactive methods including small-group exercises and discussions, role-plays, deep-learning tasks and quizzes. Each year level is built around different themes and there are downloadable teacher manuals as well as student workbooks. This program was developed collaboratively by the University of Queensland, the Victorian Centre for Adolescent Health, the South Australian Department of Education and Children's Services, and beyondblue. It draws on national and international research and the groundbreaking work conducted with schools in Australia in the past decade (beyondblue, 2016).

thedesk (University / TAFE Mental Health Education Program)

thedesk is a free online program aimed at providing Australian tertiary students with strategies and skills for success and wellbeing during their time at university or TAFE. *thedesk* includes modules to develop problem-solving and self-management skills. Topics include getting things done, staying calm, staying connected and feeling good. It also has tools to help with everyday issues such as relaxation, challenging unhelpful thoughts, using feedback constructively and problem solving. There are quizzes about different areas of life such as relationships, physical health and mental wellbeing and an online Coffee House for students to connect with other students, share experiences, music, art, recipes and more. Links are provided to information and support services to help deal with a range of common issue. All components of *thedesk* are informed by research on the prevention and treatment of mental health problems, web-based interventions and engagement. *thedesk* toolkit provides free information about *thedesk*, including the research behind it, what's involved and how schools and teachers can help promote it among their students (beyondblue, 2016).

Black Dog Institute: HeadStrong 2.0

HeadStrong 2.0 was developed by the Black Dog Institute to make it easier for teachers educating high school students about the tough topic of mental illness. The program has been linked to the Health and Physical Education curriculum for Years 9 - 10 and links directly to curriculum learning outcomes. The HeadStrong 2.0 curriculum resource is free to download and can help students better understand mental health, and how to build wellbeing and resilience. It is a unique program that equips teachers to better understand and help young people with mental health problems. HeadStrong 2.0 includes 5 modules that are split into a series of ready-to-use classroom activities and teacher development notes. Topics include depression and bipolar disorder, seeking help, helping others, and building wellbeing and resilience. It is complemented by MindStrength, a free online learning course to help young people build resilience.

Headstrong 2.0 has undergone a comprehensive research trial and is evidence based. Research has found that the program has helped improve the mental health literacy of young people which is crucial in young people seeking early help and support for a mental health problem (Black Dog Institute, 2017).

Response Ability

The Response Ability initiative was launched in 2000 by the Australian Government Department of Health and Ageing. The aim of the program was to provide free multimedia resources and practical support to universities and teacher educators, while addressing pre-service education for secondary teachers. The main target group was secondary school students with the focus being on their mental health and wellbeing. The Response Ability Project was initiated in 1997 under the Australian Federal Government's National Suicide Prevention Strategy. Its aim was to influence the pre-employment education of professional groups, so graduates could play a constructive role in addressing youth suicidal behaviour. The project represents an effective collaboration between health professionals and tertiary educators, with the team comprising staff from the Hunter Institute of Mental Health and educators from the University of Newcastle (Allen & Vincent, 2005). In 2006 the government engaged the Response Ability project team to see how this program and resources could also be implemented and rolled out in both primary and early childhood education. The main idea of the initiative was to use the resources to "encourage pre-service teachers to engage with and promote social and emotional health in their teaching practices."

Inspire "ReachOut Schools" and "ReachOut Teachers Network"

The Inspire Foundation provides a couple of different resources that can be utilised by schools for mental health education purposes. ReachOut Teachers Network provides mental health and wellbeing teaching resources and online training activities as part of an initiative of the Inspire Foundation (beyondblue, 2016).

ReachOut Schools provides free educational resources, digital tools and practical tips to encourage the development of positive mental health and wellbeing across schools and extend the impact of existing programs. The service features easy-to-understand information on a full range of mental health and wellbeing issues. The school resources include innovative digital apps and online games to help students learn to take control of their mental health. Staff and parents can use ReachOut Schools to better understand the issues young people face and as a safe place they can recommend and refer students to. School professionals can also access a range of professional development webinars and information, with resources added throughout the year. School professionals are able to register for updates (ReachOut Australia, 2017).

MIEACT (Mental Illness Education ACT)

MIEACT was founded in 1993 to deliver education sessions in schools in the Australian Capital Territory (ACT) about mental illness and was formally incorporated in 1998. MIEACT secured recurring funding from the ACT Government in 2000, and since then has expanded to deliver additional programs that reduce stigma surrounding mental illness. Whilst continuing and further developing the original Schools Education Program, MIEACT has also developed education programs for the broader community, media programs, and resources for young people (MIEACT, 2016). The School Education Program (SEP) is based on the original core program that MIEACT was founded on 25 years ago. It is best designed for students or young people in Years 9 - 12. This program is delivered by pairs of MIEACT Volunteer Educators, who are people with lived experience either themselves or as a carer of someone with a mental illness. Volunteers are trained and supported to deliver the program into schools and other youth environments. The program provides students and teachers with evidenced-based information used to broaden the student's knowledge about mental illness. Each student is provided with a resource *Hang On To This* (HOTT magazine) which contains contact information for services which can assist young people and other stories and activities aimed at engaging young people (MIEACT, 2016).

Peer Support Australia

Peer Support Australia is a peer led, evidence based mental health education program that is offered to Australian school communities. It aims to enhance the mental, social and emotional wellbeing of young people. It does this through integrating the program into the school curriculum and sustaining it by running all year groups. By doing this it looks to support a positive cultural change across the school. The program is operated in both primary and secondary schools. The Peer Support Australia program provides:

- Training and professional development for teachers and parents;
- Student leadership training and resources;
- Peer led, skills based, experiential learning modules focusing on orientation, relationships, optimism, resilience, anti-bullying and values;
- Consultancy to assist Member schools in raising awareness of the program and planning for implementation.

There are several benefits to the program. It provides students with a supportive learning environment in which to develop the skills, understandings, attitudes and strategies to improve mental wellbeing. It also helps students to develop key skills in resilience, assertiveness, decision making, problem solving and leadership and empowers young people to support each other and contribute positively to society (Peer Support Australia, 2014).

Teen Mental Health First Aid

Since 2001 there has been several variations of the original Mental Health First Aid program delivered to members of the community not only in Australia but overseas as well. The first courses however were specific in providing Mental Health First Aid by an adult to another adult. Eventually a Youth Mental Health First Aid was developed for adults who work with young people as well as for parents so that they would be equipped with the skills necessary to help out young people who might be struggling with their mental health or presenting with early mental health problems. Over the years through research conducted by Mental Health First Aid International, it became apparent that there was a need for there to be a course to be developed for young people to be trained up in having the skills and knowledge to help and support their peers who may have mental health problems or be in a mental health crisis. Thus teen Mental Health First Aid was born. teen Mental Health First Aid is a 3.5 hour mental health education program specifically designed for students in years 10 - 12 on how to provide mental health first aid to their friends.

Research and evidence found that young people have a preference for sharing their problems with peers rather than adults, be it parents, teachers, sports coaches or other significant adults in their lives. The course curriculum is based on research that was conducted on how best a young person can support their peers who might have a mental health problem. Students learn how to develop a Mental Health First Aid (MHFA) Action Plan on how to keep their peers safe, as well as information about different types of mental health problems and mental health crisis situations in young people, and the relationship between thoughts, feelings and behaviours (Mental Health First Aid Australia, 2017). Hart and colleagues (2016) said that the program would:

Focus on developing knowledge and skills in recognising warning signs that a peer is developing a mental health problem, understanding how to talk to a peer about mental health and seeking help, when and how to tell a responsible adult, where to find appropriate and helpful resources about mental illness and professional help, and how to respond in a crisis situation... teen MHFA program aims to increase mental health literacy, decrease stigmatising attitudes towards individuals with mental illness, and improve MHFA behaviours. (p.3)

MENTAL HEALTH LITERACY IN AUSTRALIAN SCHOOLS AND YOUNG AUSTRALIANS

Anthony Jorm introduced the term, 'mental health literacy' back in 1997. He defined it as "knowledge and beliefs about mental disorders which aid their recognition, management or prevention". Jorm added that Mental Health Literacy consisted of several components including:

1. The ability to recognise specific disorders or different types of psychological distress;
2. Knowledge and beliefs about risk factors and causes;
3. Knowledge and beliefs about self-help interventions;
4. Knowledge and beliefs about professional help available;
5. Attitudes which facilitate recognition and appropriate help-seeking; (and)
6. Knowledge of how to seek mental health information (Jorm, 2000).

Jorm (1997; 2007; 2011; 2012) has written much on the topic of Mental Health Literacy. He has examined it from a whole population perspective in Australia and explained the importance and need to be mental health literate in order to stay emotionally and mentally well. Some of his research in collaboration with others has focussed on Mental Health Literacy around young people of school age. He found that the lack of mental health literacy in young people is similar to that of adults. His main concern was the inability of young people to recognise mental illnesses and their failure to know what appropriate professional help and pharmacological treatment that was available. Young people have a slightly more positive attitude of receiving help from a health professional than adults but that was not necessarily reflective in their own self-help seeking preferences. Young people would still prefer to speak to a friend or family member if they have a mental health problem. Many young people also do not have positive attitudes towards the taking of psychiatric medication. His research has also found that young people are ill-equipped to provide help to peers suffering from mental illness (Jorm, & Wright, 2007). From the 2006 National Survey of Mental Health Literacy and Stigma, Jorm and Reavley (2001) in conjunction with Melbourne University uncovered some key findings about youth mental health literacy in Australia. These included:

- Only a small percentage of young people saw doctors as a source of intended help;
- There was widespread awareness among young people that the use of substances is harmful for mental health;
- When a peer had a mental health problem, it was not often recognised by a young person to encourage professional help seeking;
- Young people viewed general and informal sources of help as interventions that would be helpful rather than specialist mental health services;
- Stigma was lower in young people who had experience of mental health problems in self or others, who had been exposed to mental health campaigns, and whose parents had less stigmatising attitudes.

Following consideration of two international studies (Skre, Friborg, Breivik, Johnsen, Arnesen, & Wang, 2013; Mcluckie, Kutcher, Wei, & Weaver, 2014) it was found that after introducing mental health education and promotion programs into the curriculum that there were definite improvements in the mental health literacy of both students and staff. More research and education is needed in order to improve youth mental health literacy which in turn will improve early intervention outcomes of young people whom are developing signs of mental health problems and mental illness.

INTERNATIONAL EXPERIENCE OF MENTAL HEALTH EDUCATION IN SCHOOLS

Around the world there are literally hundreds of mental health interventions and education programs being run (Weare & Nind, 2011). From the evidence these are most popular in Western countries such as the USA, Canada, the United Kingdom, Scandinavia and parts of Europe. Most of these appear to be quite fragmented without there being one national integrated program per country. These vary in size, coverage and the amount of mental health resources that they produce and make available. Some are privately run while others have the backing of respective federal or state government money. Askell-Williams and colleagues (2009) identified several school-based mental health education programs based on the World Health Organisation (WHO) 'Health Promoting Schools' framework. These included Social and Emotional Aspects of Learning (SEAL) from the United Kingdom, the Collaborative for Academic, Social and Emotional Learning (CASEL) initiatives in the United States of America and the European Network for Socio-Emotional Competence in Children (ENSEC). Askell-Williams and colleagues (2009) noted that "each of these seeks to develop students' social, emotional and behavioural capabilities, as well as the capabilities of schools and families to support children's wellbeing". These examples show a whole-school approach not unlike MindMatters and KidsMatter in Australia.

In 2007, a secondary school mental health curriculum, the Mental Health and High School Curriculum Guide was developed in Canada in a collaboration between the Canadian Mental Health Association and mental health experts from several different organisations and universities. This has proven to be quite successful so far.

The United Kingdom have also been proactive in implementing a number of mental health education programs. These include YoungMinds, OpenMinds and Place2Be. Place2Be is the UK's leading children's mental health charity providing in-school support and expert training to improve the emotional wellbeing of pupils, families, teachers and school staff. OpenMinds is a student-led intervention, providing mental health education to school students by training medical students to deliver workshops in local schools.

The United States has an abundance of mental health education programs. Examples of these included FRIENDS, which focuses on reducing anxiety and teaching skills for managing emotions and coping with stress among students, parents and teachers. It addresses six core topic areas, including identifying feelings, understanding one's physical responses, learning to relax, linking thoughts and feelings, developing plans for coping and practicing emotion management. Other ones were Positive Action (PA), Promoting Alternative Thinking Strategies (PATHS), Cognitive-Behavioural Intervention for Trauma in Schools (CBITS) and the American Psychiatric Association Foundation's School Mental Health Program 'Typical or Troubled?'.

BARRIERS AND PROBLEMS TO IMPLEMENTING MENTAL HEALTH EDUCATION IN AUSTRALIAN SCHOOLS

Although there are many benefits for implementing Mental Health Education into school curriculum, that is not to say that it does not come with its fair share of problems, barriers and challenges. After the original audit into Mental Health Education in Australian Secondary Schools was completed in 1996 a number of barriers were discovered. These included:

- Teachers and other school staff lacked specific knowledge and skills, and thus confidence in teaching, on these issues; this lack of information was also reflected in the prejudices of staff and others in the school;
- The specified curriculum lacked a space for mental health education; there was a lack of time in an already 'packed' curriculum;
- There was a lack of relevant and reliable resources;
- Students' and parents' values;
- Within the curriculum, health generally and mental health in particular has a low status;
- There is sometimes no continuity or commitment from teachers from year to year, across and within departments, and between teachers and other staff;

- Mental health issues are often seen as crisis-driven and individual, and thus more relevant to welfare approaches than to curriculum (Youth Research Centre and Centre for Social Health, 1996).

With the introduction of MindMatters and the two variations of KidsMatter, some improvements could be seen concerning these barriers and problems. Professional development has definitely been enhanced and the resources available to schools now is much improved to what was on offer in the past. Some of these barriers however still exist today, with schools trying to fit so much into their curriculum for example. As can be seen from the findings above there are a number of challenges that present extra stresses and pressures for teachers and schools in trying to implement Mental Health Education. Additionally, some teachers and educators believe that it is not a part of their role to provide Mental Health Education or to be a role model or provide guidance around it. Another point of contention for some schools that have even been successful at embedding Mental Health Education into their curriculum is the matter of sustainability. Some schools believe that this is not possible with their many pressing demands, changes in curriculum and changes in staff. Lastly, another possible barrier is that of the attitudes and values of some teachers and educators in regard to mental health and mental illness and their willingness to pick up delivering mental health resources.

BENEFITS OF MENTAL HEALTH EDUCATION IN AUSTRALIAN SCHOOLS

There are a number of benefits and advantages for young people as well as teachers, families and the broader community with the introduction of mental health education into schools. With the high prevalence of mental illnesses such as depression and anxiety, young people are able to be provided with the skills, knowledge and understanding on how to manage these conditions as well as knowing what they can do to stay mentally and emotionally well in the first instance. Through having a greater understanding, insight and knowledge of mental illness and it's early warning signs, young people will be able to assist their peers in accessing important early help from mental health professionals and hopefully avoid a crisis situation. Education and knowledge will also help to break down the appalling stigma that still surrounds mental illness in the community and amongst young people, therefore enabling people not to feel judged and feeling comfortable to accept help for their mental health problems. Through the process of early intervention and prevention, young people will be able to learn to become more resilient and mental health conscious, which will help them to become more productive people who are better able to deal with stress and difficult and challenging life situations.

Introducing and exposing young people to mental health education at an early age will set a good precedent in raising children who are less judgmental towards people who have mental illness in the community as well as helping people to recognize the importance of maintaining their own mental health as much as their physical health. This would help in decreasing the amount of serious mental illness that exists in the community due to the fact that young people and future generations of adults would be more inclined to seek early help for either existing or emerging mental health problems or mental illness. Early identification of mental illness would help in decreasing the amount of admissions to emergency or psychiatric wards in hospitals, which is already under pressure and costs the Australian government millions of dollars each year.

Mental health education will also give young people a better understanding about the impact that drugs and alcohol can have on their mental health and recognizing that they may be self-medicating which may be masking what is an underlying mental health condition. A reduction in the use of drugs and alcohol will see an improvement in the mental health of young people which will also save the health system money and more importantly young people's lives.

Through mental health education young people will be raised to be more resilient and be able to better manage their stress from an earlier age which will prepare them better for adolescence and adulthood. This will lead to a more productive economy and save millions of dollars in tax payers money due to people taking less sick leave or filing claims for stress leave.

THE FUTURE OF MENTAL HEALTH EDUCATION IN AUSTRALIAN SCHOOLS

The future of Mental Health Education in Australian schools is looking bright after the announcement in June, 2017 by the Australian government of a new initiative to be rolled out in 2018. This new program will hopefully make it even more accessible and easier for schools to use than what is currently in place. The beyondblue Chairman at the time, Jeff Kennett, described the program as "a game-changer that would replace the current fragmented approach with a wholly integrated one" (beyondblue, 2017). From August 2018, beyondblue will lead a new National Mental Health in Education program with support from headspace and Early Childhood Australia, with funding from the Australian Government Department of Health, (beyondblue, 2016). This new initiative will transform Australia's approach to child and youth mental health care by providing a single end-to-end school-based mental health program. Covering the continuum from early childhood to secondary school, it will support mental health promotion and suicide prevention activity. The program will integrate and build on the strengths and evidence-based principles of key existing Commonwealth Government mental health initiatives being delivered in education settings.

These initiatives are:

- Response Ability
- KidsMatter Early Childhood
- KidsMatter Primary
- MindMatters
- Headspace School Support

In the meantime KidsMatter Early Childhood, KidsMatter Primary and Mind Matters will continue as normal in their current form until the new program launches in August 2018. From January 2018, headspace facilitators will deliver KidsMatter and MindMatters to primary and secondary schools, while Early Childhood Australia facilitators will deliver KidsMatter Early Childhood (beyondblue, 2016). beyondblue will continue to provide Response Ability resources to university lecturers and course facilitators who provide pre-service training to future educators, through to mid-2018. The Response Ability website will continue to be the primary information source for the pre-service training sector. In a media release from beyondblue, who were the successful bidder in a competitive tender process for the new Mental Health in Education program, their CEO, Georgie Harman affirmed that:

We will bring together the best minds from across the mental health and education sectors to build a contemporary national child and youth mental health program with the aim of helping everyone reach their full potential academically, emotionally, socially and in later life. (beyondblue, 2017)

CONCLUSION

Ever since the Australian government undertook an audit in 1996 into Mental Health Education in Australian Secondary schools, there has been a strong focus put on mental health education in schools. This is evident from the MindMatters (secondary schools) and KidsMatter (primary schools) initiatives that were successfully introduced and implemented in many schools around Australia. These initiatives also saw the introduction of other mental health education programs in Australia that have been discussed earlier. These initiatives and programs have seen Australia become one of the world leaders in school / youth mental health education as well as mental health promotion. Australia is well resourced for mental health education resources and professional development and the future is looking bright with the announcement by the government in June, 2017 of the Mental Health in Education initiative, which rolls out from 2018. This program will improve on what is already in existence by providing a seamless single end-to-end school-based mental health program from early childhood to secondary school that is wholly integrated as opposed to having separate programs in operation. From looking at the evidence that the mental health literacy of young people and students in Australia is still lacking, suggests that more needs to be done about this. Hopefully the current lack of knowledge about mental illness, mental health and seeking psychological treatment amongst young people in Australia will be improved through the new Mental Health in Education initiative and that more young people will seek out and utilize mental health services earlier. It is crucial that young people learn to recognize early presenting mental health problems and know what help and treatment options are available to both themselves and to their peers. The introduction of compulsory mental health education in Australian schools as well as forming part of the curriculum would see visible improvements in the mental health and wellbeing of young people in Australia, which in return would provide many benefits and opportunities for the broader community. For compulsory mental health education to work well would require that teachers receive good professional training and support and that schools are provided with excellent resources. It may be that the Australian government employs specialist mental health education teachers for schools to deliver the content so that the regular teachers can concentrate and focus on the rest of the curriculum. Mental health education in schools will help in decreasing the likelihood of mental health problems presenting for people when they are adults or minimizing the impact for people who have a mental illness. It will help build resilience in young people and create a society where people are more accepting of mental illness, which will lead to early help seeking. Mental health literacy will improve which will only seek to benefit Australia as a community moving forward due to the fact that more Australians in the community will be more mentally healthy.

REFERENCES

About MIEACT. (2016). Retrieved October 01, 2017, from https://www.mieact.org.au/sites/default-filesdocumentsStrat%20PlanMIEACT%20Aims%2C%20VIsion%20and%20Mission%202013%20-%20 2016.pdf

About ReachOut Schools. (2017). Retrieved October 09, 2017, from https://schools.au.reachout.com/articles/about-reachout-schools

Allen, J., & Vincent K. (2005). *Journeys: Supporting innovation in teacher education throughout Australia*. Academic Press.

Askell-Williams, H., Dix, K. L., Lawson, M. J., & Slee, P. T. (2013). Quality of implementation of a school mental health initiative and changes over time in students' social and emotional competencies. *School Effectiveness and School Improvement*, *24*(3), 357–381. doi:10.1080/09243453.2012.692697

Askell-Williams, H., Lawson, M. J., & Slee, P. T. (2009). Venturing into schools: Locating mental health initiatives in complex environments. *The International Journal of Emotional Education*, *1*(2), 14–33.

Australian partners in wellbeing for secondary schools. (2016). Retrieved October 08, 2017, from https://www.beyondblue.org.au/about-us/about-our-work/childhood-and-education-program/australian-partners-in-wellbeing-for-secondary-schools

Barry, M. M., & Jenkins, R. (2007). *Implementing Mental Health Promotion*. Philadelphia: Elsevier Limited.

Black Dog Institute. (2016). *Black Dog Institute submission in response to the 5th National Mental Health Plan*. Black Dog Institute.

Bond, L., Butler, H., Glover, S., & Patton, G. (2002). The Gatehouse Project: Mental Health Promotion Incorporating School Organisational Change and Health Education. In G. Martin, L. Rowling, & L. Walker (Eds.), *Mental Health Promotion: Concepts and Practice Young People* (pp. 128–141). Sydney: McGraw-Hill Australia Pty Limited.

Butler, H., Bond, L., Glover, S., & Patton, G. (2002). The Gatehouse Project: Mental Health Promotion Incorporating School Organisational Change and Health Education. In Mental Health Promotion and Young People: Concepts and Practice (pp. 128-141). Sydney: McGraw-Hill Australia Pty Limited.

Centre for Adolescent Health: The Gatehouse Project. (2017). Retrieved September 29, 2017, from https://www.rch.org.au/cah/research/The_Gatehouse_Project/

Commonwealth of Australia. (2009). Fourth National Mental Health Plan - An agenda for collaborative government action in mental health 2009 - 2014. Canberra: Author.

Early Childhood and Primary Schools: KidsMatter & KidsMatter Early Childhood. (2016). Retrieved October 08, 2017, from https://www.beyondblue.org.au/healthy-places/early-childhood-and-primary-schools

Hart, L. M., Mason, R. J., Kelly, C. M., Cvetkovski, S., & Jorm, A. F. (2016). 'teen Mental Health First Aid': A description of the program an initial evaluation. *International Journal of Mental Health Systems, 10*(3), 1–18. PMID:26788123

HeadStrong 2.0. (2017). Retrieved October 14, 2017, from https://www.blackdoginstitute.org.au/education-training/community-and-schools/free-school-resources/headstrong-2.0

Jorm, A. F. (2011). Mental Health Literacy: Empowering the Community to Take Action for Better Mental Health. *The American Psychologist*, 1–12. PMID:22040221

Jorm, A. F., & Kelly, C. M. (2007). Improving the public's understanding and response to mental disorders. *Australian Psychologist, 42*(2), 81–89. doi:10.1080/00050060701280565

Jorm, A. F., Kelly, C. M., & Wright, A. (2007). Improving mental health literacy as a strategy to facilitate early intervention for mental disorders. *The Medical Journal of Australia, 187*, S26–S30. PMID:17908021

Jorm, A.F., Korten, A.E., Jacomb, P.A., Christensen, H., & Rodgers, B., & Pollitt. (1997). "Mental health literacy": A survey of the public's ability to recognise mental disorders and their beliefs about the effectiveness of treatment. *The Medical Journal of Australia, 166*, 182–186. PMID:9066546

Jorm, A. F., & Wright, A. (2007). Beliefs of young people and their parents about the effectiveness of interventions for mental disorders. *The Australian and New Zealand Journal of Psychiatry, 41*(8), 656–666. doi:10.1080/00048670701449179 PMID:17620162

Kay-Lambkin, F., Kemp, E., Stafford, K., & Hazell, T. (2007, June). Mental Health Promotion and Early Intervention in Early Childhood and Primary School Setting: A Review. *Journal of Student Wellbeing, 1*(1), 31–56. doi:10.21913/JSW.v1i1.115

Kessler, R. C., Berglund, P., Demler, O., Jin, R., Merikangas, K., & Walters, E. (2005). Lifetime prevalence and age-of-onset distributions of DSM-IV disorders in the national comorbidity survey replication. *Archives of General Psychiatry, 62*(6), 593–603. doi:10.1001/archpsyc.62.6.593 PMID:15939837

KidsMatter. (n.d.). Retrieved 06 August, 2017, from http://www.pai.edu.au/content/kidsmatter-primary

Kutcher, S., Wei, Y., & Morgan, C. (2015). Successful Application of a Canadian Mental Health Curriculum Resource by Usual Classroom Teachers in Significantly and Sustainably Improving Student Mental Health. *Canadian Journal of Psychiatry, 60*(12), 580–586. doi:10.1177/070674371506001209 PMID:26720827

Lawrence, D., Johnson, S., Hafekost, J., Boterhoven De Haan, K., Sawyer, M., Ainley, J., & … . (2015). *The Mental Health of Children and Adolescents. Report on the second Australian Child and Adolescent Survey of Mental Health and Wellbeing*. Canberra: Department of Health.

McGorry, P., Purcell, R., Hickie, I., & Jorm, A. (2007). Investing in youth mental health is a best buy. *The Medical Journal of Australia, 187*(suppl. 7), S5–S7.

Mcluckie, A., Kutcher, S., Wei, Y., & Weaver, C. (2014). Sustained improvements in students' mental health literacy with use of a mental health curriculum in Canadian schools. *BMC Public Health, 14*, 379. PMID:25551789

MindMatters. (n.d.). Retrieved 06 August, 2017, from http://www.pai.edu.au/content/mindmatters

Mission Australia and Black Dog Institute. (2016). *Youth mental health report: Youth Survey 2012-16*. Sydney: Mission Australia.

Orygen Youth Health. Anxiety & Young People. (2008). Retrieved September 24, 2017, from http://oyh.org.au/sites/oyh.org.au/files/factsheets/oyh_fs_anx.pdf

Peer Support Australia. Who We Are. (2014). Retrieved September 29, 2017, from http://peersupport.edu.au/about-peer-support-australia/who-we-are/

Reavley, N. J., & Jorm, A. F. (2011). *National Survey of Mental Health Literacy and Stigma*. Canberra: Department of Health and Ageing.

Response Ability. (2012). Retrieved October 22, 2017, from http://www.responseability.org/home

Rickwood, D., Deane, F. P., Wilson, C. J., & Ciarrochi, J. (2005). Young people's help-seeking for mental health problems. *Australian e-Journal for the Advancement of Mental Health, 4*(3), 218–251. doi:10.5172/jamh.4.3.218

Sawyer, M. G., Arney, F. M., Baghurst, P. A., Clark, J. J., Graetz, B. W., Kosky, R. J., & .... (2000). *Child and adolescent component of the national survey of mental health and well-being*. Canberra: Mental Health and Special Programs Branch of the Commonwealth Department of Health and Aged Care.

Secondary schools program. (2016). Retrieved September 24, 2017, from https://www.beyondblue.org.au/healthy-places/secondary-schools-and-tertiary/secondary-schools-program

SenseAbility. (2016). Retrieved September 24, 2017, from https://www.beyondblue.org.au/healthy-places/secondary-schools-and-tertiary/senseability/download-sensibility

Sheehan, M., Cahill, H., Rowling, L., Marshall, B., Wynn, J., & Holdsworth. (2002). Establishing A Role for Schools in Mental Health Promotion: The MindMatters Project. In G. Martin, L. Rowling & L. Walker (Eds.), *Mental Health Promotion: Concepts and Practice Young People* (pp. 111 - 127). Sydney: McGraw-Hill Australia Pty Limited.

Skre, I., Friborg, O., Breivik, C., Johnsen, L. I., Arnesen, Y., & Wang, C. E. A. (2013). A school intervention for mental health literacy in adolescents: Effects of a non-randomized cluster controlled trial. *BMC Public Health, 13*, 873.

teen MHFA Course Information. (2017). Retrieved September 30, 2017, from https://mhfa.com.au/cms/teen-mhfa-course-information

The beyondblue Mental Health in Education program. (2016). Retrieved September 30 September, 2017, from https://www.beyondblue.org.au/about-us/about-our-work/childhood-and-education-program/the-i-beyondblue-i-mental-health-in-education-program thedesk. (2016). Retrieved October 15, 2017, from https://www.beyondblue.org.au/healthy-places/secondary-schools-and-tertiary/thedesk

Weare, K. & Nind, M. (2011). Mental health promotion and problem prevention in schools: what does the evidence say? *Health Promotion International, 26*(S1), i29-i69.

What is MindMatters? (n.d.). Retrieved October 09, 2017, from https://www.mindmatters.edu.au/about-mindmatters/what-is-mindmatters

Why it is needed? (n.d.). Retrieved October 21, 2017, from https://www.kidsmatter.edu.au/primary/about-kidsmatter-primary/why-it-needed-0

World Health Organisational Regional Office for Europe. (1994). *Promoting the Health of Young People in Europe: Health Education in Schools: A Training Manual for Teachers and Others Working with Young People*. Edinburgh, UK: Health Education Board for Scotland.

Youth Research Centre and Centre for Social Health. (1996). *Mental Health Education in Australian Secondary Schools*. Canberra: Australian Government Publishing Service.

Chapter 12
Encouraging Social Inclusion for Older Adults Through "Interest"-Led Technology Use

Jeanie Beh
Swinburne University of Technology, Australia

Bruno Mascitelli
Swinburne University of Technology, Australia

Sonja Pedell
Swinburne University of Technology, Australia

ABSTRACT

There are many misconceptions about older adults' capabilities and aspirations, and especially their attitudes and approach towards technology. They are often misunderstood and seen as uninterested and unmotivated to engage with use of technology. Due to an absence of an "interest" framework for older adults to learn mobile touch screen technologies, this chapter investigates the role that pre-existing interests play in older adults' adoption of technology. Can a curriculum guided only by pre-existing interests of older adults, rather than a structured curriculum have a positive influence on its adoption for mobile touch screen technologies? The results show that when older adults are taught according to requests based on their pre-existing interests, it encouraged long-term adoption of technology including building up their confidence in usage of mobile touch screen technologies.

INTRODUCTION

As technology of all varieties becomes more accessible to the totality of society across all generations and as an outcome of increased life expectancy, older adults are leading lives that are more active in their third age. While the world was embracing the shift with touch screen technology and the Internet in our everyday lives, people were actually living longer compared to their predecessors (DESA, 2015). The developed countries were the first to undergo this major shift and currently, it is a worldwide phenomenon.

DOI: 10.4018/978-1-5225-7402-6.ch012

Although this brings about societal and economical challenges (Sander, Oxlund, Jespersen, Krasnik, Mortensen, Westendorp, Rasmussen, 2015) it also presents a new array of opportunities. Older adults do this in creating for themselves opportunities to learn new skills and pursue new interests and hobbies to challenge themselves. At the same time, there are many misconceptions about older adults' capabilities and aspirations, especially their attitudes towards technology (Cherry, Brigman, Lyon, Blanchard, Walker, & Smitherman, 2016). They are often misunderstood and seen to lack interest and motivation in the use of technology even though studies have shown otherwise (Anderson & Perrin, 2017). What has become evident to government authorities is that there is low-level uptake of technology amongst older adults (Chen, McGaughey, Zeltmann, Lu, Hsin-Ke, &, Maria, 2018). Not being able to use technology is isolating and makes it difficult for older adults to conduct their everyday lives (Quan-Haase, Guang & Wellman, 2018). Hence, it is imperative for older adults to participate in technology use. Thus, the aim of this chapter is to seek out ways and means in which social and digital inclusion for older adults can occur. This chapter aims to explore the relationship of older adults to pre-existing "interests" and their interest in technology with reference to Hidi and Renninger's Four-Phase Model of Interest Development (2006). In order to better understand the subject matter of this theme, the definition of terms such as "older adults" and "interest" will be required. Older adults generally refers to people 65 years old and over, mainly to represent a benchmark of life stage, whereby it is considered a legal retirement age and eligibility for pension (OECD, 2018). In Australia, in order to be eligible to apply for senior's card, the minimum age is 60 years and working less than 35 hours per week (DHS, 2018). The use of the term "interest" refers to older adults' individual interests and hobbies in general. However, in order to avoid confusion, it will be referred to as *pre-existing interests*. When *interest* is described as a verb, the word will be presented in italic, whereas in the case of a noun, it will not be italicised.

The topic of interest was first explored within the field of psychology as far back as 1891. It then disappeared for a few decades and resurfaced in the 1980s falling into the subcategory of educational psychology (Silvia, 2006). Most studies today gravitate towards technology uptake and younger children and in the case of the elderly mostly in a classroom setting. To date, there has been very little research about how technology could support older adults' pre-existing interests. The main factor for adoption of new technology is constructed around the notion of interest. An effective and sound theoretical and motivation approach framework is contained in the three models referred to here: The Four-Phase Model of Interest Development (Hidi & Renninger, 2006), Self-Determination Theory (Deci & Ryan, 1985) and Socioemotional Selectivity Theory (Carstensen, 1992). These models have assisted studies in the exploration of the factors that can stimulate interest in use of mobile touch screen technologies by older adults and consequently improve the quality of their lives. While it can be imperative to provide technologies to the elderly that are easy to learn, there is also the specific pre-existing interests of older adults in order to facilitate a successful learning environment. This approach allows for a better understanding of the relationship of how interest can best complement and support their pre-existing interests in their everyday activities and also make use of old age learning capabilities.

MOTIVATIONAL THEORIES

Self-Determination Theory

There needs to be a paradigm shift with identification of issues related to older adults' motivation towards the adoption of technologies. At this junction, motivation according to some is considered to be another relevant concept for understanding how people learn. According to Ryan and Deci (2000) to be motivated means "to be moved to do something" (p.54). An example provided by Graham and Weiner (1996), is when a person is oblivious to all else, through being engaged in a particular activity, that is considered interesting, captivating and involving to an individual, then motivation is considered high. Bernard and colleagues (2005) state that 'motivation is what animates us, what prompts our initiation, choice and persistence in particular behaviours in particular environments' (p.137). On the one hand, motivation can be considered a unitary phenomenon, when a person either has very little motivation to act or a great deal of it. Alternatively, although, by nature, human beings are curious and possess the desire to learn (Niemiec & Ryan, 2009), they can be considered to have different amounts and different kinds of motivation. In other words, they vary not only in levels of motivation but also in orientation for that motivation (Deci & Ryan, 2008). Numerous studies related to Self-Determination Theory (SDT) were conducted for children, adolescents and younger adults. In high schools, studies included academic subjects such as physical education (Standage, Duda & Ntoumanis, 2005). Within the higher education sector (e.g. universities), subjects such as organic chemistry (Black & Deci, 2000), second languages (Noels, Pelletier, Clement, & Vallerand, 2000), law (Sheldon & Krieger, 2007) and medicine (Williams & Deci, 1996) use this approach. In workplaces, for instance corporate and charity organisations (Deckop & Cirka, 2000) SDT is also used. According to Ryan and Deci (2000), 'although motivation is often treated as a singular construct, even superficial reflection suggests that people are moved to act by very different types of factors, with highly varied experiences and consequences. People can be motivated because they value an activity or because there is strong external coercion' (p.69). Deci and Ryan (1985) define the three important elements that make up SDT to be: (1) autonomy; (2) competence, and; (3) relatedness. These three elements are the essential foundation towards the development of personal well-being and social development (Ryan & Deci, 2000). Both autonomy and competence are classified as basic psychological needs and necessary for sustained motivation (Niemiec & Ryan, 2009). Sound learning outcomes are more likely if determined by individuals who feel that they have a certain amount of control over their learning (Hagay, Baram-Tsabari, Ametler, Cakmakci, Lopes, Moreira, & Pedrosa-de-Jesus, 2013). Motivation can be classified along a continuum from intrinsic or extrinsic (Reeve, 2005). Deci and Ryan (2008) reported that the latter theory was indeed a stable idea due to the abundance of research. Since the mid-1980s, Deci and Ryan (1985) have been leaders in motivational research in education. There has been little research conducted of relevance with older adults using Self-Determination Theory (SDT).

Socioemotional Selectivity Theory

Socioemotional Selectivity Theory (SST) is of relevance to older adults. It is also known as life-span theory of motivation, and maintains that as people start to age, they realise that their time horizons shrink (Carstensen, 1992). SST was developed by Laura Carstensen, an American psychologist (1992).

In SST, time remaining is viewed as a constraint. Older adults become very aware that they are running out of time. Perception of time plays a vital role in decision making towards the selection and pursuit of individual goals (Carstensen, Isaacowitz & Charles, 1999). Therefore, older adults tend to be more selective about making the right choices so as not to waste their precious time. Carstensen and her colleagues (1999) claim that SST plays an important role; it determines the motivational shift leading older adults' to invest their time to select and pursue goals and activities that are emotionally meaningful. Charles and Carstensen (2009) state that ageing brings changes to social and emotional life. Besides motivational shifts, ageing also influences personal goals. Studies show that younger adults perceive their future as open-ended and therefore they prioritise their goals towards knowledge-related goals. They concentrate on acquisition of knowledge in order to plan for endeavours that would pay off in the future such as applying for a job promotion. On the other hand, older adults shift their focus towards emotion-related goals directing their attention towards goal-relevant information to deepen existing relationships and fulfil personal satisfaction. A number of studies show that older adults with strong social connections are less likely to experience decline in their cognitive functioning. Social networks also contribute towards regaining higher cognitive functioning (Glymour, Weuve, Martha, Glass & Berkman, 2008).

An Ageing Australia and Associated Issues

In the 19th century, fuelled by Gold Rush, Australia's population reached nearly 4 million by 1901 (ABS, 2006). At the beginning of the 20th century, natural increase was the main contributor towards population growth though later migration would provide the greater level of population replenishment. For the first time, birth rates outnumbered death rates. Over the past century, life expectancy increased gradually due to the improvement of living conditions, advances in food quality, better health education and public sanitation and lower mortality levels. With the advancement of medical science such as immunization and antibiotics, Australians are expected to live considerably longer than those from last century (Harvey & Thurnwalk, 2009). The current population of Australia is over 24.8 million and continues to increase through births and migration (ABS, 2018) as seen in Figure 1. In 1891, the life expectancy

Figure 1. Australia's population (millions) from 1901 to 2101(reproduced from ABS, 2017)

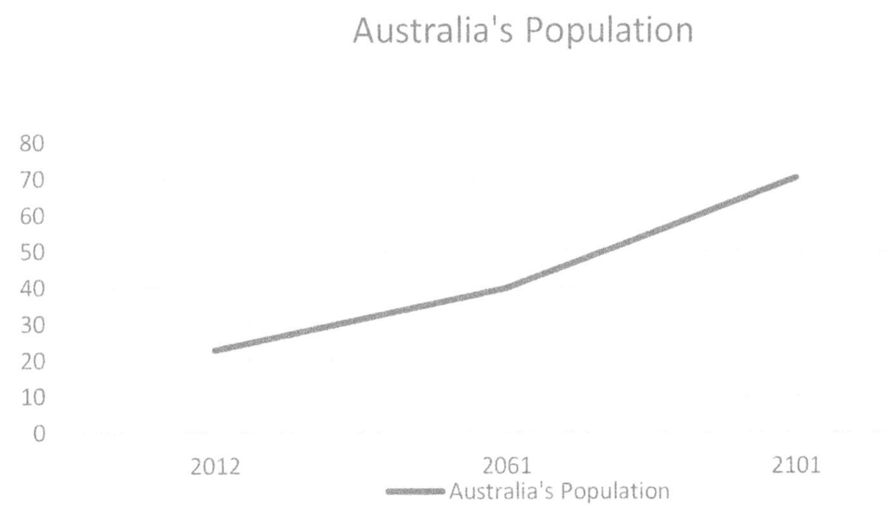

rate for men was 33.3 years and women at 33.7 years (ABS, 2017). According to ABS (2017), a person born in 2015, would have the average life expectancy of 84.5 years for women and 80.4 years for men giving an average of 82 years. This, therefore, ranks Australian life expectancy amongst the highest in the world (WEF, 2017) as seen in Table 1.

Between the period of 1996 and 2016, the aged 65 years and over group increased from 12 per cent to 15.3 per cent of the Australian population (ABS, 2016). In 2015, older Australians made up of 14 per cent, approximately 3.5 million individuals (ABS, 2015), an increase of 1 per cent since 2013 (CEPAR, 2014). By 2050, the projected number of Australians above the age of 65 is estimated to reach 7.2 million (CEPAR, 2014). According to ABS (2016), over the past two decades, the number of persons aged 85 years and over increased by 141.2 per cent, compared with a total population growth of 32.4 per cent over the same period.

Population ageing is a significant factor into the future heralding both challenges and opportunities. The Australian Government is seeking solutions for funding and managing its current healthcare and pension systems to support the growing ageing population (ABS, 2016). According to CEPAR (2014), in 2050, the projected public expenditure on health proportion to Gross Domestic Product (GDP) is 10.3 per cent, an increase of 6 per cent from 2010. Compulsory contribution to superannuation started in 1983. It was an initiative by the Australian Government for people to accumulate funds that will provide them with a source of income to sustain them through retirement. In 2013, when the first baby boomers reached 65 years with retirement in the near horizon, ideally, one of the government's key policy focus was people's ability to support themselves financially, funding their own retirement through superannuation, investments and other personal income sources (ABS, 2017). But in actual fact, older adults were reliant upon government pension as their main source of income (ABS, 2017). According to Uren (2017), 80

Table 1. Average life expectancy of 15 nations with highest levels of life expectancy (reproduced from World Economic Forum, 2017)

Ranking	Country	Life Expectancy
1	Hong Kong	84.3
2	Japan	83.8
3	Italy	83.5
3	Spain	83.4
5	Switzerland	83.2
6	Iceland	82.9
7	France	82.7
8	Singapore	82.6
9	Sweden	82.6
10	Australia	82.5
11	Luxembourg	82.2
12	Korea, Rep.	82.2
13	Canada	82.1
14	Norway	82.1
15	Israel	82.1

per cent of older adults are still relying on at least a part pension. A report by Roy Morgan (2016) stated that the average retirement funding is insufficient to be categorised as "self-funded". The number of people intending to retire has increased 27 per cent from 327,000 in 2008 compared to 415,000 in 2016. Edgar (2013) suggests that the Australian Government is mistaken in measuring older Australian's worth in the economy in terms of productivity that contributes directly towards the nation's GDP (DCCSDS, 2012). It was stated that the majority of Australians are predicted to be better educated, healthier and wealthier. Older Australians are saving the Australian Government considerable expenditure through social and volunteer activities (Edgar, 2013). According to Betts (2014) in 2010, 45 per cent of those aged 65 years and older volunteered their services. In 2015, volunteering by older adults is estimated to have added $A3.1 billion dollars to the Australian economy (Perrier, 2015).

Older Adults and Technology

Older adults are often seen as being excluded from the digital world, possibly because of misconceptions that they are not capable of adopting the technology or interested and/or motivated to use new technologies (Durick, Robertson, Brereton, Vetere & Nansen, 2013). In fact, globally, older adults are consuming more technology products, such as mobile touch screen technologies (smartphones and tablets) and appear to want to participate more actively in social life (OECD, 2015) than previous generations at this stage of life (Ianculescu, Lupeanu, Alexandru, Tudora, Coman, & Coman, 2011). There are more opportunities available for generations of older adults in the developed world. This happens because they are more educated, healthier and skilled, and therefore remain more active in the workforce compared to their predecessors (OECD, 2015). Computing technology not only bring benefits to the young but also to older generations and can increase the social inclusion of older adults and improve the quality of their lives (Phiriyapokan, 2011). For this to occur it is therefore useful to understand what motivates older adults to use technology (Doyle, Skrba, McDonnell & Arent, 2010). Studies have shown that learning occurs most rapidly when an individual is generally the happiest and to obtain optimum results, time spent on learning is best distributed across many shorter sessions (Amthor, 2012). Advantages associated with use of the internet and computers for the elderly could include increase in self-confidence, ability to learn and memory retention (OECD, 2015). Nevertheless, despite older adults' willingness to learn the use of computers, they are usually faced with difficulties such as understanding technical terms, remembering steps to perform a task and using technology, such as the mouse (Sayago & Blat, 2011).

Some of the main barriers that prevent the uptake of technologies by older adults could include physical and/or financial constraints, difficulty with transportation and/or mobility, health and ageing issues (OECD, 2015). There are also issues associated with digital literacy and educational levels where older adults may not have been taught good conceptual models related to the workings of technologies (Sayago & Blat, 2011). A number of technological devices rely on a person's ability to keep information active over time in memory that could be an unrealistic expectation for older adults unless they are proficient users (Caprani, O'Connor & Gurrin, 2011). Studies have shown that there are similarities with the use of technologies between younger and older adults, but at different usage rates. It is also necessary to take into consideration that there are many cognitive differences between younger and older adults. For example, the slowing down of the working memory (short-term memory) and thought processing. Older adults may interact with computer devices differently when faced with trying to use new computer products (Phiriyapokan, 2011). Older adults do not necessarily gain the support required to help with their learning of technology but if there is a learning model that is both engaging and attainable, it could keep older adults interested and motivated in learning technology. Mobile touch screen devices is one of the options that could enable older adults to access the internet. Recently, there has been increased interest in researching the use of mobile touch screen devices for older adults. Mobile touch screen devices can have advantages over traditional keyboard/ mouse/ screen interfaces for older adults because of ease of use, thus enhancing communications and improving their quality of lives. Mobile touch screen devices can be easier to use than some equivalent technologies as they accommodate some of the age-related physical and cognitive limitations faced by older adults (Caprani, O'Connor, & Gurrin, 2011). The close proximity of keyboard to information on the screen could increase spatial contiguity and reduce cognitive load (Doubé & Beh, 2012). In addition, mobile touch screen devices enables items such as buttons and texts to be enlarged, making them: (1) easier to see and; (2) easier to select accurately (Caprani, O'Connor, & Gurrin, 2011). One of the key aspects towards successful ageing is to remain actively engaged in leisure activities (Nimrod, 2010). It has proven to be vital through fostering of social communications (Doyle, Skrba, McDonnell, & Arent, 2010). Technologies are also able to create new opportunities and stretch potential towards development of new activities for older adults (OECD, 2015). In addition, older adults' quality of lives have been enhanced through the use of technologies and simultaneously enables them to remain connected in an inexpensive and flexible way (Satariano, Scharlach & Lindeman, 2014). Boulton-Lewis (2009) suggests that it is not only important to provide technologies that are easy to learn, but to also consider the specific interests of older adults in order to facilitate a successful learning environment and make use of learning capabilities of older adults.

Interest

The notion of "interest" is further separated into situational interest and individual interest. Situational interest is fleeting, once triggered, it could either be maintained or disappear altogether. Ainley and colleagues contend that situational interest is usually associated with individuals who do not have any pre-existing individual interests (Ainley, Hidi & Berndorff, 2002). Situational interest is associated with support from the environment and the people around an individual (Renninger, 2009), usually – momentary and may or may not last over time. According to Tin (2013), situational interest acts as a bridge in order for more stable individual interests to develop. Hidi and Renninger (2006) maintained that there is a misconception that situational interest cannot be developed if it is non-existent. On the contrary, it could actually be nurtured over a period of time. Individual interest could be referred to as personal interest, that resides in individuals and is considered relatively stable, that indicates that individuals are able to re-engage with contents after a certain time (Hidi & Renninger, 2006). While individuals are engaged with the experience and seek opportunities to engage in a particular activity, he or she will expand their knowledge of that activity (Ainley, Hidi, & Berndorff, 2002). Individual interest is associated with intrinsic motivation because it is considered a stable predisposition, content-specific as it develops over time, through the interaction between an individual and his or her object of interest (Tin, 2013). The Four-Phase Model of Interest Development developed by Hidi and Renninger (2006) and illustrated and adapted by the authors (See Figure 2), extends and expands on their earlier three-phase model (Krapp, 2002). The Four-Phase Model of Interest Development consists of the following: (1) phase one – triggered situational interest; (2) phase two – maintained situational interest; (3) phase three – emerging individual interest and; (4) phase four – well-developed individual interest.

Hidi and Renninger (2011) have suggested that triggered situational interest could be sparked by either environmental or textural features, as a psychological state resulting from short-term changes in

Figure 2. The four-phase model of interest development (adapted from Hidi & Renninger, 2006)

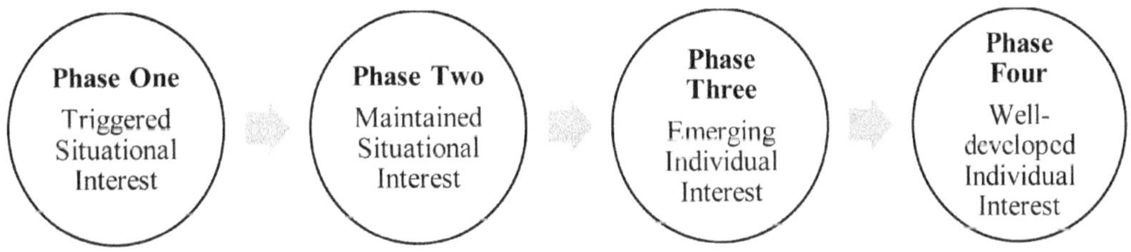

both affective and cognitive processing. Maintained situational interest is described as subsequent to a triggered state. It typically occurs over an extended period of time, reoccurs persistently and involves focused attention. In maintained situational interest, learners are drawn to understand more about particular content, and are inclined to ask questions about it, thus marking a shift in phases of interest (Renninger & Su, 2011). Emerging individual interest refers to the beginning phases of an endearing predisposition indicated by seeking repeated engagement with particular content over time. Well-developed individual interest is defined as showing a relatively enduring predisposition toward engaging with the particular content over time. Renninger and Su (2011) reported that 'learners at all ages with varying experiences can develop new interest at any time but age also affected how and whether interest is likely to develop' (p.171). Related to the current research, the authors proposed that it is important to know about pre-existing interests of older adults in order to leverage them in technology learning. As a first step it is important to better understand the relationship between individual interest and technology uptake by older adults. This is partly because the Four-Phase Model of Interest Development suggested neither focus on older adults nor on technology learning. At the end of this chapter, there will be a case study and its findings examining the role of interest in creating a positive environment for older adults' uptake of mobile touch screen technologies.

Lifelong Learning

In order for the progression of a knowledge society to occur and in keeping up with this volatile environment, the ability to learn is considered one of the most basic skills required for success (Chan, 2010). According to Lachman (1997), learning refers to a relatively permanent change in behaviour as a result of practice or experience (p.477). Learning is seen as adaptation of an individual's lifetime to its environment. It is viewed as a process of skill transference and Chan (2010) also recommends that in order to engage students in active learning towards acquiring practical skills, the instructor should tailor contents with activities by applying anagogical principles. Regardless of age, active learning can be more effective than passive learning (Chan, 2010). According to Hebb (1949), in order to be remembered, new learning should be transferred into everyday life. Stimulating and real-life experiences can be crucial for learning to occur, since the brain can be compared to a muscle, use it or lose it (Amthor, 2012). As humans age, there is a need to find dynamic flexibility in the brain. With the development of neuroplasticity theory, the long held belief that the brain becomes rigid has been overturned (Doidge, 2016). Throughout adult life, synapses can be modified by further activities, thus, demonstrating a connection between adult development and learning processes (Wilson, 2011). In addition, older adults have different individual characteristics shaped by personal life experiences (De Houwer, Barnes-Holmes & Moors, 2013), different life patterns (Jeong, 2011), memories and habits (Chropa & Tanzi, 2012). Learning is not entirely an intellectual activity, but something that has been embedded in human ability to accomplish tasks and challenges that can be overcome (Amthor, 2012).

Learning has a lifespan trajectory; it can be easy when young, difficult after adolescence and very challenging for most older adults (Amthor, 2012). Arrowsmith-Young (2012) argued that despite opposing learning theories, including obsolete conjecture that the brain is fixed, whereby education was based on pouring content into a fixed system – the brain, has major implications towards education and learning. This learning theory is still embedded in many educational systems and will therefore continue to play a role in the teaching and learning process (Chan, 2010). In contrast, a new paradigm of "neuroplasticity" has emerged. Neuroplasticity advocates that each human brain has the ability to create a map of its own workings – a map based on knowledge and training. The concept of the neuroplastic brain with a map, in relation to education has yet to be fully understood and implemented in education systems. In the course of a lifetime, the human brain can remap itself and grow new neural connections (Doidge, 2016). In other words, the brain has circuitry but no wires. The circuits consist of living tissues and constantly rewire themselves with new thoughts, memories, desires and experiences (Doidge, 2016). The brain is plastic, capable of change and is constantly adapting to the environment in order to optimise behaviour. Doidge (2008), stated that humans are able to change the structure of the brain itself and increase its capacity to learn because unlike a computer, the brain is constantly adapting itself, suggesting that it is capable of being flexible and dynamic. Learning and memory work together because learning changes the brain, changing the synaptic weights thereby allowing learning to take place rapidly compared to adding new neurons and connections (Amthor, 2012). Merzenich stated in an interview with Doidge (2008), that when learning occurs in a way consistent with the laws that govern brain plasticity, the mental machinery of the brain can be improved so that we learn and perceive with greater precision, speed and retention. This research shows that brain health can improve. In addition, intellectual abilities increase and the brain reserve gets larger due to more education (Wilson, 2011). According to Wilson (2011), brain-based learning is a new paradigm but very little interest has been given to it in the field of andragogy. As the brain is not definitive but open to change, the main interest of brain-based learning is to continue to discover how the brain was designed to learn in its natural form (Wilson, 2011); it also improves individuals' future responses to situations that are similar to situations that triggered the learning (Amthor, 2012). Our understanding from these studies is that older brains function just as well as their younger counterparts (Doidge, 2008). According to DCCSDS (2012), older adults are keen to continue to learn and 'many have an interest in learning about new things' (p.17). The main issue is to find out about older adults' motivations towards learning. Their needs and prior experiences should also be considered during the learning process.

CASE STUDY: THE INTEREST-BRIDGE MODEL

Older adults can differ greatly in general background, level of technical experience and knowledge. Consequently, it would be very difficult to conduct quantitative research with control groups to investigate singular variables. Subsequently, over 131 older adults, 5 staff members and 8 teachers participated in the studies. Quantitative methods comprised of background demographics, pre, mid and post-study questionnaires. Qualitative methods such as observations and interviews (one-to-one and focus group) provided a deeper insight into teachers' experiences and teaching approaches. Older adults were not

Table 2. Elements and summary of self-determination theory for older adults. Source: (adapted from Reeve, 2005).

Elements	Explanations
Life-satisfaction	Fulfil purposes, using and sharing of interest, existing knowledge, life experiences and providing peer-support
Autonomy	Listens and allows others to work in their own individual way Nurtures inner motivational resources Promotes valuing
Self-confidence	Feeling of being respected, valued as an individual and being part of the community

always able to articulate their attitudes and problems with technology and therefore, observations were often a more effective means of data gathering. Finally, an Action Research approach was taken to trialling the concepts and tools developed in the course of the investigation.

The research has recognised the importance of structuring curriculum that catered towards older adults' pre-existing interests in order to facilitate their learning of technology. Two out of the three existing elements in SDT did not correspond with the researchers' findings towards the role of learning in mobile touch screen technologies for older adults. "Autonomy" remained the same. Those two elements replaced were "competence" and "relatedness". They were substituted by "self-confidence" and "life-satisfaction" respectively as seen in Table 2. According to Reeve (2005), "autonomy" represents listening and allowing others to work in their own individual way, while nurturing their inner motivational resources and thus promoting valuing. When older adults embarked on their journey towards learning of technology, they are not obsessed with the thought of being "competent" per se, because the building up of "self-confidence" is the foundation towards being competent over time as they practice the use of technology outside of classroom hours. In addition, as people get older, they want to remain a part of their local community. The sense of connectedness, having the ability to continue to contribute their knowledge and experiences makes them feel valued and respected as an individual, also contributing to building up their self-confidence. Consequently, older adults place emphasis on emotional goals that lead to high level of "life-satisfaction" instead of knowledge-based goals that lead to, for instance building of career towards promotion at work. In other words, older adults find that fulfilling of purposes in their lives lead to life-satisfaction. The other factors that contributed to it comprised of, taking into consideration older adults' pre-existing interests and building upon these by utilising their existing knowledge and life experiences. These three elements formed the recommendations for the running of mobile touch screen classes for older adults (See Table 3). Classes were based on interest-led curriculum, whereby participants had full autonomy to decide on how they wanted to plan their own curriculum. The findings led to the extension of the *Four-Phase Model of Interest Development* (See Figure 2) and was named the *Interest-Bridge Model* (See Figure 3).

Participants were divided into two classes of eight and nine participants. Before the commencement of classes, participants were asked about their pre-existing interests. The activities requested by participants varied from group to group (See Table 3). Some of the differences observed were based on participants' lifestyles and background. The majority of participants from group one had family and friends living overseas, therefore their activity requests were to learn more about communication apps such as Skype and Face-time, in order to stay in touch. Due to the different time zones, most participants try to keep in touch through emails. Participants from group two requested to learn about photography; photography comprised of use of still camera and video camera and photo gallery. Participants were also interested

Figure 3. The Interest-Bridge Model (adapted by Beh, Pedell & Doubé, 2015, p. 443 and informed by Hidi & Renninger, 2006; Deci & Ryan, 1985; Carstensen, 1992)

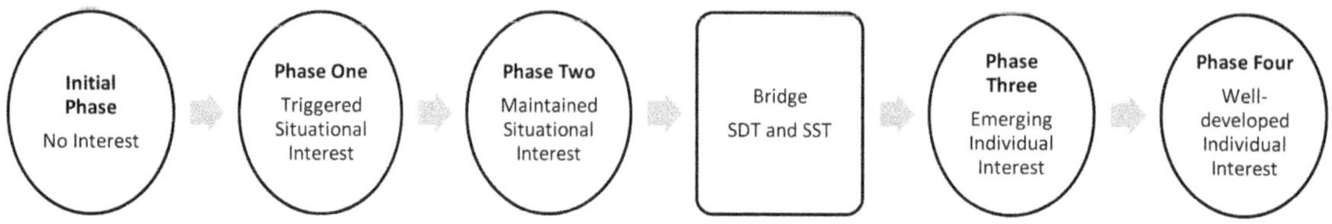

Table 3. Activities requested by participants to be taught based on individual groups

Group	Activities Requested
1	Skype, Face-time, emails, sync with other device (smartphones and laptops)
2	Camera, video camera, camera roll, photo stream, delete photos
3	Downloading photographs from email attachments, contact lists, photo transfers
4	iCloud, e-books, newspapers, email attachments, organise photos
5	e-books, newspapers, backing up of data, YouTube, iCloud, email
6	Organise photos, online banking, share portfolio, online shopping, ad-blocks
7	iCloud, backing up of data, calendar, online shopping, updating of operating systems
8	Bookmarks (webpages), iCloud, online shopping, backing up of data, podcast
9	e-books, pay bills, online shopping, Microsoft Word, search history, iCloud
10	Camera, camera roll, photo transfers, photo stream, Facebook, printing

to acquire skills such as transferring of photographs from their mobile touch screen tablets to desktop computers and/or laptops as backups. They also requested to learn about sorting of photographs such as creating folders, renaming folders and categorising. A few participants were committee members of U3As. Their roles included organising meetings and allocating spaces for courses, so they requested skills to learn about Microsoft Word in order to keep track of meeting minutes and to create newsletters for other members. In the study, based on participants' activity requests, they were introduced to equivalent apps that were paired with their pre-existing interests (See Table 4). Based on the positive written and verbal feedback provided by a large number of participants, there was a consensus view that

Table 4. Pairing of participants' pre-existing interests with equivalent apps

Pre-Existing Interests	Equivalent Apps
Emails	Yahoo mail, Gmail, Hotmail
Entertainment	ABC iView, Plus 7, 9 Now, 10 Play, SBS on Demand
Newspapers	The Age, Herald Sun, The Australian, The Guardian, The Financial Review
Searching	Google Chrome, Safari, Mozilla Firefox
Travel	Skyscanner, Expedia, TripAdvisor, Google Translate, TramTracker, Public Transport Victoria (PTV), Google Maps
Weather	Weatherzone, AUS Weather

the workshops were a success (Beh, Pedell & Doubé, 2016). Participants enjoyed the workshops and gained increased knowledge and skills in mobile touch screen technology use. This is reflected in the following participant comments:

Being open-ended has been fabulous. I have come with my own query list and tutor has cheerily upskilled me greatly!'; 'I have enjoyed the relaxed nature of the class – able to ask questions and find a solution to problems'; 'Very useful for travel'; 'I was starting from base – I didn't even own tablet when I started.' (Beh, Pedell & Doubé, 2016)

Reference to Real Life

Participants felt that in order to motivate themselves to keep up with technology, they needed to be able to learn about new technologies and the various apps available. Most of them commented on the use of apps such as Internet search using Google, checking emails and taking photographs. These activities were already relevant to their everyday lives but as the class curriculum was based on participants' pre-existing interests, therefore, they could see a relevance of learning technology as it was already incorporated into their everyday lives.

Curriculum and Contents

Participants said that they now have a better understanding about mobile touch screen technologies and its functions. However, to a certain extent, the teacher did not expect her classes to be conducted on an ad-hoc basis. She was improvising as the classes moved forward. Some of the contents requested by participants included basic gesture interactions, information about privacy settings and viruses, and most importantly, advice about purchasing of mobile touch screen devices.

Learning of Basic Tablet Interactions

Participants using desktop computers and laptops were accustomed to input devices such as keyboard and mouse. Mobile touch screen devices function in a different way. The input and output components are amalgamated into a single hardware component that is operated through gestures that older adults were unfamiliar with at the start of the workshop. Participants were able to acquire basic tablet interaction gestures such as tap, swipe, pinch, zoom and drag through activities that were developed in the context of real world applications. Activities include use of a wide range of apps that required participants to familiarise themselves with use of basic gestures.

Repetitions and Reinforcement

The flexibility of an interest-driven curriculum provided participants with the freedom to choose and build their own workshop contents. They were able to ask the teacher to repeat activities and explanations regardless of timeframe. This technique helped with their learning and also built up their level of self-confidence as they had opportunities to practice the tasks in workshop sessions. Course materials were distributed and participants were encouraged to practice at home as they now had a point of reference.

Number of Students

Participants said that some of the classes they have attended previously had too many students. At times, the classroom ration was one teacher to 20 students. Therefore, they were not able to gain much out of it. Ideally, class size should not have more than eight people at a time. This is to ensure that the teacher was able to move around the classroom and provide participants with more one-on-one assistance with weekly activities, while accompanied with demonstrations and further explanations. Participants welcomed the attention placed upon them in classes with less numbers of students.

Purchase Advice

Participants also queried about price differences between similar devices, as they were unfamiliar with technical specifications such as storage capacity, processor chips and connectivity (Wi-Fi only or Wi-Fi and 3G/4G enabled devices). Participants that did not own any mobile touch screen devices made their purchase either while still attending classes or upon completion of classes.

Bring Along Technical Questions

Participants commented on being able to bring along their technical problems and issues to workshop sessions. They were able to learn how to tackle these problems and issues they faced without having to turn to their children and grandchildren who most of the time lack the patience to provide older adults with a teaching approach that is jargon free and easy to understand. Also, participants enjoyed the peer-supported environment whereby they feel safe and are able to share their problems and issues without being judged.

Adoption Outside Classes

Course materials were distributed and this encouraged participants to practice at home as mentioned previously, they now had a point of reference including their own notes. A fortnight after the completion of the pilot classes, two of the participants contacted the researcher via email to share their experiences. A participant upgraded her existing mobile phone to a smartphone and another participant purchased an iPad at the end of the pilot classes. They have since used their mobile touch screen devices even while travelling.

CONCLUSION

The Interest-Bridge Model was employed to conduct technology classes while teaching older adults based on their pre-existing interests. The chapter has shown that the interest-led approach plays a crucial role in older adults' uptake and inclusion of technology. The results found with 131 older adults, have confirmed that interest in technology and pre-existing interests could be fostered as older adults progressed through the interest phases supported by the two motivational theories of Self-Determination Theory and Socioemotional Selectivity Theory. When it comes to the teaching of technology, the authors suggest that older adults should be considered as individuals and not as a homogenous cohort because everybody learns differently. Older adults should not be prescribed with a structured curriculum based on what we think they should learn, on the contrary older adults should be consulted on what they need and want to learn. In addition, the study results support the effectiveness of theory when put into practice. The results show that when older adults are taught according to requests based on their pre-existing interests, it encourages long-term engagement of technology uptake and the ability to integrate technology into their everyday lives, thus achieving social and digital inclusion amongst older adults.

ACKNOWLEDGMENT

The authors would like to acknowledge the assistance given by staff members and members of U3A (University of the Third Age) Hawthorn and Box Hill whom without their support this research project would not have been possible.

REFERENCES

Ainley, M., Hidi, S., & Berndorff, D. (2002). Interest, learning and the psychological processes that mediate their relationship. *Journal of Educational Psychology, 94*(3), 545–561. doi:10.1037/0022-0663.94.3.545

Amthor, F. (2012). *Neuroscience for Dummies*. John Wiley & Sons Ltd.

Anderson, M., & Perrin, A. (2017). *Tech adoption climbs among older adults*. Washington, DC: Pew Research Centre.

Arrowsmith-Young, B. (2012). *The Woman Who Changed Her Brain: Unlocking the Extraordinary Potential of the Human Mind*. Pty Ltd.

Australian Bureau of Statistics. (2006). *2001 Census of population and housing – 00 1901 A snapshot of Australia 1901*. Retrieved from: http://www.abs.gov.au/websitedbs/D3110124.NSF/24e5997b9bf2ef35ca2567fb00299c59/c4abd1fac53e3df5ca256bd8001883ec!OpenDocument#Table%201.%201901%20Population%20Counts%20f

Australian Bureau of Statistics. (2015). *Australian Demographic Statistics, Jun 2015 (3101.0)*. Retrieved from: http://www.abs.gov.au/ausstats/abs@.nsf/featurearticlesbyCatalogue/7A40A407211F35F4CA257A2200120EAA?OpenDocument

Australian Bureau of Statistics. (2016). *Census of Population and Housing: reflecting Australia – Stories from the Census, 2016 (2071.0)*. Retrieved from: http://www.abs.gov.au/ausstats/abs@.nsf/Lookup/by%20Subject/2071.0~2016~Main%20Features~Ageing%20Population~14

Australian Bureau of Statistics. (2017). *Australian Demographic Statistics, June 2017 (3101.0)*. Retrieved from: http://www.abs.gov.au/ausstats/abs@.nsf/mf/3101.0

Australian Bureau of Statistics. (2017). *Retirement and Retirement Intentions, Australia, July 2016 to June 2017 (6238.0)*. Retrieved from: http://www.abs.gov.au/ausstats/abs@.nsf/mf/6238.0

Beh, J., Pedell, S., & Doubé, W. (2015). *Where is the "I" in iPad?: The role of interest in older adults' learning of mobile touch screen technologies. In Proceedings of OzCHI 2015: Being Human* (pp. 437–445). Melbourne, Australia: ACM Press.

Beh, J., Pedell, S., & Doubé, W. (2016). *Evaluation of interest-bridge model: Older adults meditated learning of mobile technology. In Proceedings of OzCHI 2016: Connected Futures* (pp. 293–302). Tasmania, Australia: ACM Press.

Bernard, L. C., Mills, M., Swenson, L., & Walsh, R. (2005). An evolutional theory of human motivation. *Genetic, Social, and General Psychology Monographs, 131*(2), 129–184. doi:10.3200/MONO.131.2.129-184 PMID:16779946

Betts, K. (2014). *The ageing of the Australian population: triumph or disaster?* Melbourne, Australia: Monash Center for Population and Urban Research, Monash University.

Black, A., & Deci, E. (2000). The effects of instructors' autonomy support and students' autonomous motivation on learning organic chemistry: A Self-Determination Theory perspective. *Science Education, 84*(6), 740–756. doi:10.1002/1098-237X(200011)84:6<740::AID-SCE4>3.0.CO;2-3

Boulton-Lewis, G. (2009). Issues in Learning and Education for the Ageing. Education and Learning for the Elderly: Why, How and Why. *Educational Gerontology, 36*(3), 213–228. doi:10.1080/03601270903182877

Caprani, N., O'Connor, N., & Gurrin, C. (2011). Touch Screens for the Older User. In *Assistive Technologies* (pp. 95–118). Rijeka, Croatia: In-Tech.

Carstensen, L. (1992). Social and Emotional Patterns in Adulthood: Support for Socioemotional Selectivity Theory. *Psychology and Aging, 7*(3), 331–338. doi:10.1037/0882-7974.7.3.331 PMID:1388852

Carstensen, L., Isaacowitz, D. & Charles, S. (1999). Taking time seriously: A theory of socioemotional selectivity. *American Psychological Association, 54*(3) 165-181.

Centre of Excellence in Population Ageing Research. (2014). *Older Australian fact sheet: a statistical portrait of the older Australian.* Sydney, Australia: University of New South Wales.

Chan, S. (2010). Applications of Andragogy in Multi-Disciplined Teaching and Learning. *Journal of Adult Education, 39*(2).

Charles, S., & Carstensen, L. (2009). Social and emotional aging. *Annual Review of Psychology, 61*(1), 383–409. doi:10.1146/annurev.psych.093008.100448 PMID:19575618

Chen, A., McGaughey, R., Zeltmann, S., Lu, H.-K., & Lee, M. R. (2018). How seniors in Taiwan use Information Technology: Computer and cell phones. *International Journal of Human-Computer Interaction, 34*(2), 166–176. doi:10.1080/10447318.2017.1335445

Cherry, K., Brigman, S., Lyon, B., Blanchard, B., Walker, E., & Smitherman, E. (2016). Self-reported ageism across the lifespan: Role of aging knowledge. *International Journal of Aging & Human Development, 83*(4), 366–380. doi:10.1177/0091415016657562 PMID:27380779

Chopra, D., & Tanzi, R. E. (2012). *Super Brain: Unleash the Explosive Power of Your Mind.* Rider Books.

De Houwer, J., Barnes-Holmes, D., & Moors, A. (2013). What is learning? On the nature and merits of a functional definition of learning. *Psychonomic Bulletin & Review*, *20*(4), 631–642. doi:10.375813423-013-0386-3 PMID:23359420

Deci, E. L., & Ryan, R. M. (1985). The general causality orientations scale: Self-determination in personality. *Journal of Research in Personality*, *19*(2), 109–134. doi:10.1016/0092-6566(85)90023-6

Deci, E. L., & Ryan, R. M. (2008). Facilitating optimal motivation and psychological well-being across life's domain. *Canadian Psychology*, *49*(1), 14–23. doi:10.1037/0708-5591.49.1.14

Deckop, J., & Cirka, C. (2000). The Risk and Reward of a Double-Edgedsword: Effects of a Merit Payprogram on Intrinsic Motivation. *Nonprofit and Voluntary Sector Quarterly*, *29*(3), 400–418. doi:10.1177/0899764000293003

Department of Communities, Child Safety and Disability Services. (2012). *Ageing: Myth and reality*. Brisbane, Queensland: Queensland Government, Department of Communities, Child Safety and Disability Services.

Department of Economic and Social Affairs. (2017). *World population ageing*. New York: United Nations.

Department of Health and Human Services. (2018). *Concessions and benefits*. Melbourne, Australia: Victorian State Government.

Doidge, N. (2015). *The Brain's Way of Healing*. London: Penguin Books Ltd.

Doubé, W., & Beh, J. (2012). *Typing Over Auto Complete: Cognitive Load in Website Use by Older Adults*. Melbourne, Australia: ACM Press.

Doyle, J., Skrba, Z., McDonnell, R., & Arent, B. (2010). Designing a Touch Screen Communication Device to Support Social Interaction amongst Older Adults. In *BCS '10 Proceedings of the 24th BCS Interaction Specialist Group Conference* (pp. 177-185), Swindon, UK: BCS Learning and Development Ltd.

Durick, J., Robertson, T., Brereton, M., Vetere, F., & Nansen, B. (2013). *Dispelling Ageing Myths in Technology Design*. Adelaide, Australia: OzCHI.

Edgar, P. (2013). *In Praise of Ageing*. Melbourne, Australia: Text Publishing.

Glymour, M., Weuve, J., Martha, E., Glass, T., & Berkman, L. (2008). Social ties and cognitive recovery after stroke: Does social integration promote cognitive resilience? *Neuroepidemiology*, *31*(1), 10–20. doi:10.1159/000136646 PMID:18535395

Graham, S., & Weiner, B. (1996). *Theories and Principles of Motivation. Cognition and Motivation*. New York: Prentice Hall.

Hagay, G., Baram-Tsabari, A., Ametller, J., Cakmakci, G., Lopes, B., Moreira, A., & Pedrosa-de-Jesus, H. (2013). The Generalizability of Students' Interests in Biology across Gender, Country and Religion. *Research in Science Education*, *43*(3), 895–919. doi:10.100711165-012-9289-y

Harvey, P., & Thurnwald, I. (2009). Ageing Well, Ageing Productively: The Essential Contribution of Australia's Ageing Population to the Social and Economic Prosperity of the Nation. *Health Sociology Review*, *18*(4), 379–386. doi:10.5172/hesr.2009.18.4.379

Hebb, D. O. (1949). *The organization of behaviour*. New York: Wiley.

Hidi, S., & Renninger, K. A. (2006). The four-phase model of interest development. *Educational Psychologist*, *41*(2), 111–127. doi:10.120715326985ep4102_4

Ianculescu, M., Lupeanu, E., Alexandru, A., Tudora, E., Coman, O. & Coman, L. (2011). Strengthening the Role of Medical Informatics in Promoting a Successful Positive Ageing. *Recent Advances in Applied & Biomedical Informatics and Computational Engineering in Systems Applications*, 305-310.

Jeong, H. (2011). *The Skill of Communication in Aged Care (Master of Science)*. Aged and Community Services.

Krapp, A. (2002). An Educational-Psychological Theory of Interest and its Relation to Self-Determination Theory. In E. Deci & R. Ryan (Eds.), *The Handbook of Self-determination Research* (pp. 405–427). New York: University of Rochester Press.

Lachman, S. (1997). Learning is a process: Toward an improved definition of learning. *The Journal of Psychology*, *131*(5), 477–480. doi:10.1080/00223989709603535

Morgan, R. (2016). *Over 400,000 Australians intend to retire in the next 12 months, increasing burden on government funding*. Melbourne, Australia: Roy Morgan Research.

Niemiec, C., & Ryan, R. (2009). Autonomy, Competence and Relatedness in the Classroom: Applying Self-Determination Theory to Educational Practice. *Theory and Research in Education*, *7*(2), 133–144.

Nimrod, G. (2010). Seniors' online communities: A quantitative content analysis. *The Gerontologist*, *50*(3), 382–392. doi:10.1093/geront/gnp141 PMID:19917645

Noels, K., Pelletier, L., Clement, R., & Vallerand, R. (2000). Why are you learning a second language? Motivational orientations and Self-Determination Theory. *Journal of Research in Language Studies*, *50*(1), 57–85.

Organisation for Economic Co-operation and Development. (2015). *Ageing in Cities*. Paris, France: OECD Publishing.

Organisation for Economic Co-operation and Development. (2018). *Definition of elderly population*. Retrieved from: https://data.oecd.org/pop/elderly-population.htm

Perrier, E. (2015). *Positive disruption: Healthcare, ageing and participation in the age of technology*. Sydney, NSW: McKell Institute.

Phiriyapokan, T. (2011). *Is a Big Button Interface Enough for Elderly Users? Towards User Interface Guidelines for Elderly Users* (Master's thesis). Eskilstuna, Sweden: Malardalen University.

Quan-Haase, A., Guang, Y., & Wellman, B. (2018). Connected seniors: How older adults in East York exchange social support online and offline. *Information Communication and Society*, *20*(7), 967–983. doi:10.1080/1369118X.2017.1305428

Renninger, K. A., & Su, S. (2012). *Interest and Its Development. In Handbook of Human Motivation*. Oxford University Press.

Ryan, R., & Deci, E. (2000). Intrinsic and Extrinsic Motivations: Classic Definitions and New Directions. *Contemporary Educational Psychology*, *25*(1), 54–67. doi:10.1006/ceps.1999.1020 PMID:10620381

Sander, M., Oxlund, B., Jespersen, A., Krasnik, A., Mortensen, E., Westendorp, R., & Rasmussen, L. (2015). The challenges of human population ageing. *Age and Ageing*, *44*(2), 185–187. doi:10.1093/ageing/afu189 PMID:25452294

Satariano, W., Scharlach, A., & Lindeman, D. (2014). Aging, place, and technology: Toward improving access and wellness in older populations. *Journal of Aging and Health*, *26*(8), 1373–1389. doi:10.1177/0898264314543470 PMID:25502245

Sayago, S., & Blat, J. (2011). An Ethnographical Study of the Accessibility Barriers in the Everyday Interactions of Older People with the Web. *Universal Access in the InfoPrmation Society*, *10*(4), 359–371. doi:10.100710209-011-0221-4

Sheldon, K., & Krieger, L. (2007). Understanding the negative effects of legal education on law students: A longitudinal test of Self-Determination Theory. *Personality and Social Psychology Bulletin*, *33*(6), 883–897. doi:10.1177/0146167207301014 PMID:17483395

Silvia, P. J. (2006). *Exploring the psychology of interest*. Melbourne, Australia: Oxford University Press. doi:10.1093/acprof:oso/9780195158557.001.0001

Standage, M., Duda, J., & Ntoumanis, N. (2005). A test of self-determination theory in school physical education. *The British Journal of Educational Psychology*, *75*(3), 411–433. doi:10.1348/000709904X22359 PMID:16238874

Tin, T. B. (2013). Exploring the Development of 'Interest' in Learning English as a Foreign/Second Language. *RELC Journal*, *44*(2), 129–146. doi:10.1177/0033688213488388

Uren, D. (2017). *A super fail: 80pc retire on pension benefits. The Australian. 12.00am, August 26.* Canberra, Australia: News Corp Australia.

Williams, G., & Deci, E. (1996). Internalization of biopsychosocial values by medical students: A test of Self-Determination Theory. *Journal of Personality and Social Psychology*, *70*(4), 767–779. doi:10.1037/0022-3514.70.4.767 PMID:8636897

Wilson, C. (2011). *Neuroandragogy: Making the Case for a Link with Andragogy and Brain-Based Learning. In Midwest Research-to-Practice Conference in Adult, Continuing, Community and Extension Education* (pp. 21–23). St. Charles, MO: Lindenwood University, September.

World Economic Forum. (2017). *Life expectancy*. Washington, DC: The World Bank.

Chapter 13
Natural Environments, Ecosystems, Conflict, and Wellbeing:
Access to Water

Fatih Bodzemir
RMIT University, Australia

Jennifer Martin
Swinburne University, Australia

ABSTRACT

This chapter examines the correlation between environmental issues and wellbeing. A broad literature review illustrates that changing climate, increasing populations, and degrading natural environments have negative impacts on health and wellbeing. The focus of this chapter is on conflicts arising from the limited supply of natural resources and competing needs, interests, and demands. This can create high levels of tension and division within communities that erodes community spirit, support, and connectedness as people compete for limited resources. The conflict arising from such disputes has negative impacts on social cohesion and the high levels of stress experienced, without adequate supports, can trigger mental ill health. The example of basin level water conflict in Turkey is used to illustrate this.

INTRODUCTION

In recent years, scholars commenced looking at the impact of environmental issues on wellbeing. However, definitions of "the environment" and "wellbeing" still remain limited thereby hindering the capacity to develop evidence-based interventions to influence policy makers. In this chapter the term "environment" is paired with "ecosystems" as the concept of "natural environment and ecosystems" is deemed the most appropriate way of identifying environmental issues that corelate with wellbeing. It is broadly acknowledged that the natural environment is degrading in many regions of the world, and this dates back, at least, to the industrial revolution. In the context of changing climate, increasing population and

DOI: 10.4018/978-1-5225-7402-6.ch013

limited natural resources, sustainability has been at the core and center of political debates and scientific studies. However, the impacts of this emerging phenomenon are often ignored. Water-induced conflicts are pertinent examples for obtaining insights into how the wellbeing of people is detrimentally affected by such conflicts. According to a European Environment Agency, (2014) report, climate change cannot be considered as a single environmental issue as it also creates health issues. They provide an example of the pollen movement resulting from the spread of Common Ragweed (*Ambrosia artemisiifolia*), a flowering native plant of the Americas. Currently, the plant is seen in Europe as climate change has allowed the plant to extend its range northwards. Ragweed also harms ecosystems and reduces crop yields. This invasive plant has pronounced health effects. The pollen is one of the most aggressive causes of allergic reactions; one in five Europeans suffers from allergies, one in seven experiences allergic rhinitis and one in eleven lives with asthma. This example shows that health and wellbeing is clearly connected with environmental issues, as does the case study on access to water provided in this chapter. The chapter identifies key issues related to the degradation of the environment. A focus is on conflict that develops when resources are scarce or limited and there are subsequent health and wellbeing impacts upon communities. The resource focused upon is water and the underlying factors causing basin water conflicts in developing nations. The chapter highlights a gap in knowledge on the correlation between health and wellbeing and degrading natural environments and eco-systems. The aim is to bring this environmental correlation to the attention of policy makers in setting the future agenda when looking at possible solutions in mitigating deteriorating health and wellbeing.

BACKGROUND

Water is a precious commodity that we cannot afford to see depleted. Developing and developed nations are experiencing a high demand for water for different uses depending on the needs of the particular country (Hinrichsen & Tacio, 2011). Water has many uses ranging from agricultural purposes, manufacturing, fresh water for drinking and cooking, water for construction, water for washing clothes and many other uses (Wolf, Kramer, Carius & Dabelko, 2005). It is important to note that the earth is a watery place where approximately 71% of the earth's surface is covered with water, with 96.5% of this in the oceans. Water can also be found in rivers and lakes, in the air as water vapour, in the soil as moisture, in glaciers and icecaps in addition to being found within human beings and animals. The vast majority of water in the surface of the earth, which is held in oceans, is saline, while fresh drinking water is sourced from rivers and lakes in addition to water that falls as rain.

All the sources of water in the world that produce fresh water account for only 2.5% of global water reserves, which makes fresh water unevenly distributed across the globe (Central Intelligence Agency, 2015). Approximately 1 billion people are not able to access clean, safe drinking water, while only 10 countries share 60% of the entire global renewable and natural water resources (FAO, 2011). It is estimated that the total volume of water on the Universe is 333 million cubic miles (Loucks & Beek, 2005).

According to the United Nations, to support and feed the future global population the world economy will have to experience considerable growth with water a critical factor (FAO, 2011). The United Nations has proposed the need for sustainable management of water to reduce the risks associated with water shortage (FAO, 2011). The global water consumption is experiencing high demand pressures, which have been brought about by the increase in population and adoption of behaviours that have seen high consumption of water. In addition to this, climate changes have largely contributed to the decrease in water supplies causing tensions between communities and countries. These trends have led to water stress often exhibited by political and economic conflicts. Economic and population growth have both contributed to rising water stress. Approximately 36% of the global population (2.5 billion people) resides in areas experiencing water stress (UNESCO, 2015). In addition, 20% of the total global domestic product (GDP) emanates from areas that are risky and experience water scarcity. This affects production and corporate reputations as competition for available water escalates (UNESCO, 2015). The United Nations notes that the slow process of managing water resources and the accelerated pace of human development presents future water challenges that are knocking on the global door. By the year 2050, if changes to how water is managed are not made, water stress will put the world population at risk especially due to less agriculture production (UNESCO, 2015). It is therefore important to waste less water, pollute less, and reuse more water. Effective management of water resources is required collectively and individually and in particular water used for industrial and agricultural purposes (FAO, 2011).

WATER CONFLICTS AND CONFLICT TYPES

Water conflict has been defined as conflict which arises between states, groups or countries because of access to water resources (Ohlsson, 2000). According to the United Nations, water disputes result from opposing interests. Historically, water has been a source of tension and a catalyst for other conflicts, which may be related to other circumstances, such as border conflicts (Wolf, Kramer, Carius, & Dabelko, 2005). Water conflicts arise for varied reasons including fighting for resources, need to gain strategic advantage and territorial disputes. Water conflicts happen over both salt water and fresh water and between nations, with the latter most common. The availability of water in a country affects the economic and living conditions. In the event of a water crisis in a region, all water users are put under severe pressures whether they be government, corporate or individuals, which leads to tension and sometimes aggression (Vuković, 2008). Some humanitarian catastrophes such as the war in the Sudanese Darfur and genocide in Rwanda have been linked to water conflicts (Pacific Institute, 2015). Where countries have active cooperation, in terms of water management, the likelihood of war is reduced. For all human activities, water is a vital component, and therefore its unavailability can easily result in disagreements, which often explode into full-blown conflicts that cause war. When demand exceeds supply it is difficult to manage disputes arising from the need to access and share the available water. Between years 1950-2000, there were approximately 1,831 water conflicts (Wolf, Yoffe & Giordano, 2003).

Water conflicts exist in all continents from Asia to Africa, North America to South America and from Europe to Australia. There have been notable water conflicts that have existed for decades. Water conflicts can only exist at interstate or intrastate levels. Interstate conflicts are those that occur between neighbouring countries, which share a trans-boundary source of water such as a lake, sea or river (Weinthal, 2006). For instance, in the Middle East, 5% of the world population shares 1% of the world's fresh water (Pacific Institute, 2015). On the other hand, intrastate conflicts involve two or more parties residing in the same nation (Weinthal, 2006).

Current interstate water conflicts are mainly in the Middle East. These include the dispute involving Turkey, Iraq and Syria stemming from the Tigris and Euphrates Rivers as well a dispute involving Jordan, Lebanon, Israel and the state of Palestine stemming from the Jordan River (Jongerden, 2010). In Africa, the most notable water conflict stems from River Nile and involves the Sudan, Egypt and Ethiopia. In Central Asia there has been conflict between Turkmenistan, Kazakhstan, Kyrgyzstan, Tajikistan and

Uzbekistan over the Aral Sea (Kameri-Mbote, 2007). The United Nations has reported that an increase in the consumption of water resources will lead to constant water conflicts in the future (UNESCO, 2015). In a bid to understand the connections between water systems, resources and international conflict and security, the Pacific Institute (2015) started a project in the 1980s to categorize and track events, which are related to conflict and water.

Water conflicts exists because the parties involved in a conflict have goals which are incompatible, and their behaviours, attitudes and perceptions encourage them to participate in competitive action (FAO, 2011). In most cases, conflicts arise because the users of downstream water normally incur additional costs to improve the water security to be able to access water at the right time in the desired quality and quantity. Additionally, conflicts arise when people have to forego benefits that they ought to have accrued from water resources. The actions of upstream users and/ or polluters largely contribute to the reduced access and control of water as per the desire of the downstream users (Gichuki, 2002). The intensity and level of water conflicts often varies depending upon the season and region where the basin is located. Potential conflicts arise when the dispute between parties is not addressed with unresolved grievances (Carius, Debelko & Wolf, 2004). Potential conflict is low when water resources are plentiful. Normally, this happens during the rainy season however, when the water resources become scarce one party, mainly in the upstream region, often starts using these resources more than others do, exposing others to negative economic or social impacts. This leads to the escalation of existing low-level disputes to a level the aggrieved party feels this behaviour can no longer be tolerated (Gichuki, 2002). At this heightened level of conflict, the aggrieved party often demands that necessary action be taken by the other party to alleviate the negative impacts on others. The parties in conflict often resolve to meet to strike an agreement however, if they fail third parties are called in to assist. If the situation remains unresolved, the conflict may escalate to violent acts (Gichuki, 2002). Water conflicts can be classified into a number of categories as summarized in Table 1.

The causes of water conflicts have been largely attributed to attempts by nations to increase their water supply, which results in competitions between various groups in society or between two or more neighbouring countries. Water disputes have resulted in hundreds of agreements and treaties over the last few decades, which shows the need to have unique strategies to manage water conflicts. The increase in water conflicts has seen some people refer to water as being the oil of the 21st century (Morrisette & Borer, 2004).

Table 1. Type of water conflicts (adapted from: Pacific Institute, 2015)

Type of Water Conflict	Explanation
Control of water resources	The access to water supplies causes tensions
Military tool	Water resources are used by nations as a weapon
Political tool	In this case, water resources are used by nations/ states to gain political goals
Terrorism	Non-state actors use water resources as a tool of coercion or violence
Military Target	State actors use water resources systems to act as military actions
Development disputes	In this case, water resources are major sources of disputes in the context of social and economic development

Local Level Water Conflicts

Water conflicts happen internationally and are locally driven by almost the same forces but under different circumstances. Conflicts at the local level are quite different to international water conflicts predominantly due to the water uses involved (Ohlsson, 1999). Examples of water conflicts at the local level include tensions brought by the efficient and effective use of water and between pastoralists or communities practicing modern agricultural activities. Failure to manage local level water conflicts can often turn into violence and it is therefore important to use conflict management systems to calm the situation. History has it that in Africa conflicts between agri-business and agro-pastoralists have been fuelled by the access to water points and green grazing land, which has led to loss of life on both sides (Ohlsson, 1999). Local level water conflicts have included parties such as tribes, states, rural and urban populations and water using sectors (UNESCO, 2013). As the geographic level decreases, the intensity and likelihood of violence increases. Local level water conflicts often revolve around water issues that have dominated the conflict for decades and generations (Kramer, Wolf, Carius & Dabelko, 2013). People who care for the environment, the Indigenous people and the irrigators believe that water is their way of life and therefore it is being threatened by the development of cities and hydropower developments. Internal water conflicts have seen acts such as civil disobedience, violent protests and acts of sabotage between local members of different communities. It is important to note that local level water conflicts can influence the destabilization of a country as people fight for the water supplies that are constantly declining as witnessed in Pakistan (Mustafa, Akhter & Nasrallah, 2013). For instance, when a group of young people depend on a certain source of water for irrigation and it is turned off, they will often find their way into cities and neighbouring towns causing havoc as their source of livelihood is cut from them. Essentially, at the local level, poor governance and management of water, rather than lack of water, normally bring about conflicts over water (Kramer, Wolf, Carius, & Dabelko, 2013).

A Local Water Conflict in Tokat, Turkey

Back in 2009, there was horrifying news of five people killed in a water conflict in Tokat, a small town in Turkey. The deceased people were relatives and practicing agriculture in a village on the outskirts of Tokat. Similarly, the murderer was also a farmer, but surprisingly also the neighbouring landlord who was in desperate need of irrigation water for his wheat crop at the time of incident. The friends of the deceased said that the region has limited water resources and that the locals fully rely upon to provide for their socio-economic activities. This is similar to many parts of the world today, and is the main factor of conflicts if the water is not available on time for the farmers to irrigate their crops. In sum, the murderer noticed that the available water being used by the deceased people would be unavailable and confronted them over this. He was not convinced by his neighbour's arguments and committed the crime putting him in jail for life, while five middle aged people passed away. At the first look, the incident clearly illustrates a lack of efficient tools for conflict management in a region where irrigation unions, the chamber of agriculture, district directorates of the Turkish Ministry of Agriculture and several relevant NGOs are available. Despite these existing bodies, the question of how this incident took place remained unanswered. Unfortunately, similar water-induced, preventable conflicts often occur in many parts of the country and many lose their lives. In terms of mental health and wellbeing, the authors are not suggesting that mental illness was a factor in these incidents. However, we do argue that such conflict will necessarily inflict trauma on the populations affected and in accordance with the stress diathesis model for the development of mental illness, those who are vulnerable may develop mental health issues (Jones & Fernyhough, 2007). Effective conflict management strategies will promote the strengthening of positive community relationships as a protective factor against developing mental health issues, as well as providing an environment conducive to recovery and living well for those with mental health issues (Tew, Ramon, Slade, Bird, Melton, & Le Boutillier, 2011).

Conflicts in Agricultural Basins in Developing Nations

Developing Nations are under pressure to feed their citizens and grow their economy with agricultural basins critical for achieving this purpose. The main problem has been how to share the limited agricultural basins locally and with neighbouring countries and regions who all want a piece of the water resources (FAO, 2011). In almost all agricultural basins, the usage of water through various investments such as industrial, urban and agricultural growth to serve human beings is approaching if not exceeding the amount or water that is renewable. This has led to the over commitment of water resources caused by disregarding the environment, water rights that lack clarity, lack of hydrological knowledge and agricultural projects that are politically motivated. This has resulted in the overuse of agricultural basins and sometimes closure of the basins, which escalates into ongoing conflicts over the remaining water in the basins (Mollie, 2009).

Most developing countries have discovered that agriculture can play an important role in the growth of their economies and because of this, they strive to safeguard any agricultural basin they regard as their own. Developing nations are committing huge amounts of money in engaging in large agricultural projects which often have less economic impact due to poor planning to establish the viability of engaging in a particular project. This has led to water shortages contributing to increasing internal and external conflicts (Daily & Ehrlich, 1992). Internally, these countries are facing conflicts which are caused by local communities residing around the agricultural basins and wanting to take control of the basin, while externally, conflicts are viewed as a state's conflict on how to share the water resources from the agricultural basins. As countries develop, often the water resources in the agricultural basins become increasingly used, controlled and diverted (Mollie, 2009).

The demand for agricultural water from basins in developing countries is increasing rapidly. The inability of basins to satisfy the various water demands often results in conflicts. Water resources in the agricultural basins are being consumed at a rate more than what these basins can get from their feeders such as lakes and oceans (Donkor & Wolde, 2012). In addition to this, in many developing nations, agricultural basins are faced with the problem of industries setting up along these basins, which often results in sanitation, pollution and sewage problems. The lack of efficient planning has resulted in poor quality water from the basins, which escalates already rising conflicts (Agwata, 2006). The continued shortage of water has seen the trend of building dams and streams particularly from the source of the basin for irrigation purposes which affects other areas the basin feeds. In many instances this has resulted in conflicts between neighbouring developing states and conflicts between communities who depend on the same water for irrigation purposes. An example of an agricultural basin in a developing country, which has constant conflicts between the local communities, is the Tana Basin located in Kenya. With the country having a large agro-based economy, in addition to an industrial sector which is growing rapidly, the demand for water resources is rising constantly and basins such as the Tana Basin experience internal conflicts as it is unable to meet the growing demand (Agwata, 2006).

The population increase in developing countries also plays a role in the conflicts, as water resources experience shortages. Additionally, the aspect of urbanization has contributed to the need for more agricultural products pressuring agricultural basins to produce more crops. This builds the basis of ongoing conflicts, as communities fight for the limited resources to earn a living through irrigation to feed the many upcoming urban areas in these countries (Donkor & Wolde, 2012). While water resources are causing conflicts internally because of increasing demand from the local communities, often the same pressure emanates from the neighbouring nations, which also depend on the same basins for irrigation. Conflicts over water resources arising from agricultural basins in developing countries are therefore continuously increasing with calls for the need for conflict management policies to avoid future water wars (Agwata, 2006). Another agricultural basin, which has caused constant conflicts, is the Jordan River Basin, which affects Lebanon, Israel, Syria, Jordan and the West Bank (Wolf, 1998). With this region experiencing an arid climate, water resources have become valuable resources for the residents and governments of these countries. Some of these countries in this basin are among the poorest in the world and due to their natural environment, they depend on this water for serving their agricultural purposes. The conflict has been focused on how the water from the basin should be distributed equally to all nations that share the basin. Israel uses the largest amount of water, followed by Jordan, despite the river basin originating in Lebanon (Villiers, 2000). The patterns of the usage of water, territorial issues caused by politics and water overuse have led to disagreements over the distribution of water.

A further example of water conflicts that surround agricultural basins in developing countries, is in the Nile River Basin. The Nile River is the longest in the world serving water to nine countries before reaching the Mediterranean Sea. For centuries, the sea has been the source of livelihood for people of Sudan and Egypt (El-Fadel, El-Sayegh, El-Fadl, & Khorbotly, 2003). Since the Egyptians have no other source of water except the Nile, the country has resorted to using military force to control the Nile headwaters. The annual withdrawals of the water resources from the Nile Basin have continued to increase as countries engage in building mega-projects along the basin continually increasing the shortage of water (El-Fadel, El-Sayegh, El-Fadl, & Khorbotly, 2003). In Asia, conflicts over agricultural basins have also been on the increase as demand for water to serve various purposes has risen. Developing countries in South Asia deal with constant conflicts caused by sharing basin water supplies in upstream and downstream regions. In Central and Southeast Asia, the distribution of water resources has turned into a political issue as tensions rise on how supplies from the river basins should be shared among the nations (Izquierdo, Stangerhaugen, Castillo, Nixon, & Jimenez, 2010). As the populations in Asia grow, the demand for water is increasing, becoming a catalyst for conflicts propagated by political and ethnic disputes (Allouche & Thèse, 2004). Additionally, the idea of sharing river basin water resources has not been fully understood in Asian countries, contributing to constant conflicts.

Water conflicts in agricultural basins in India present both economic and social threats, as the country finds itself in disputes with neighbouring countries such as China (Williams, 2013). Throughout Pakistan, India, Bangladesh and Nepal, increasing shortages of water from the agricultural basins poses new forms of conflict (Mustafa, Akhter, & Nasrallah, 2013). The inability of these countries to have proper mechanisms to distribute the available waters from their basins attributes to the making of conflicts (Bernauer, & Siegfried, 2012). The conflict between India and Pakistan over the Indus River Basin has been in existence for many years. The River Basin with its tributaries makes one of the largest irrigation canals in the entire universe (Mustafa, Akhter, & Nasrallah, 2013). The Indus River Basin provides millions of people in Pakistan and India with water for irrigation and other purposes, however, the canals and dams which have been built along the basin have led to the drying up of some of the Indus River stretches (Wolf, 1998). These and other projects have largely led to the displacement of people contributing to the destruction of the eco-system in the plains of Indus. Divisions which emanate from river basin waters have led to frictions being created between countries of South Asia as well as among provinces and states. Accusations of water resources overdrawing by certain regions have led other regions experiencing water resource shortages resulting in escalation of tensions (Wolf, 1998). Tables 2 and 3 show basins in dispute and those at risk of future conflicts at the beginning of this century.

UNDERLYING FACTORS OF BASIN LEVEL WATER CONFLICTS

There are several factors causing basin level water conflicts in different parts of the world. These factors are interconnected in one way or another, as they are integrally linked as well as mutually reinforcing. Three broad factors contributing to the basin level water conflicts include; socio-economic factors, political/ institutional factors and physical and geographic issues (Bandaragoda, 2000).

Table 2. Basins in conflicts/negotiations/disputes (adapted from: Yoffe, Wolfe & Giordano, 2001, pp. 95-100)

Basins Currently in Conflicts/Negotiations/Disputes	Countries Involved
Aral Sea	Afghanistan, China, Kazakhstan, Kyrgyzstan, Tajikistan, Turkmenistan, Uzbekistan
Jordan	Israel, Jordan, Lebanon, Palestine, Syria
Nile	Burundi, Congo (Kinshasa), Egypt, Eritrea, Ethiopia, Kenya, Rwanda, Sudan, Tanzania, Uganda
Tigris-Euphrates	Iran, Iraq, Jordan, Saudi Arabia, Syria, Turkey

Table 3. Basins at risk of future conflicts (adapted from: Yoffe, Wolfe & Giordano, 2001, pp. 95-100)

Basins at Risk of Future Conflicts	Countries Involved
Tigris and Euphrates	Lebanon, Syria, Turkey
Ganges-Brahmaputra-Meghan	Bangladesh, Bhutan, Burma, China, India, Nepal
Han	North and South Korea
Indus	Afghanistan, China, India, Pakistan
Kunene	Angola, Namibia
Lake Chad	Algeria, Cameroon, Central African Republic, Chad, Libya, Niger, Nigeria, Sudan
Mekong	Burma, Cambodia, China, Laos, Thailand, Vietnam
Okavango	Angola, Botswana, Namibia, Zimbabwe
Salween	Myanmar, China, Thailand
Senegal	Guinea, Mali, Mauritania, Senegal

Socio-Economic Factors

According to Gehrig and Rogers (2009), socio-economic factors contributing to the increase in water conflicts are an increase in affluence and demand for water, impoverishment and poverty, economic disparities and competing interests at the local/community level. To start with, the demand for water resources increased six times in the 20th century as a result of the world population increasing thrice. More water is being needed for serving different human purposes such as irrigation, drinking and the production of hydropower, among other uses. Mega projects are being set up along basins to provide power for the growing consumer demands, which results in millions of people being relocated into other areas. This increases tensions between communities as well as between nations. According to Postel and Wolf (2001), the new source of water conflicts is the transfers and changes in the ownership/ management of water basins from public authorities to private multinationals. Additionally, according to the World Bank, many of the water projects, which were privatized, were under distress or were cancelled because of the failure to manage the conflicts arising from the privatization. Furthermore, the United Nations Development Program's *Human Development Report* (2006a, p. 21) acknowledged that the idea that privatization would lead to efficiency and equity in the proper use of water resources in basins was misplaced and ill advised. Economic disparities among the states, countries/provinces or communities sharing water resources from particular basins often contribute to water conflicts as one party uses force to control the water resources from the water basin while the other party feels agitated and seeks to find ways to retaliate.

Abuse of power and money has been attributed to the increase in conflicts an example being the case of Egypt and its neighbours where the country has resulted in using military force to gain control of the Nile basin (El-Fadel, El-Sayegh, El-Fadl, & Khorbotly, 2003). On the other hand, another socio-economic factor that contributes to conflict is the competing interests at the local level between communities residing near the basins. The lack of a common understanding of how to plan and organize how water resources should be shared equally between the communities within the basin often leads to conflicts (Bandaragoda, 2000).

Another major socio-economic cause of conflicts in water basins is largely associated with food security and agriculture. The largest source of water consumption globally is agriculture, which accounts for 70% of the total world consumption (UNESCO, 2013). The competition for using water resources from basins normally leads to an increase in conflicts. As the world population increases, countries need to do more irrigation to feed their citizens as well as preserve for others in the form of food security for the future (Hanjra, & Qureshi, 2010). Since everyone wants a share of the water resources, the problem of the shortage is often experienced, and when the competition for the remaining resources escalates, without proper mechanisms being put in place to manage how the resources should be managed, conflicts between involved parties arises. In the agricultural basins, irrigation concerns have largely contributed to the rise in conflicts as every state/province/country and/or region aims at producing more to secure food for their residents. Finally, developing countries with agricultural basins are experiencing conflicts because of the needs of modernization and infrastructure development. Some countries are being involved in the construction of mega development projects sourcing water resources from the basins without agreements with other parties, particularly those countries downstream of these basins, which results in conflicts as others feel aggrieved (USAID, 2014).

Political/Institutional Factors

Beyond the increasing scarcity of water, conflicts in water basins are also being attributed to the governance of water and its uses. The lack of coordination within and between states, in addition to institutional structures which are fragmented, significantly contribute to increasing basin water conflicts (Ravnborg, 2004). One of the main causes of conflicts associated with political factors is the making of public policies, which are politically motivated and, therefore, unable to address the competing interests in these water basins. Many public officials who are charged with enforcing the laws and regulations set on sharing water resources (regulating agencies, judicial officers and the police) engage in corrupt activities, which often sway the expected outcomes aggrieving some of the parties (Gehrig, & Rogers, 2009). A global corruption report, by Transparency International (2008, p. 16), focusing on corruption in the water sector revealed that the impact of corruption in constructing water networks raised access to water resources by 25% to 45%. The lack of transparency in dealing with sharing of water resources in basin regions often leads to conflicts, which are hard to manage at times causing violent wars between the parties involved.

In addition to this, basin water conflicts are also caused by trans-boundary tensions that exist between the various parties with an interest in the water resources from the basin. Many regional, national and local borders are drawn in accordance with watercourses, which makes water a critical issue when dealing with trans-boundary issues (Wolf, Kramer, Carius, & Dabelko, 2005). Therefore, differing perspectives on issues related to water governance by political entities from neighbouring countries can lead to conflicts on issues such as water sharing and diversion, infringed water rights and poor quality of water among others. Often these conflicts between neighbour states hinder sustainable development. These tensions often result in claims of "National Security" where other nations use military force with an excuse of violation of rights to natural resources to invade countries while the aim is to grab the resources (Gehrig & Rogers, 2009). Such acts cause tensions between nations and conflicts which have led to violent wars. The need to control water basins contributes to the conflicts in water basin regions. An example of this type of conflict is a single basin between Israel and Palestine, which has existed for decades. Palestinians have continued to face injustices caused by the Israeli military forces as they seek to control the Palestinian water resources (Mustafa, Akhter, & Nasrallah, 2013). Israel has gone a step further in arranging to build a separation wall to control the water resources. The separation wall is, however, being built on the Palestinians' land which has caused some of the Palestinian villages to experience water shortages (Center for Economic and Social Rights and Palestinian Hydrology Group, 2003, p. 37-38). Further, the conflicts which are associated with flow diversions and dams generate international tensions along trans-boundary basins such as the Nile basin, which has ten countries sharing the water resources, the Tigris and Euphrates that involves Turkey, Iraq and Syria together with the Indus Basin which is shared by Pakistan and India. The building of dams along basins comes with huge environmental and social costs, among them the displacement of millions of people from their villages. People who live downstream of constructed dams and source their livelihood from fishing and irrigation activities can suffer serious harm (World Commission on Dams, 2000).

Physical and Geographical Issues

In addition to socio-economic and politically related factors, physical and geographical issues also contribute to water conflicts. One of these issues is upstream and downstream flows (Gehrig, & Rogers, 2009). Depending on the physical location of the region within the water basin, users will experience either disadvantages or benefits. For instance, upstream diversions, whether for hydropower or agriculture, cause downstream impacts on local users affecting their health and livelihood. Without mutually acceptable agreements on how resources will be shared, conflicts between the downstream users and upstream users will arise constantly. Another issue causing conflicts in water basin areas is pollution and contamination of water by industries based within the basins. Pollution of water affects the ecosystems endangering food supplies as it threatens the health of crops as well as fishing (Pimentel, Berger, Filiberto, Newton, Wolfe, Karabinakis, ... & Nandagopal, 2004). During conflicts which are constant, contamination is often experienced as groups may engage in reverse intentional damage of the water resources with an aim to cause harm to another group. This makes communities living downstream vulnerable to effects caused by the contamination of the water. Without having proper management of the water resources in the basin, these conflicts can escalate to violent wars. A further cause of conflicts in the water basins is attributed to human-induced climate change. The continued availability of water in the river basins will be determined by patterns of global warming (Link, Piontek, Scheffran, & Schilling, 2012). Most basins in the world will see gradual decline in their water reserves, due to extreme weather events caused by climate change and ongoing human-activities. Change in the climate often leads to a rise in sea levels, which can negatively affect freshwater resources. For instance, the river delta systems in Bangladesh could become saline, which would affect the livelihoods of millions of residents in this region. As more changes in climate are experienced, water resources are expected to continue to become scarce leading to increased tensions along the major water basins (UNDP, 2006b).

In summary, the underlying factors that cause water basin conflicts are varied. Timely responses and interventions are required to prevent the escalation of conflicts. The factors contributing to conflicts between states/regions/countries and provinces are often interconnected and require goodwill from all parties involved in resolving the disputes. Millions of people living downstream or upstream of water basins depend on the water resources provided by these basins to sustain their lives. It is therefore important to have equitable sharing arrangements in place among all parties involved. Looking into the future it is important to mitigate the underlying factors that cause conflicts in the water basins for the benefit of all people involved.

DYNAMICS OF LOCAL LEVEL WATER CONFLICT

The dynamics of local water conflicts in many parts of the world can be seen as similar, yet occurring under different circumstances and situations. Often conflicts at the local level involving water are motivated by competing interests of communities living upstream and downstream of the basin (Wolf, 1998). A lack of common vision between the communities residing locally contributes to constant disputes (Mehta, Veldwisch, & Franco, 2012). Local conflicts are also motivated by histories of simmering and unresolved disputes between the locals sharing the water. Often, these disputes date back many decades without any efficient and effective plan to manage them. This results in conflicts between local people as they try to settle these water disputes themselves. Natural resources may be used as an excuse or shield for other conflicts, with local people forced to evict other communities/locals building a permanent rivalry between the locals (Matthew, Halle & Switzer, 2002). Democracy is an important agent for resolving conflicts and living in harmony. However, if dictatorship is the style of leadership practiced by locals often they will be motivated to seek control of the water resources from their neighbouring communities. When a local community learns that one group is being favoured when sharing the water resources because they corrupted a public officer, conflicts will start to appear with demonstrations by locals likely to escalate (Evans, 1999). Corruption is one dynamic in water conflicts in local areas that has persistently led to conflicts between the locals at times causing violent wars (Kramer, Wolf, Carius, & Dabelko, 2013).

In communities whose sources of livelihood vary (for instance where one might practice agriculture and the other is pastoral), conflict on how to share water resources equitably will frequently arise. This has occurred in many local water conflicts in African countries as locals engage and dispute how water resources should be shared in an equitable manner (Donkor & Wolde, 2012). The dynamics of water conflicts in local areas are not that different with factors motivating conflicts at the international level. This is because often in both situations the lack of proper management of these conflicts leads to violent wars causing loss of lives. Another dynamic to water conflicts in the local areas is based on the aspect of discrimination against age, group, tribe and ethnicity, among other forms of discrimination. This dynamic affects how local communities are willing to share water resources between themselves. If a group of people learn they are being discriminated against by others, resulting in a smaller share of the water resources, they will often feel agitated causing conflict between local groups within a community. Lack of employment and basic resources among the locals is a further source of conflict (Shamir & Kutner, 2003). When many members of a local society, particularly the youth, are unemployed, constant conflicts will often arise. Even when small disputes arise, idle people are often willing to fight back using all means to prove a point. Generally, the dynamics of local water conflicts has not evolved much when compared with the dynamics of international water conflicts. Local water dynamics continue to have the same motivating factors across generations as unresolved conflicts are carried forward to the generation after generation causing constant disputes between some locals.

THEORETICAL FRAMEWORKS OF BAISN LEVEL WATER CONFLICTS

This section clarifies the main concepts in basin level water conflicts, namely: conflicts, cooperation and sharing and water shortage/scarcity.

Conflict

Conflict is defined as a social situation where a minimum of two parties aim to acquire the same scarce resources (Wallensteen, 2002, p. 15). It is important to note that for a commodity to be scarce, it does not necessarily mean that resources are limited. Basin level water conflicts can be understood by applying a "conflict triangle". The conflict triangle has three features: (1) incompatibilities and attitudes; (2) actors and; (3) parties. Often "attitudes" are replaced with "interests" making it more evident that actual parties are involved in a specific conflict. The dynamics or the actions show how the conflicts evolve either in a violent manner or not. The intensity of conflicts often changes over time and may disappear or possibly be transformed into political issues that escalate the nature of the conflict (Thomasson, 2004, p. 9). As noted earlier in this chapter, some conflicts are recurrent, originating from decades ago caused by a lack of equitable sharing of water resources.

Basin level water conflicts originate from different perceptions related to the use, access and management of the available water resources. There are specific underlying factors that cause water conflicts in the basin areas where the lack of effective and efficient policies to manage these water resources often leads to violent wars. Factors that cause basin level water conflicts are related to politics, the society and the physical and environmental aspects. In many water basins globally, problems between upstream users of water and downstream users have continued to cause constant conflicts between states/provinces and regions (Böge, 2003). While conflicts are known to bring change, changes are also capable of triggering conflicts. Managing or resolving a conflict normally leads to more positive changes, as grievances and incompatibilities between the parties involved in a conflict lessen (Thomasson, 2004). It is therefore important to note that conflicts can be used either constructively or destructively, depending on how the current parties involved in the conflict behave. How conflicts evolve will often depend on whether there are mechanisms put in place to manage the disputes. Perceptions of parties contributes to how conflicts are viewed and understood. For instance, a downstream province may not necessarily see that an upstream province is using more water resources. In this kind of scenario, conflict is unlikely to arise, as neither party sees any form of problem in the sharing of resources.

Cooperation and Sharing

Cooperation is defined as doing something together towards a shared aim. On the other hand, sharing is defined as the portion which is given or allotted to an individual (Wehmeier, 2000, p. 276). In many water basins around the world, cooperation and sharing have been the trend for many years. For instance, the water resources from the River Nile Basin have been shared by some countries such as Kenya and Uganda without conflicts as the cooperation between the two countries has been enhanced creating mechanisms for sharing and solving conflicts as soon as they arise. The aspect of sharing and forming cooperation between states within a basin is important to avoid and resolve conflicts which have existed for years. This will also reduce the use of military force by powerful nations to oppress developing nations, such as the conflict between Israel and Palestine where the Israelites continue to oppress the Palestinians in their own land because of water resources (Shuval, 1992). Cooperation is not able to solve all problems. However, the aim of sharing water resources is a step in the right direction towards reaching an amicable solution between the parties involved.

Water Scarcity/ Water Demand

Water scarcity is defined as the diminishing of water resources or the incremental pressure of supplying water resources, due to rise in demand. According to Ohlsson (1999, p. 2), there are three types of water scarcity: (1) demand induced due to increased population pressures; (2) supply induced caused by reduced availability of water resources, and; (3) structural scarcity caused by the confiscation of large parts of water resources by more powerful groups, as shown in the Table 4.

These three types of water scarcity are present in many countries where water basins exist. These forms of scarcity lead to water basin conflicts, which affect the political, social and economic stability

Table 4. Type of scarcity (adapted from: Ohlsson, 1999, p. 2)

Type of Scarcity	Definition
Demand-induced scarcity	Because of the increase in populations the need of more water resources from the basins increases
Supply induced scarcity	This has been caused by the drying up of river basins, water tables that are lowering and pollution of the available water basins
Structural scarcity	This is caused by powerful segments of the basin water users confiscate large parts of the basins via the use of force resulting in marginalization of the less powerful users

of the region. It is therefore important to note that conflicts in water basins are caused by factors which are interrelated, and require the cooperation of the involved parties to design proper mechanisms, which will lead to equitable sharing of the scarce water resources.

CONFLICT MANAGEMENT IN WATER CONFLICTS

It has been proclaimed that the most likely source of social and political unrest in some parts of the world like the Middle East into the future will be not be warfare but rather water (Lesser, Nardulli & Arghavan, 1998). The population in these and many other countries is continuing to increase demands for water to perform human activities such as agriculture, drinking, sourcing hydropower, industry and water for building (FAO, 2011). As the supply of water is decreasing, the rising demand causes competition for the available water resources between local and international communities. Water conflicts are spread across many parts of the world and because of this reason it is important to have conflict management and resolution strategies to facilitate solutions to the conflicts. Through conflict management and resolution strategies, parties are able to easily agree on some of the issues such as how to share the water resources effectively and equitably (Shamir & Kutner, 2003). By employing conflict management and resolution strategies, parties involved in conflicts are able to avoid the escalation of the conflicts to levels which lead to violent wars causing the loss of innocent lives. Conflict management and resolution strategies are therefore important aspects of reducing the impacts of water conflicts between local and international communities. This section explores some basin level conflict management and resolution strategies in irrigated agriculture. Additionally, conflict management policies in developing nations are explored.

Basin Level Conflict Management and Resolution in Irrigated Agriculture

Conflict management and resolution is a process which normally guides conflicts into constructive outcomes. It is a process that promotes dialogue and negotiation in irrigated agriculture activities where conflicts are experienced (Shamir, & Kutner, 2003). Basin level conflict management and resolution in irrigated agriculture serves three purposes. First, is to ensure that issues which cause disagreements between parties are resolved before they become hostile. Second, they help the different actors involved in the conflict to find alternative methods that can minimize the conflicts and guide them to the selection of the most suitable option that all parties involved in the basin level conflict can live with comfortably. Third, the management and resolution process in basin level conflicts helps in the identification of the underlying factors causing the conflict aiming to address them to prevent their occurrence in the future

(Babbit, Gutlove & Jones, 1994). The United Nations has developed a management process to be followed in managing water resources in irrigated agriculture to avoid conflicts. This process includes pro-active conflict management strategies and post-conflict resolution strategies. Conflict management is a continuous process in irrigated agriculture areas aimed at preventing an occurrence of conflict and reducing tensions by solving the underlying contributing causes as early as possible. In irrigated agriculture, often water and land go hand in hand and conflict management will involve resolving water and land issues.

Integrated water resources management (IWRM) is a process that promotes coordinated management and development of land, water and resources with a view to maximizing social and economic equitability without compromising the sustainability of ecosystems. According to Cap-Net (2005), IWRM is a systematic process for sustainable development, monitoring and allocation of the uses of water in irrigated agricultural areas in the context of achieving economic, social and environmental objectives. This means that in irrigated agriculture areas, the needs of most of the people will be considered together with other uses of water resources for the minority groups that do not use water for irrigation. Water management and allocation decisions in irrigated agriculture areas should consider and take account of other users in the region. Conflict management strategies aim to prevent conflicts from occurring and to identify potential conflicts and mitigate these before they escalate (Cap-Net, 2008).

A conflict management strategy in irrigated agriculture involves raising awareness of the continued water scarcity in the basin in addition to information on appropriate coping strategies to undertake. In areas where irrigation is the livelihood of communities, water conflicts are bound to happen when communities in the upstream regions engage in activities that affect water flow in the basin (Gichuki, 2002). People who rely on irrigation for their livelihood often fail to accept any mode of conflict resolution due to a lack of knowledge and understanding that basins are experiencing water shortages because of factors such as climate change. Development initiatives that raise awareness of the increase in demand for water compared to the available water supply would help in supporting equitable and fair water sharing. Through this strategy, stakeholders using the same water resources are given an opportunity to engage in dialogue and come up with possible interventions that benefit all parties. For instance, if problems are found to arise from irrigators in the upstream regions interventions can be initiated to ensure that downstream users are able to access water resources from the basin (Gichuki, 2002).

Conflict management in irrigated agriculture is an ongoing process where all stakeholder work together to creating conditions, which discourage dysfunctional conflicts while at the same time, promoting conflict resolution methods to ensure that all parties involved achieve a win-win outcome (Cap-Net, 2008). Conflict management will normally use tools, that will respond, anticipate and prevent basin level water conflicts in irrigated agriculture. Using these tools, the parties involved are encouraged to open up and discuss the issues causing the conflicts and find "win-win" solutions (Wolf, 1998). However, a "win-win" outcome is much harder to achieve when the parties involved have a long history of entrenched conflict. For a viable outcome to be achieved compromise and trade-off will be necessary thereby requiring parties to give up something in the process. An important aspect in conflict management is changing communities positively by creating an environment where people can practice their agricultural skills peacefully while sharing the available resources in a fair and equitable manner (Cap-Net, 2008; Dinar, 2006).

DISPUTE RESOLUTION PROCESSES

Conflict resolution at the basin level in irrigated agriculture can be carried out in a number of ways.

It is important to note that there is no clear preferred method for solving basin water level conflicts. However, an enabling environment for all parties involved is a step in the right direction (Tanner, 2000).

It is important for conflict resolution methods to create synergy between the parties in conflict. Some of the conflict resolution methods that have been explored in the past in irrigated agriculture, and others that are available but have not been explored by parties in water conflicts, are detailed below. Apart from litigation all of these processes are alternative dispute resolution strategies. Table 5 outlines the key differences between the conflict resolution techniques of negotiation and litigation.

Litigation

Parties in basin water level conflicts in irrigated agriculture areas often turn to the legal system of their countries or the international criminal court (ICC), like in the case of Israel and Palestine (Mustafa,Akhter, & Nasrallah, 2013). Litigation is the most formal process of conflict resolution. The parties in dispute present their arguments and cases in a court of law that decides the case based on the international laws or country laws. In many instances, litigation is the most common form of conflict resolution mechanism. This is particularly so in instances where multiple parties are involved who use common water basin resources with no single party clearly having a superior legal claim (Cap-Net, 2008).

Table 5. Comparison of conflict resolution techniques of negotiation and litigation adapted from: Cap-Net, 2008)

Technique	Negotiation	Litigation
Result sought	A mutually acceptable agreement	Court Judgement
Voluntary/Involuntary	Voluntary	Involuntary
Binding-Non-binding	Agreement enforceable as contract	Binding
Private/Public	Private	Public
Participants	Parties only	Judge and parties
Third Party Involvement	Parties have direct communication	None
First Steps	Flexible	One party initiates the proceedings
Approach/Methodology	Non-adversarial It is unstructured and informal	• Adversarial • Structure is set by rules which are predetermined • Formal
Advantages	• Cheaper and quicker • Parties have control of the outcome and policy • To find a win-win situation parties have to work together • Decisions can be matched to the needs of th parties • The agreements made are more likely to be implemented	Power imbalances can be addressed with legal rules
Disadvantages	• This is not the best method in complex cases • Failure to implement agreements may lead to litigation	• It is an expensive and slow process • There are chances of further litigation • The decision made is limited to narrow legal parameters

Arbitration

Arbitration is a less formal approach to basin water conflict than litigation with a neutral third person giving an award to one party. This process is not often used in solving water conflicts and is often not successful as the losing party does not follow the decision handed down. However, when parties involved in a conflict choose an arbitrator via consensus, while at the same time setting rules and conditions that govern the process, the outcome of arbitration is more likely to be accepted by all parties. The conflict will be resolved if the parties honour their commitment to agreeing to the award (Cap-Net, 2008). Before engaging in conflict resolution methods for water-related conflicts in irrigated agriculture areas, it is important to build consensus/ stakeholder involvement between the involved parties. Stakeholder involvement is critical to sustainable management of basin water resources. In the context of basin conflicts, it is important to provide an environment where stakeholders can meet from time to time and communicate with each other their needs, interests and concerns.

Conciliation

Conciliation involves a conciliator, who meets with the parties separately or together with the aim to resolve their differences. This may help the conflicting parties to lower tensions, improve communications, interpret issues, encourage parties to explore potential solutions and assist them to find a mutually acceptable outcome. The conciliator can provide expert advice to the parties. The conciliation process, in and of itself, has no legal standing, and the conciliator usually is not given an authority to seek evidence or call witnesses. Further, the conciliator does not make any decision or award to any party (Cap-Net, 2008).

Mediation

In the recent times, the increase in basin level water conflicts has seen the mediation process of settling conflicts become more frequently used by parties in conflict. Mediation is a process where outside parties oversee the negotiations between two or more parties, who are involved in a conflict. The parties in the conflict often agree to the mediator who will guide their negotiations as well as assist in reaching a mutually acceptable agreement. The mediators create an environment, which is safe for the parties in the conflict to share information and seek solutions to the underlying problems affecting the sharing of water resources equitably. Unlike the conciliator, the mediator does not have an advisory role. This is considered to be the perfect mechanism for resolving conflicts when parties have reached a standoff (Mason & Blank 2013).

Negotiation

In negotiation, each of the parties presents their own interests without the intervention of a third party, unless assistance is required. Parties in water conflicts are often invited to participate in negotiations which aim at coming up with new policies and regulations to govern how the water resources are shared. Through negotiations, parties can agree on water pollution caused by dumping of agricultural related chemicals into the water among other issues that may have attributed to the conflicts (Cap-Net, 2008). Negotiation is the final stage of mediation and conciliation.

Facilitation

Facilitation is a conflict resolution strategy where a conductive environment is provided for parties in a conflict to discuss the way forward. In this process, the facilitator does not provide any ideas to solve the conflicts but leaves the involved parties to come up with implementable ideas which they can all agree on. Often, facilitation is the first step towards creating or identifying a dispute resolution process that will be acceptable by all parties (Cap-Net, 2008).

SOLUTIONS AND RECOMMENDATIONS

Conflict Management Policies in Developing Nations

In developing nations, water conflicts have been on the rise due to increasing demands from population growth and declining fresh water resources. In the past governments of developing nations have often engaged in projects without adequately assessing the impacts on surrounding communities. More recently, policies on water projects have been effective in providing clear directions on whether to engage in certain kind of projects. These policies on water projects help to reduce corruption and interference by donor agencies (Conca, 2006). Many developing nations have established conflict management policies that provide guidance on water conflicts and the prevention of internal or external conflicts. Some of these conflict management policies in developing nations have resulted in the incorporation of knowledge on the most current dynamics of local water conflicts with a view to establishing proper mechanisms to prevent, manage and resolve disputes arising from water conflicts. Below are some of the main aspects included in these conflict management policies in developing nations to mitigate water-related conflicts.

Policies That Strengthen Human Rights to Water

Developing nations are making policies, which have strong laws on human rights to water, which creates the notion that each person has the right to use water regardless of their affiliation. By strengthening human rights to water, developing nations are removing the traditional ownership of water basins or water resources by certain communities. Through these reforms, it is easy to share resources equitably without having major disagreements (Conca, 2006).

Policies Acknowledging Environmental Aspects

Developing nations are realizing that environmental factors are critical attributes to water conflicts and because of this, they are making policies which provide for solving environmental disputes between communities. By having policies that govern activities affecting the environment, which in turn affect the water basins, developing nations are reducing the future chances of conflicts between organizations and local communities. For instance, by having policies that control pollution of water by industries along water basins developing countries are reducing conflicts between industry and members of the local community (Agwata, 2006).

Policies Regulating the Apportionment and Utilization of Water

Developing nations are realizing the need to have water sharing bodies whose function is to regulate how water is utilized and apportioned among members of society. The creation of bodies that are responsible for overseeing how water is utilized in developing countries is ensuring that minimal conflicts are experienced (Agwata, 2006).

Policies Geared Towards Funding for Water Resources Management

Developing nations have realized the need of increasing their funding to efforts geared to the management of the water resources. Water is an essential commodity for developing nations and it must be used in a manner that promotes sustainable development. Agriculture is one of the essential drivers of many economies in developing nations. Policies, that fund efforts to manage water resources contributes largely to fewer water conflicts in the future (Donkor & Wolde, 2012). Water in developing countries plays an important role in industrial development, agricultural development and the production of hydropower. It is therefore important to have effective and efficient water resource management tools that are able to deal with water disputes within the less time possible (Agwata, 2006). Conflict management policies for water-related disputes in developing nations are critical in securing the future development of these countries (Tanner, 2000). While different developing nations face different types of conflicts, often these are interconnected and policies that are effective on a country level can reduce rising cases of international water conflicts. Conflict management policies, that are drafted by water conflict professionals, are necessary to safeguard water resources from threats that are continually reducing the availability of water resources globally. Conflict management policies on water resources will ensure equitable and fair utilization of resources by locals contributing to the social, economic and political stability of these developing nations (Conca, 2006).

FURTHER RESEARCH

Further research is required aimed at developing more detailed knowledge and understandings of disputes at a local basin level using both quantitative and qualitative research methods. A key objective is to identify the underlying factors that causes basin conflicts in the eastern region of Turkey and what resolution and management measures can be put in place to guide an equitable and fair sharing of water resources. Theoretical frameworks best suited to this type of research are the mutual gains approach as well as game theory.

CONCLUSION

Limited access to resources, in this case basin level water, creates stress and tension that necessarily impacts in varying degrees on the health and wellbeing of those directly affected. In cases of extreme stress and conflict, when applying the stress diathesis model for the development of mental health issues, those who are genetically vulnerable are most certainly at risk of developing mental health issues as well as physical health problems related to prolonged stress and anxiety. Dominant paradigms in relation to mental health and wellbeing emphasise "recovery" and "living well" in the community. In cases of protracted conflict this is not easy to achieve. Effective conflict management policies and strategies are required at governmental, organizational and local levels to reduce water conflicts and promote community inclusion to support health and wellbeing through strength of community and at the same time protect our precious natural resources for current and future generations.

REFERENCES

Agwata, J. F. (2006). Resource potential of the Tana Basin with particular Focus on the Bwathonaro Watershed, Kenya. *FWU*, *5*, 1–15.

Allouche, J., & Thèse, N. (2004). *Water nationalism: An explanation of past and present conflicts in Central Asia, The Middle East and The Indian Subcontinent*. Geneva: University of Geneva.

Babbit, E., Gutlove, P., & Jones, L. (1994). *Handbook of Basic Conflict Resolution Skills: Facilitation, Mediation and Consensus Building*. Cambridge, MA: The Balkans Peace Project.

Bandaragoda, D. J. (2000). *A framework for institutional analysis for water resources management in a river basin context*. Working Paper 5. Colombo, Sri Lanka: International Water Management Institute.

Bernauer, T., & Siegfried, T. (2012). Climate change and international water conflict in Central Asia. *Journal of Peace Research*, *49*(1), 227–239. doi:10.1177/0022343311425843

Böge, V. (2003). *Water governance in Southern Africa – cooperation and conflict prevention in transboundary river basins (Brief series no. 33)*. Bonn, Germany: Bonn International Centre for Conversion.

Cap-Net. (2005). *Tutorial on basic principles of integrated water resources management (Version 2)*. New York: United Nations Development Fund Program.

Cap-Net. (2008). *Conflict resolution and negotiation skills for integrated water resources management*. New York: United Nations Development Fund Program.

Carius, A., Debelko, G., & Wolf, A. T. (2004). Water, conflict, and cooperation. *Environmental Change and Security Project Report*, *10*, 60–66.

Center for Economic and Social Rights and Palestinian Hydrology Group. (2003). *Thirsting for justice: Israeli violations of human right to water in the Occupied Palestinian Territories: Parallel report to the 30th session of the United Nations CESR*. Brooklyn, NY: Center for Economic and Social Rights.

Central Intelligence Agency. (2015). *The World Factbook 2015*. Central Intelligence Agency.

Conca, K. (2006). The new face of water conflict. In Navigating Peace 3. Washington DC: Woodrow Wilson International Center for Scholars' Environmental Change and Security Program.

Daily, G. C., & Ehrlich, P. R. (1992). Population, sustainability, and earth's carrying capacity. *Bioscience*, *42*(10), 761–771. doi:10.2307/1311995

Donkor, S. M. K., & Wolde, Y. E. (2012). *Integrated Water Resources Management in Africa: Issues and Options. The United Nations Water Development Report*. Washington, DC: United Nations Economic Commission for Africa.

El-Fadel, M., El-Sayegh, Y., El-Fadl, K., & Khorbotly, D. (2003). The Nile River Basin: A case study in surface water conflict resolution. *Journal of Natural Resources and Life Sciences Education*, *32*, 107–117.

European Environment Agency. (2015). *Annual Report 2014*. Luxembourg: European Union.

Evans, B. R. (1999). *The cost of corruption*. Teddington, UK: Tearfund.

FAO. (2011). *The state of the world's land and water resources for food and agriculture (SOLAW): Managing systems at risk*. Earthscan.

Gehrig, J., & Rogers, M. (2009). *Water and conflict: incorporating peacebuilding into water development*. Baltimore, MD: Catholic Relief Services.

Gichuki, F. (2002). Water conflicts in the Upper Ewaso Ngiro North Basin: causes, impacts and management strategies. E-conference paper.

Hanjra, M. A., & Qureshi, M. E. (2010). Global water crisis and future food security in an era of climate change. *Food Policy*, *35*(5), 365–377. doi:10.1016/j.foodpol.2010.05.006

Hinrichsen, D., & Tacio, H. (2011). *Finding the source: The coming freshwater crisis is already here*. Washington, DC: Woodrow Wilson International Center for Scholars.

Huggins, R., Izushi, H., Prokop, D., & Thompson, P. (2014). *The global competitiveness of regions: Regions and cities*. London, UK: Routledge.

Izquierdo, L., Stangerhaugen, M., Castillo, D., Nixon, R., & Jimenez, G. (2010). *Water Crisis in Central Asia: Key Challenges and Opportunities*. New York: Graduate Program in International Affairs, New School University.

Jeffrey, C., & Craig, D. (2011). Application of Environmental Conflict Resolution to Public Interest Issues in Water Disputes. International Journal of Rural Law and Policy, 1, 1-13.

Jones, S., & Fernyhough, C. (2007). A new look at the neural diathesis stress model of schizophrenia: The primacy of social evaluative and uncontrollable situations. *Schizophrenia Bulletin*, *33*(5), 1171–1177. doi:10.1093chbulbl058 PMID:17105966

Jongerden, J. (2010). Dams and politics in Turkey: Utilizing water, developing conflict. *Middle East Policy*, *17*(1), 137–143. doi:10.1111/j.1475-4967.2010.00432.x

Kameri-Mbote, P. (2007). Water, conflict, and cooperation: Lessons from the Nile river basin 4. Washington, DC: Woodrow Wilson International Center for Scholars' Conflict Resolution and Peacebuilding Program.

Kramer, A., Wolf, A., Carius, A. & Dabelko, G. (2013). The key to managing conflict and cooperation over water. *A World of Science, 11*(1), 4-12.

Lesser, I. O., Nardulli, B. R., & Arghavan, L. A. (1998). Sources of conflict in the Greater Middle East. In *Sources of conflict in the 21st century: Regional futures and U. S. strategy*. Santa Monica, CA: RAND.

Link, P. M., Piontek, F., Scheffran, J., & Schilling, J. (2012). *On foes and flows: Water conflict and co-operation in the Nile River Basin in times of climate change*. Hamburg, Germany: CLISEC, University of Hamburg.

Loucks, D. P., & van Beek, E. (2005). *Water resources systems planning and management: Facts about water*. Paris, France: UNESCO Publishing Company.

Mason, S. J., & Blank, D. (2013). *Mediating Water Use Conflicts in Peace Processes*. Zurich, Switzerland: Center for Security Studies, Swiss Federal Institute of Technology, ETH Zurich.

Matthew, R. A., Halle, M., & Switzer, J. (2002). *Conserving the peace: Resources, livelihoods and security*. Winnipeg, Canada: International Institute for Sustainable Development.

Mehta, L., Veldwisch, G. J., & Franco, J. (2012). Introduction to the Special Issue: Water grabbing? Focus on the (re) appropriation of finite water resources. *Water Alternatives*, *5*(2), 193–207.

Mollie, F. (2009). River basin planning and management: The social life of a concept. *Geoforum*, *40*(3), 484–494. doi:10.1016/j.geoforum.2009.03.004

Morrisette, J. J., & Borer, D. A. (2004). Where Oil and Water Do Mix: Environmental Scarcity and Future Conflict in the Middle East and North Africa. *Parameters*, *34*, 94–96.

Mustafa, D., Akhter, M., & Nasrallah, N. (2013). *Understanding Pakistan's water-security nexus. Peaceworks, No. 88*. Washington, DC: United States Institute of Peace.

Ohlsson, V. L. (1999). Water scarcity and conflict. *International Security Challenges in a Changing World*, *3*, 211.

Ohlsson, V. L. (2000). Water conflicts and social resource scarcity. *Physics and Chemistry of the Earth. Part B: Hydrology, Oceans and Atmosphere*, *25*(3), 213–220. doi:10.1016/S1464-1909(00)00006-X

Pacific Institute. (2015). *Water conflict: The world's water*. Retrieved from: http://worldwater.org/water-conflict/

Pimentel, D., Berger, B., Filiberto, D., Newton, M., Wolfe, B., Karabinakis, E., ... Nandagopal, S. (2004). Water resources: Agricultural and environmental issues. *Bioscience*, *54*(10), 909–918. doi:10.1641/0006-3568(2004)054[0909:WRAAEI]2.0.CO;2

Postel, S. L., & Wolf, A. T. (2001). Dehydrating conflict. *Foreign Policy*, *126*(126), 60–67. doi:10.2307/3183260

Ravnborg, H. M. (2004). *Water and conflict: Conflict prevention and mitigation in water resources management. DIIS REPoRT 2004:2*. Copenhagen: Danish Institute for International Studies.

Shamir, Y. & Kutner, R. (2003). *Alternative dispute resolution approaches and their application*. PCCP, UNESCO-IHP, Series 7, 1-43.

Shuval, H. I. (1992). Approaches to resolving the water conflicts between Israel and her neighbors: A regional water-for-peace plan. *Water International, 17*(3), 133–143. doi:10.1080/02508069208686133

Tanner, F. (2000). Conflict prevention and conflict resolution: Limits of multilateralism. *Revue Internationale de la Croix-Rouge. International Review of the Red Cross, 82*(839), 541–559. doi:10.1017/S1560775500184615

Tew, J., Ramon, S., Slade, M., Bird, V., Melton, J., & Le Boutillier, C. (2011). Social factors and recovery from mental health difficulties: A Review of the evidence. *British Journal of Social Work, 42*(3), 443–460. doi:10.1093/bjsw/bcr076

Thomasson, F. (2004). *Water and local conflict: A brief review of the academic literature and other sources.* Stockholm, Sweden: Conflict and Water Group, Swedish Waterhouse.

Transparency International. (2008). *Global corruption report 2008: Corruption in the water sector.* New York: Cambridge University Press.

United Nations Development Program. (2006a). *Human development report 2002: Deepening democracy in a fragmented world.* New York: Oxford University Press.

United Nations Development Program. (2006b). *Annual report 2006: Global partnership for development.* New York: UNDP.

United Nations Educational, Scientific, and Cultural Organization. (2013). Water for people, water for life (The United Nations World Water Development Report). Paris, France: UNESCO Publishing and Berghahn Books.

United Nations Educational, Scientific and Cultural Organization. (2015). *The United Nations World Water Development Report 2015.* Paris: UNESCO Publishing.

United States Agency for International Development. (2014). *The Conflict Early Warning and Response Mechanism (CEWARN).* Washington, DC: USAID.

Villiers, M. D. (2000). *Water: The fate of our most precious resource.* New York: Mariner Books.

Vuković, M. (2008). The identification of water conflict and its resolution. *FACTA UNIVERSITATIS, Series Philosophy, Sociology. Psychology and History, 7*(1), 81–93.

Wallensteen, P. (2002). *Understanding Conflict Resolution, War, Peace and the Global System.* London: Sage Publications.

Wehmeier, S. (2000). *Oxford Advanced Learner's Dictionary of Current English* (6th ed.). New York: Oxford University Press.

Weinthal, E. (2006). Water Conflict and Cooperation in Central Asia. *Human Development Report Occasional Paper, 32*, 1-36.

Williams, J. (2013). *The international implications of China's water policies.* Bristol, UK: E-International Relations (E-IR). Retrieved from: http://www.e-ir.info/2013/02/15/chinas-water-policies-and-their-international-implications/

Wolf, A., Yoffe, S. & Giordano, M. (2003). *International waters: Indicators for identifying basins at risk*. PCCP, UNESCO-IHP, 1-24.

Wolf, A. T. (1998). Conflict and cooperation along international waterways. *Water Policy*, *1*(2), 251–265. doi:10.1016/S1366-7017(98)00019-1

Wolf, A. T., Kramer, A., Carius, A., & Dabelko, G. D. (2005). Managing water conflict and cooperation: State of the world 2005. In Redefining global security (pp. 80-95). Washington, DC: The World Watch Institute.

World Commission on Dams. (2000). *Dams and development: A new framework for decision-making*. London: Earthscan.

Yoffe, S., Wolfe, A. T., & Giordano, M. (2001). *Conflict and cooperation over international freshwater resources: Indicators and findings of the Basins at Risk project*. Retrieved from: http://transboundarywaters.science.oregonstate.edu/sites/transboundarywaters.science.oregonstate.edu/filesDatabase/ResearchProjects/BAR/BAR_chapter4.pdf

Compilation of References

Abdullah, Md. A. S. (2015). Muslims in pre- and post-9/11 contexts. *International Journal of Comparative Literature & Translation Studies*, *3*(3), 52–59.

Aboriginal Healing Foundation (Canada). (2006). *Final report of the Aboriginal Healing Foundation*. Ottawa: Aboriginal Healing Foundation.

About MIEACT. (2016). Retrieved October 01, 2017, from https://www.mieact.org.au/sites/defaultfilesdocumentsStrat%20 PlanMIEACT%20Aims%2C%20VIsion%20and%20Mission%202013%20-%202016.pdf

About ReachOut Schools. (2017). Retrieved October 09, 2017, from https://schools.au.reachout.com/articles/about-reachout-schools

Acrey, P. L. (2004). *Social work research and disability: Does research emphasize strengths or deficits?* (Unpublished master's thesis). University of Texas, Arlington, TX.

Adams, M. P. J. (2011). *Social work field instructors' perceptions of core attributes. Implications for leadership and gatekeeping* (Unpublished doctoral dissertation). Bowling Green State University, Bowling Green, OH.

Adams, R., Jones, A., Lefmann, S., & Sheppard, L. (2016). Service Level Decision-making in Rural Physiotherapy: Development of Conceptual Models. *Physiotherapy Research International*, *21*(2), 116–126. doi:10.1002/pri.1627 PMID:25899820

Agani, F., Landau, J., & Agani, N. (2010). Community-building before, during, and after times of trauma: The application of the LINC Model of community resilience in Kosovo. *The American Journal of Orthopsychiatry*, *80*(1), 143–149. doi:10.1111/j.1939-0025.2010.01017.x PMID:20397999

Agwata, J. F. (2006). Resource potential of the Tana Basin with particular Focus on the Bwathonaro Watershed, Kenya. *FWU*, *5*, 1–15.

Ainley, M., Hidi, S., & Berndorff, D. (2002). Interest, learning and the psychological processes that mediate their relationship. *Journal of Educational Psychology*, *94*(3), 545–561. doi:10.1037/0022-0663.94.3.545

Akinyela, M. M. (2014). Narrative therapy and cultural democracy: A testimony view. *Australian and New Zealand Journal of Family Therapy*, *35*(1), 46–49. doi:10.1002/anzf.1041

Alakeson, V. (2008). Self-directed care for adults with serious mental illness: The barriers to progress. *Psychiatric Services (Washington, D.C.)*, *59*(7), 792–794. doi:10.1176/ps.2008.59.7.792 PMID:18586997

Albuquerque, G. A., de Lima Garcia, C., da Silva Quirino, G., Alves, M. J. H., Belém, J. M., dos Santos Figueiredo, F. W., ... de Abreu, L. C. (2016). Access to health services by lesbian, gay, bisexual, and transgender persons: Systematic literature review. *BMC International Health and Human Rights*, *16*(1), 2. doi:10.118612914-015-0072-9 PMID:26769484

Aldridge, D., & Somerville, C. (2014). *Your Services Your Say: LGBT people's experiences of public services in Scotland.* Stonewall.

Al-Krenawi, A., & Graham, J. R. (2000). Culturally sensitive social work practice with Arab clients in mental health settings. *Health & Social Work, 25*(1), 9–22. doi:10.1093/hsw/25.1.9 PMID:10689599

Allen, D. M. (2013). Invalidation in Families: What Are The Hidden Aspects? *Psychology Today.* Retrieved from: https://www.psychologytoday.com/us/blog/matterpersonality/201309/invalidation-in-families-what-are-the-hidden-aspects

Allen, J., & Vincent K. (2005). *Journeys: Supporting innovation in teacher education throughout Australia.* Academic Press.

Allied Health Professionals Federation. (2013). *Details of AHP Professions, their roles and Numbers.* Author.

Allouche, J., & Thèse, N. (2004). *Water nationalism: An explanation of past and present conflicts in Central Asia, The Middle East and The Indian Subcontinent.* Geneva: University of Geneva.

Alves, H.C., de Oliveira, N.P., & Chaves, A.D. (2016). "We want to show our face, man": Hip hop helping to build identity, awareness and social participation of young people in a socially vulnerable situation. *Cadernos de Terapia ocupacional, 24*(1), 39-52. doi: 10.4322/0104-4931.ctoAO0637

American Psychiatric Association. (1952). *Diagnostic and statistical manual of mental disorders* (1st ed.). Washington, DC: APA.

American Psychiatric Association. (2004). *Practice guidelines for the treatment of psychiatric disorders.* Washington, DC: APA.

American Psychological Association. (2009). ICD vs. DSM. *Monitor on Psychology, 40*(9), 65.

Amthor, F. (2012). *Neuroscience for Dummies.* John Wiley & Sons Ltd.

Anderson, M., & Perrin, A. (2017). *Tech adoption climbs among older adults.* Washington, DC: Pew Research Centre.

Anderson, P., & Tilton, E. (2017). *Bringing them home: 20 years on: An action plan for healing.* Barton, ACT: Aboriginal and Torres Strait Healing Foundation.

Andersson, T., & Liff, R. (2012). Does patient-centred care mean risk aversion and risk ignoring? Unintended consequences of NPM reforms. *International Journal of Public Sector Management, 25*(4), 260–271. doi:10.1108/09513551211244098

Andrade, A. (2015). *Community college students' experiences of mental-health stigma: A phenomenological study* (Unpublished doctoral dissertation). Colorado State University, Fort Collins, CO.

Aneshensel, C. S., Phelan, J. C., & Bierman, A. (2013). *Handbook of the sociology of mental health.* New York: Columbia University. doi:10.1007/978-94-007-4276-5

Angelis, A., Kanavos, P., & Montibeller, G. (2017). Resource Allocation and Priority Setting in Health Care: A Multi-criteria Decision Analysis Problem of Value? *Global Policy, 8*(S2), 76–83. doi:10.1111/1758-5899.12387

Anthony, W. A. (1993). Recovery from mental illness: The guiding vision of the mental health service system in the 1990s. *Psychosocial Rehabilitation Journal, 16*(4), 11–23. doi:10.1037/h0095655

Arens, E. A., Grabe, H. J., Spitzer, C., & Barnow, S. (2011). Testing the biosocial model of borderline personality disorder: Results of a prospective 5-year longitudinal study. *Personality and Mental Health, 5*(1), 29–42. doi:10.1002/pmh.143

Armstrong, S., Buckley, S., Lonsdale, M., Milgate, G., Kneebone, L. B., Cook, L., & Skelton, F. (2012). *Starting school: a strengths-based approach towards Aboriginal and Torres Strait Islander children*. Melbourne: Australian Council for Educational Research.

Arntz, A., Stupar-Rutenfrans, S., Bloo, J., van Dyck, R., & Spinhoven, P. (2015). Prediction of treatment discontinuation and recovery from Borderline Personality Disorder: Results from an RCT comparing Schema Therapy and Transference Focused Psychotherapy. *Behaviour Research and Therapy*, *74*, 60–71. doi:10.1016/j.brat.2015.09.002 PMID:26432172

Arrowsmith-Young, B. (2012). *The Woman Who Changed Her Brain: Unlocking the Extraordinary Potential of the Human Mind*. Pty Ltd.

Askell-Williams, H., Dix, K. L., Lawson, M. J., & Slee, P. T. (2013). Quality of implementation of a school mental health initiative and changes over time in students' social and emotional competencies. *School Effectiveness and School Improvement*, *24*(3), 357–381. doi:10.1080/09243453.2012.692697

Askell-Williams, H., Lawson, M. J., & Slee, P. T. (2009). Venturing into schools: Locating mental health initiatives in complex environments. *The International Journal of Emotional Education*, *1*(2), 14–33.

Asthana, S., Gibson, A., & Halliday, J. (2013). The medicalisation of health inequalities and the English NHS: The role of resource allocation. *Health Economics, Policy, and Law*, *8*(2), 167–183. doi:10.1017/S1744133112000126 PMID:22947257

Australia Human Rights Commission (AHRC). (2010). *In our own words: African Australians: A review of human rights and social inclusion issues*. Retrieved October 20, 2017 from https://www.humanrights.gov.au/our-work/race-discrimination/projects/our-own-words-african-australians-review-human-rights-and

Australian Association of Social Workers (AASW). (2010). *Code of Ethics*. Canberra, Australia: AASW.

Australian Association of Social Workers (AASW). (2012a). *Australian Social Work Education and Accreditation Standards (ASWEAS) V1.4*. Canberra: Australian Association of Social Workers.

Australian Association of Social Workers (AASW). (2012b). *Australian Social Work Education and Accreditation Standards (ASWEAS) 2012: Guideline 1.2: Guidance on field education programs*. Canberra: Australian Association of Social Workers.

Australian Association of Social Workers (AASW). (2013). *Practice Standards*. Canberra: Australian Association of Social Workers.

Australian Association of Social Workers (AASW). (2014). *Practice standards for mental health social workers*. Retrieved October 20, 2017 from https://www.aasw.asn.au/document/item/6739

Australian Broadcasting Commission. (2014). Mental illness – a history. *Rear vision*. Available at http://www.abc.net.au/radionational/programs/rearvision/mental-illness---a-history/5611268

Australian Bureau of Statistics. (1995). *National health survey: use of medications, Australia, 1995. cat No. 4377.0*. Canberra: ABS.

Australian Bureau of Statistics. (2006). *2001 Census of population and housing – 00 1901 A snapshot of Australia 1901*. Retrieved from: http://www.abs.gov.au/websitedbs/D3110124.NSF/24e5997b9bf2ef35ca2567fb00299c59/c4abd1fac53e3df5ca256bd8001883ec!OpenDocument#Table%201.%201901%20Population%20Counts%20f

Australian Bureau of Statistics. (2015). *Australian Demographic Statistics, Jun 2015 (3101.0)*. Retrieved from: http://www.abs.gov.au/ausstats/abs@.nsf/featurearticlesbyCatalogue/7A40A407211F35F4CA257A2200120EAA?OpenDocument

Australian Bureau of Statistics. (2016). *Census of Population and Housing: reflecting Australia – Stories from the Census, 2016 (2071.0)*. Retrieved from: http://www.abs.gov.au/ausstats/abs@.nsf/Lookup/by%20Subject/2071.0~2016~Main%20 Features~Ageing%20Population~14

Australian Bureau of Statistics. (2017). *Australian Demographic Statistics, June 2017 (3101.0)*. Retrieved from: http:// www.abs.gov.au/ausstats/abs@.nsf/mf/3101.0

Australian Bureau of Statistics. (2017). *Retirement and Retirement Intentions, Australia, July 2016 to June 2017 (6238.0)*. Retrieved from: http://www.abs.gov.au/ausstats/abs@.nsf/mf/6238.0

Australian Government Solicitor. (2012). *Express Law*. Retrieved October 2, 2017, from http://www.ags.gov.au/publications/express-law/el178.pdf

Australian Government. (2011). *Clinical Practice Guideline for the Management of Borderline Personality Disorder (BPD)*. Canberra, ACT: National MedicalResearch Council.

Australian Human Rights Commission (AHRC). (2011). *Federal Discrimination Law - Chapter 5. The Disability Discrimination Act*. Australian Human Rights Commission. Retrieved 16 May, 2016, from https://www.humanrights.gov.au/sites/default/files/content/legal/FDL/2011/5_DDA.pdf

Australian Institute of Health and Welfare (AIHW). (2016). *Australian Burden of Disease Study: Impact and causes of illness and death in Australia 2011. Australian Burden of Disease Study Series no. 3. BOD 4*. Canberra: Australian Institute of Health and Welfare.

Australian Law Reform Commission. (2017). *Inquiry into the Incarceration Rates for Aboriginal and Torres Strait Islander Peoples (ALRC Report 133)*. Canberra, ACT: Australian Law Reform Commission, Australian Government.

Australian partners in wellbeing for secondary schools. (2016). Retrieved October 08, 2017, from https://www.beyondblue.org.au/about-us/about-our-work/childhood-and-education-program/australian-partners-in-wellbeing-for-secondary-schools

Australian Psychological Society (APS). (2012). *Stress and Wellbeing in Australia in 2012: A State-of-the-Nation Survey*. Melbourne: The Australian Psychological Society.

Australian Psychological Society Ltd. (2010). *Evidence-based Psychological Interventions in the Treatment of Mental Disorders: A Literature Review*. Melbourne: Australian Psychologcal Society.

Australia, O. I. I. (2012). *Intersex for allies*. Melbourne: OII Australia. Retrieved from https://oii.org.au/21336/intersex-for-allies

Babbit, E., Gutlove, P., & Jones, L. (1994). *Handbook of Basic Conflict Resolution Skills: Facilitation, Mediation and Consensus Building*. Cambridge, MA: The Balkans Peace Project.

Bærøe, K. (2008). Priority setting in health care: On the relation between reasonable choices on the micro-level and the macro-level. *Theoretical Medicine and Bioethics*, *29*(2), 87–102. doi:10.100711017-008-9063-3 PMID:18528781

Baird, L. (2008). Childhood Trauma in the Etiology of Borderline Personality Disorder: Theoretical Considerations and Therapeutic Interventions. *Hakomi Forum, 19*(20-21), 31-42.

Baltussen, R., & Niessen, L. (2006). Priority setting of health interventions: The need for multi-criteria decision analysis. *Cost Effectiveness and Resource Allocation*, *4*(1), 14. doi:10.1186/1478-7547-4-14 PMID:16923181

Bambra, C., Garthwaite, K., & Hunter, D. (2014). All Things Being Equal: Does it Matter for Equity How You Organize and Pay for Health Care? A Review of the International Evidence. *International Journal of Health Services*, *44*(3), 457–477. doi:10.2190/HS.44.3.c PMID:25618985

Bandaragoda, D. J. (2000). *A framework for institutional analysis for water resources management in a river basin context*. Working Paper 5. Colombo, Sri Lanka: International Water Management Institute.

Banks, C., Muhajarine, N., Waygood, K., Duczek, L., & Hellquist, G. (2003). *The cost of homophobia: Literature review on the human impact of homophobia in Canada*. Gay & Lesbian Health Services of Saskatoon.

Barczyk, A. N., & Lincove, J. A. (2010). Cash and counseling: A model for self-directed care programs to empower individuals with serious mental illnesses. *Social Work in Mental Health*, *8*(3), 209–224. doi:10.1080/15332980903405298

Barham, P. (1992). *Closing the asylum: the mental patient in modern society*. London: Penguin.

Barlow, C., & Coleman, H. (2003). Suitability for practice guidelines for students: A survey of Canadian social work programmes. *Social Work Education*, *22*(2), 151–164. doi:10.1080/0261547022000058206

Barnard-Brak, L., Lechtenberger, D., & Lan, W. Y. (2010). Accommodation strategies of college students with disabilities. *Qualitative Report*, *15*(2), 411.

Barnes, B. (1977). *Interests and growth of knowledge*. London: Routledge and Kegan Paul.

Bar-On, A. (1999). Social work and the 'Missionary zeal to whip up the heathen along the path of righteousness'. *British Journal of Social Work*, *29*(1), 5–26. doi:10.1093/oxfordjournals.bjsw.a011440

Barrett, C., & Crameri, P. (2015). *An extra degree of difficulty. An evidence based guide to the experiences and needs of older LGBTI carers and the carers of older LGBTI people. Australian Research Centre in Sex, Health and Society*. Melbourne, Australia: La Trobe University.

Barrett, C., Turner, L., & Leonard, L. (2013). *Beyond a rainbow sticker. A report on How² create a gay, lesbian, bisexual, transgender and intersex (GLBTI) inclusive service 2012-2013*. Melbourne: Gay and Lesbian Health Victoria.

Barrett, C., Whyte, C., Comfort, J., Lyons, A., & Crameri, P. (2015). Social connection, relationships and older lesbian and gay people. *Sexual and Relationship Therapy*, *30*(1), 131–142. doi:10.1080/14681994.2014.963983 PMID:25544830

Barry, M. M., & Jenkins, R. (2007). *Implementing Mental Health Promotion*. Philadelphia: Elsevier Limited.

Bastien, J. (1992). *Drum & stethoscope*. Salt Lake City, UT: University of Utah Press.

Bateman, A., & Fonagy, P. (2010). Mentalization-based treatment for borderline personality disorder. *World Psychiatry; Official Journal of the World Psychiatric Association (WPA)*, *9*(1), 11–15. doi:10.1002/j.2051-5545.2010.tb00255.x PMID:20148147

Bates, E. M. (1977). *Models of madness*. St Lucia: University of Queensland Press.

Beatson, J., & Rao, S. (2014). Psychotherapy for borderline personality disorder. *Australasian Psychology*, *22*(6), 529–532. doi:10.1177/1039856214555531 PMID:25319122

Beck, U. (2008). Global generations in world risk society. *Revista CIDOB d'Afers Internacionals,* (82/83), 203-216.

Beck, U. (1992). *Risk society: Towards a new modernity*. London: Sage.

Beck, U. (2002). The terrorist threat: World risk society revisited.(State of Emergency). *Theory, Culture & Society*, *19*(4), 39–55. doi:10.1177/0263276402019004003

Beck, U. (2009). *World at risk*. Cambridge, UK: Polity.

Beh, J., Pedell, S., & Doubé, W. (2015). *Where is the "I" in iPad?: The role of interest in older adults' learning of mobile touch screen technologies. In Proceedings of OzCHI 2015: Being Human* (pp. 437–445). Melbourne, Australia: ACM Press.

Beh, J., Pedell, S., & Doubé, W. (2016). *Evaluation of interest-bridge model: Older adults meditated learning of mobile technology. In Proceedings of OzCHI 2016: Connected Futures* (pp. 293–302). Tasmania, Australia: ACM Press.

Belgrave, F. Z., Cherry, V. R., Cunningham, D., Walwyn, S., Letlaka-Rennert, K., & Phillips, F. (1994). The influence of Afrocentric values, self-esteem, and Black identity on drug attitudes among African American fifth graders: A preliminary study. *The Journal of Black Psychology*, *20*(2), 143–156. doi:10.1177/00957984940202004

Bell, K. (2012). Towards post-conventional philosophical base for social work. *British Journal of Social Work*, *42*(3), 408–423. doi:10.1093/bjsw/bcr073

Bendit, N. (2014). Reputation and science: Examining the effectiveness of DBT in the treatment of borderline personality disorder. *Australasian Psychology*, *22*(2), 144–148. doi:10.1177/1039856213510959 PMID:24191293

Bennet, B. (2014). "Stop deploying your white privilege on me!": Aboriginal and Torres Strait Islander Engagement with the Australian Association of Social Workers. *Australian Social Work*, 1–13. doi:10.1080/0312407X.2013.840325

Bennett, B. (2013). The importance of Aboriginal and Torres Strait Islander history for social work students and graduates. In B. Bennet, S. Green, & D. Bessarab (Eds.), *Our voices: Aboriginal and Torres Strait Islander social work* (pp. 1–25). Melbourne: Palgrave McMillan.

Beresford, P., Croft, S., & Adshead, L. (2008). 'We don't see her as a social worker': The importance of the social worker's relationship and humanity. *British Journal of Social Work*, *38*(7), 1388–1407. doi:10.1093/bjsw/bcm043

Berliner, L., & Kolko, D. J. (2016). Trauma Informed Care: A Commentary and Critique. *Child Maltreatment*, *21*(2), 168–172. doi:10.1177/1077559516643785 PMID:27152025

Bernard, L. C., Mills, M., Swenson, L., & Walsh, R. (2005). An evolutional theory of human motivation. *Genetic, Social, and General Psychology Monographs*, *131*(2), 129–184. doi:10.3200/MONO.131.2.129-184 PMID:16779946

Bernauer, T., & Siegfried, T. (2012). Climate change and international water conflict in Central Asia. *Journal of Peace Research*, *49*(1), 227–239. doi:10.1177/0022343311425843

Bessant, J. (2012). 'Measuring Up'? Assessment and students with disabilities in the modern university. *International Journal of Inclusive Education*, *16*(3), 265–281. doi:10.1080/13603116.2010.489119

Betts, K. (2014). *The ageing of the Australian population: triumph or disaster?* Melbourne, Australia: Monash Center for Population and Urban Research, Monash University.

Bialocerkowski, A., Johnson, A., Allan, T., & Phillips, K. (2013). Development of physiotherapy inherent requirement statements–an Australian experience. *BMC Medical Education*, *13*(1), 1. doi:10.1186/1472-6920-13-54 PMID:23590219

Bigby, C. (2013). A National Disability Insurance Scheme—challenges for social work. *Australian Social Work*, *66*(1), 1–6. doi:10.1080/0312407X.2013.771602

Biskin, R. S. (2015). The Lifetime Course of Borderline Personality Disorder. *Canadian Journal of Psychiatry*, *60*(7), 303–308. doi:10.1177/070674371506000702 PMID:26175388

Black Dog Institute. (2016). *Black Dog Institute submission in response to the 5th National Mental Health Plan*. Black Dog Institute.

Black, A., & Deci, E. (2000). The effects of instructors' autonomy support and students' autonomous motivation on learning organic chemistry: A Self-Determination Theory perspective. *Science Education*, *84*(6), 740–756. doi:10.1002/1098-237X(200011)84:6<740::AID-SCE4>3.0.CO;2 3

Blignault, I., Ponzio, V., Rong, Y., & Eisenbruch, M. (2008). A qualitative study of barriers to mental health services utilisation among migrants from mainland China in South East Sydney. *The International Journal of Social Psychiatry*, *54*(2), 180–190. doi:10.1177/0020764007085872 PMID:18488410

Boeckxstaens, P., De Smedt, D., De Maeseneer, J., Annemans, L., & Willems, S. (2011). The equity dimension in evaluations of the quality and outcomes framework: A systematic review. *BMC Health Services Research*, *11*(1), 209. doi:10.1186/1472-6963-11-209 PMID:21880136

Böge, V. (2003). *Water governance in Southern Africa – cooperation and conflict prevention in transboundary river basins (Brief series no. 33)*. Bonn, Germany: Bonn International Centre for Conversion.

Bond, L., Butler, H., Glover, S., & Patton, G. (2002). The Gatehouse Project: Mental Health Promotion Incorporating School Organisational Change and Health Education. In G. Martin, L. Rowling, & L. Walker (Eds.), *Mental Health Promotion: Concepts and Practice Young People* (pp. 128–141). Sydney: McGraw-Hill Australia Pty Limited.

Bonyhady, B. (2014, Summer). Tides of change: the NDIS and its journey to transform disability support. *Newparadigm: The Australian Journal on Psychosocial Rehabilitation,* 7-9.

Borg, C., & Hallberg, I. R. (2006). Life satisfaction among informal caregivers in comparison with non-caregivers. *Scandinavian Journal of Caring Sciences*, *20*(4), 427–438. doi:10.1111/j.1471-6712.2006.00424.x PMID:17116152

Bott, E. (1976). Hospital and society. *The British Journal of Medical Psychology*, *49*(2), 97–140. doi:10.1111/j.2044-8341.1976.tb02357.x PMID:821510

Boulton-Lewis, G. (2009). Issues in Learning and Education for the Ageing. Education and Learning for the Elderly: Why, How and Why. *Educational Gerontology*, *36*(3), 213–228. doi:10.1080/03601270903182877

Bourque Bearskin, R. L. (2011). A critical lens on culture in nursing practice. *Nursing Ethics*, *18*(4), 548–559. doi:10.1177/0969733011408048 PMID:21673120

Bracken, P., & Thomas, P. (2001). Postpsychiatry: A new direction for mental health. *British Medical Journal*, *322*(7288), 724–727. doi:10.1136/bmj.322.7288.724 PMID:11264215

Bracken, P., Thomas, P., Timimi, S., Asen, E., Behr, G., Beuster, C., ... Downer, S. (2012). Psychiatry beyond the current paradigm. *The British Journal of Psychiatry*, *201*(6), 430–434. doi:10.1192/bjp.bp.112.109447 PMID:23209088

Braveman, P. (2006). Health disparities and health equity: Concepts and measurement. *Annual Review of Public Health*, *27*(1), 167–194. doi:10.1146/annurev.publhealth.27.021405.102103 PMID:16533114

Braveman, P. A., Kumanyika, S., Fielding, J., LaVeist, T., Borrell, L. N., Manderscheid, R., & Troutman, A. (2011). Health disparities and health equity: The issue is justice. *American Journal of Public Health*, *101*(S1), S149–S155. doi:10.2105/AJPH.2010.300062 PMID:21551385

Braveman, P., & Gruskin, S. (2003). Poverty, equity, human rights and health. *Bulletin of the World Health Organization*, *81*(7), 539–545. PMID:12973647

Brett, M. (2014). Equity policy and knowledge in Australian higher education. In T. Fitzgerald (Ed.), *Advancing Knowledge in Higher Education: Universities in Turbulent Times: Universities in Turbulent Times, 44*. Hershey, PA: IGI Global. doi:10.4018/978-1-4666-6202-5.ch004

Briskman, L. (2007). *Social work with Indigenous communities*. Annandale, NSW: Federation Press.

Broady, T., & Aggar, C. (2017). Carer interventions: An overview of service effectiveness. *Journal of the Australasian Rehabilitation Nurses Association, 20*(2), 5.

Brooke, N. (2011). Needs of Aboriginal and Torres Strait Islander clients residing in Australian residential aged-care facilities. *The Australian Journal of Rural Health, 19*(4), 166–170. doi:10.1111/j.1440-1584.2011.01207.x PMID:21771156

Brophy, L., Bruxner, A., Wilson, E., Cocks, N., Stylianou, M., & Mitchell, P. (2015). People making choices: the support needs and preferences of people with psychosocial disability: project summary. *newparadigm*, 14-15.

Brown, A. R., & Mulley, G. P. (1997). Injuries sustained by caregivers of disabled elderly people. *Age and Ageing, 26*(1), 21–23. doi:10.1093/ageing/26.1.21 PMID:9143433

Brown, G. K., Ten Have, T., Henriques, G. R., Xie, S. X., Hollander, J. E., & Beck, A. T. (2005). Cognitive therapy for the prevention of suicide attempts: A randomized controlled trial. *Journal of the American Medical Association, 294*(5), 563–570. doi:10.1001/jama.294.5.563 PMID:16077050

Brown, R. (2001). Australian Indigenous mental health. *The Australian and New Zealand Journal of Mental Health Nursing, 10*(10), 33–41. doi:10.1046/j.1440-0979.2001.00189.x PMID:11421971

Bruun, A., & Hynan, C. (2006). Where to from here? Guiding for mental health for young people with complex needs. *Youth Studies Australia, 25*(1), 19–27.

Buchanan, J. L. (2012). Prevention of depression in the college student population: A review of the literature. *Archives of Psychiatric Nursing, 26*(1), 21–42. doi:10.1016/j.apnu.2011.03.003 PMID:22284078

Burns, E., & Martin, A. J. (2014). ADHD and Adaptability: The Roles of Cognitive, Behavioural, and Emotional Regulation. *Australian Journal of Guidance & Counselling, 24*(2), 227–242. doi:10.1017/jgc.2014.17

Burwick, A., Gates, G., Baumgartner, S., & Friend, D. (2014). *Human Services for Low-Income and At-Risk LGBT Populations: The Knowledge Base and Research Needs. Project Brief. OPRE Report Number 2014-84*. Washington, DC: Office of Planning, Research and Evaluation, Administration for Children and Families, U.S. Department of Health and Human Services.

Bury, M. R. (1986). Social constructionism and the development of medical sociology. *Sociology of Health & Illness, 8*(2), 137–169. doi:10.1111/1467-9566.ep11340129

Butler, H., Bond, L., Glover, S., & Patton, G. (2002). The Gatehouse Project: Mental Health Promotion Incorporating School Organisational Change and Health Education. In Mental Health Promotion and Young People: Concepts and Practice (pp. 128-141). Sydney: McGraw-Hill Australia Pty Limited.

Butler, S. S. (2017). Older lesbians receiving home care: Formal and informal dimensions of caregiving. *Journal of Women & Aging*, 1–20. PMID:28632089

Campo, M., & Tayton, S. (2015). *Intimate partner violence in lesbian, gay, bisexual, trans, intersex and queer communities*. Retrieved from https://aifs.gov.au/cfca/publications/intimate-partner-violence-lgbtiq-communities

Cap-Net. (2005). *Tutorial on basic principles of integrated water resources management (Version 2)*. New York: United Nations Development Fund Program.

Cap-Net. (2008). *Conflict resolution and negotiation skills for integrated water resources management*. New York: United Nations Development Fund Program.

Caprani, N., O'Connor, N., & Gurrin, C. (2011). Touch Screens for the Older User. In *Assistive Technologies* (pp. 95–118). Rijeka, Croatia: In-Tech.

Carius, A., Debelko, G., & Wolf, A. T. (2004). Water, conflict, and cooperation. *Environmental Change and Security Project Report, 10*, 60–66.

Carroll, A., & Mendos, L. R. (2017). *State-Sponsored Homophobia 2017: A World Survey of Sexual Orientation Laws: Criminalisation, Protection and Recognition*. Retrieved from https://ilga.org/downloads/2017/ILGA_State_Sponsored_Homophobia_2017_WEB.pdf

Carstensen, L., Isaacowitz, D. & Charles, S. (1999). Taking time seriously: A theory of socioemotional selectivity. *American Psychological Association, 54*(3) 165-181.

Carstensen, L. (1992). Social and Emotional Patterns in Adulthood: Support for Socioemotional Selectivity Theory. *Psychology and Aging, 7*(3), 331–338. doi:10.1037/0882-7974.7.3.331 PMID:1388852

Cavazzi, T., & Becerra, R. (2014). Psychophysiological Research of Borderline Personality Disorder: Review and Implications for Biosocial Theory. *Europe's Journal of Psychology, 10*(1), 185–203. doi:10.5964/ejop.v10i1.677

Cayleff, S. (2008). Feeding the hand that bit you: Lesbian daughters at mid-life negotiating parental caretaking. *Journal of Lesbian Studies, 12*(2-3), 237–254. doi:10.1080/10894160802161398 PMID:19042735

Center for Economic and Social Rights and Palestinian Hydrology Group. (2003). *Thirsting for justice: Israeli violations of human right to water in the Occupied Palestinian Territories: Parallel report to the 30th session of the United Nations CESR*. Brooklyn, NY: Center for Economic and Social Rights.

Central Intelligence Agency. (2015). *The World Factbook 2015*. Central Intelligence Agency.

Centre for Adolescent Health: The Gatehouse Project. (2017). Retrieved September 29, 2017, from https://www.rch.org.au/cah/research/The_Gatehouse_Project/

Centre of Excellence in Population Ageing Research. (2014). *Older Australian fact sheet: a statistical portrait of the older Australian*. Sydney, Australia: University of New South Wales.

Chanen, A., McCutcheon, L., Jovev, M., Jackson, H., & McGorry, P. (2007). Prevention and early intervention for Borderline Personality Disorder. *The Medical Journal of Australia, 187*(7), 18–21. PMID:17908019

Chan, S. (2010). Applications of Andragogy in Multi-Disciplined Teaching and Learning. *Journal of Adult Education, 39*(2).

Chappell, P. (2015). Queering the social emergence of disabled sexual identities: Linking queer theory with disability studies in the South African context. *Agenda (Durban, South Africa), 29*(1), 54–62.

Charles, S., & Carstensen, L. (2009). Social and emotional aging. *Annual Review of Psychology, 61*(1), 383–409. doi:10.1146/annurev.psych.093008.100448 PMID:19575618

Chehil, S., & Kutcher, S. (2012). *Suicide risk management a manual for health professionals*. Chichester, UK: Wiley.

Chen, A., McGaughey, R., Zeltmann, S., Lu, H.-K., & Lee, M. R. (2018). How seniors in Taiwan use Information Technology: Computer and cell phones. *International Journal of Human-Computer Interaction, 34*(2), 166–176. doi:10.1080/10447318.2017.1335445

Chen, N. (2015). Predicting vaccination intention and benefit and risk perceptions: The incorporation of affect, trust, and television influence in a dual-mode model. *Risk Analysis, 35*(7), 1268–1280. doi:10.1111/risa.12348 PMID:25808562

Cherry, K., Brigman, S., Lyon, B., Blanchard, B., Walker, E., & Smitherman, E. (2016). Self-reported ageism across the lifespan: Role of aging knowledge. *International Journal of Aging & Human Development*, *83*(4), 366–380. doi:10.1177/0091415016657562 PMID:27380779

Chew-Graham, C. A., Rogers, A., & Yassin, N. (2003). 'I wouldn't want it on my CV or their records': Medical students' experiences of help-seeking for mental health problems. *Medical Education*, *37*(10), 873–880. doi:10.1046/j.1365-2923.2003.01627.x PMID:12974841

Choon, L. H., Teo, E., Choo, C. T. I., Mun, L. C., Beng, L. H., Chua, M., . . . Wong, G. (2015). Allied Health Professionals. *'Singapore's Health Care System': What 50 Years Have Achieved*, 155.

Chopra, D., & Tanzi, R. E. (2012). *Super Brain: Unleash the Explosive Power of Your Mind.* Rider Books.

Christiana, J., Gilman, S., Guardino, M., Mickelson, K., Morselli, P., Olfson, M., & Kessler, R. (2000). Duration between onset and time of obtaining initial treatment among people with anxiety and mood disorders: An international survey of members of mental health patient advocate groups. *Psychological Medicine*, *30*(03), 693–703. doi:10.1017/S0033291799002093 PMID:10883723

Clancy, L., & Happell, B. (2014). Tensions of difference: Reconciling organisational imperatives for risk management with consumer-focused care from the perspectives of clinicians and managers. *Journal of Clinical Nursing*, *23*(21-22), 3177–3187. doi:10.1111/jocn.12564 PMID:25453122

Clarkin, J. F., Hull, J. W., & Hurt, S. W. (1993). Factor structure of borderline personality disorder criteria. *Journal of Personality Disorders*, *7*(2), 137–143. doi:10.1521/pedi.1993.7.2.137

Clarkson, C., Jacobs, Z., Marwick, B., Fullagar, R., Wallis, L., Smith, M., . . . Pardoe, C. (2017). Human occupation of northern Australia by 65,000 years ago. *Nature, 547*(7663), 306–310. doi:. ISSN 0028-0836.10.1038/nature22968

Collins, S. (2006). Mental health difficulties and the support needs of social work students: Dilemmas, tensions and contradictions. *Social Work Education*, *25*(5), 446–460. doi:10.1080/02615470600738809

Commonwealth of Australia. (2009). Fourth National Mental Health Plan - An agenda for collaborative government action in mental health 2009 - 2014. Canberra: Author.

Conca, K. (2006). The new face of water conflict. In Navigating Peace 3. Washington DC: Woodrow Wilson International Center for Scholars' Environmental Change and Security Program.

Connolly, M., & Healy, K. (2013). Social work practice theories and frameworks. In M. Connolly & L. Harms (Eds.), *Social work: Context and Practice* (pp. 19–33). South Melbourne, Australia: OUP.

Conrad, P. (2007). *The medicalization of society: on the transformation of human conditions into treatable disorders.* Baltimore, MD: The John Hopkins University Press.

Conrad, P., & Schneider, J. W. (1992). *Deviance and medicalization: from badness to sickness.* Philadelphia: Temple University Press.

Coon, D. W. (2007). Exploring interventions for LGBT caregivers: Issues and examples. *Journal of Gay & Lesbian Social Services*, *18*(3-4), 109–128. doi:10.1300/J041v18n03_07

Cooper, N., Stevenson, C., & Hale, G. (1996). *Integrating perspectives on health.* Buckingham, UK: Open University Press.

Cornell, S. E., & Taylor, J. B. (2000). *Sovereignty, devolution, and the future of tribal-state relations.* Cambridge, MA: Harvard University.

Cox, C. B., & Ephross, P. H. (1998). *Ethnicity and social work practice*. Oxford, UK: Oxford University press. doi:10.1093/acprof:oso/9780195099317.001.0001

Crimes Act. 1958. (Vic) (Austl.)

Croft, B., & Parish, S. (2016). Participants' assessment of the impact of behavioral health self-direction on recovery. *Community Mental Health Journal*, *52*(7), 781–792. doi:10.100710597-016-9999-0 PMID:26911369

Croghan, C. F., Moone, R. P., & Olson, A. M. (2014). Friends, family, and caregiving among midlife and older lesbian, gay, bisexual, and transgender adults. *Journal of Homosexuality*, *61*(1), 79–102. doi:10.1080/00918369.2013.835238 PMID:24313254

Crooke, A., & Travis, R. (2017). *Hip Hops healing power*. Retrieved October 20 from https://pursuit.unimelb.edu.au/articles/hip-hop-s-healing-power

Crowell, S. E., Beauchaine, T. P., & Linehan, M. M. (2009). A Biosocial Developmental Model of Borderline Personality: Elaborating and Extending Linehan's Theory. *PMC*, *135*(3), 495–510. PMID:19379027

Crowe, M. (2004). Never good enough–part 1: Shame or Borderline Personality Disorder? *Journal of Psychiatric and Mental Health Nursing*, *11*(11), 327–334. doi:10.1111/j.1365-2850.2004.00732.x PMID:15149381

Cruz, T. M. (2014). Assessing access to care for transgender and gender nonconforming people: A consideration of diversity in combating discrimination. *Social Science & Medicine*, *110*, 65–73. doi:10.1016/j.socscimed.2014.03.032 PMID:24727533

Culyer, A. J., & Wagstaff, A. (1993). Equity and equality in health and health care. *Journal of Health Economics*, *12*(4), 431–457. doi:10.1016/0167-6296(93)90004-X PMID:10131755

Currer, C., & Atherton, K. (2008). Suitable to remain a student social worker? Decision making in relation to termination of training. *Social Work Education*, *27*(3), 279–292. doi:10.1080/02615470701381343

Curtice, M. J., & Exworthy, T. (2010). FREDA: A human rights-based approach to healthcare. *The Psychiatrist*, *34*(4), 150–156. doi:10.1192/pb.bp.108.024083

Cvetkovski, S., Jorm, A. F., & Reavley, N. J. (2012). The prevalence and correlates of psychological distress in Australian tertiary students compared to their community peers. *The Australian and New Zealand Journal of Psychiatry*, *46*(5), 457–467. doi:10.1177/0004867411435290 PMID:22535294

Czaja, S. J., Sabbag, S., Lee, C. C., Schulz, R., Lang, S., Vlahovic, T., ... Thurston, C. (2016). Concerns about aging and caregiving among middle-aged and older lesbian and gay adults. *Aging & Mental Health*, *20*(11), 1107–1118. doi:10.1080/13607863.2015.1072795 PMID:26247917

Da Roit, B., & Le Bihan, B. (2010). Similar and yet so different: Cash-for-care in six European countries' long-term care policies. *The Milbank Quarterly*, *88*(8), 286–309. doi:10.1111/j.1468-0009.2010.00601.x PMID:20860573

Daily, G. C., & Ehrlich, P. R. (1992). Population, sustainability, and earth's carrying capacity. *Bioscience*, *42*(10), 761–771. doi:10.2307/1311995

Daley, A. E., & MacDonnell, J. A. (2011). Gender, sexuality and the discursive representation of access and equity in health services literature: Implications for LGBT communities. *International Journal for Equity in Health*, *10*(1), 40. doi:10.1186/1475-9276-10-40 PMID:21957894

Daniel Davis, F. (2000). Friendship as an ideal for the patient-physician relationship: A critique and an alternative. In D. C. Thomasma & J. L. Kissell (Eds.), *The health care professional a friend and healer: Building on the work of Edmund D. Pellegrino* (pp. 24–34). Washington, DC: Georgetown University Press.

Daniels, N. (1985). *Just health care.* Cambridge University Press. doi:10.1017/CBO9780511624971

Daniels, N. (1999). Decisions about access to health care and accountability for reasonableness. *Journal of Urban Health, 76*(2), 176–191. doi:10.1007/BF02344674 PMID:10924028

Daniels, N., & Sabin, J. E. (2008). *Setting limits fairly: learning to share resources for health.* Oxford University Press.

Darlington Statement: Joint consensus statement from the intersex community retreat in Darlington, March 2017. (2017). Working Paper. Sydney, NSW: QUT.

Darlington, A. (2011). Raising a critical consciousness for the reformation of health care culture. *Canadian Journal of Respiratory Therapy, 47*(3), 6–12.

Davies, K., & Gray, M. (2015). Mental health service users' aspirations for recovery: examining the gaps between what policy promises and practice delivers. *British Journal of Social Work, 45*(suppl 1), i45-i61.

Day, L. (2012). Journeying to a new understanding of cultural safety. *Kai Taiki Nursing New Zealand, 18*(4), 14–15. PMID:22866462

De Bortoli, L., Ogloff, J., Coles, J., & Dolan, M. (2017). Towards best practice: Combining evidence-based research, structured assessment and professional judgement. *Child & Family Social Work, 22*(2), 660–669. doi:10.1111/cfs.12280

De Houwer, J., Barnes-Holmes, D., & Moors, A. (2013). What is learning? On the nature and merits of a functional definition of learning. *Psychonomic Bulletin & Review, 20*(4), 631–642. doi:10.375813423-013-0386-3 PMID:23359420

Deacon, B. J. (2013). The biomedical model of mental disorder: A critical analysis of its validity, utility, and effects on psychotherapy research. *Clinical Psychology Review, 33*(7), 846–861. doi:10.1016/j.cpr.2012.09.007 PMID:23664634

Deci, E. L., & Ryan, R. M. (1985). The general causality orientations scale: Self-determination in personality. *Journal of Research in Personality, 19*(2), 109–134. doi:10.1016/0092-6566(85)90023-6

Deci, E. L., & Ryan, R. M. (2008). Facilitating optimal motivation and psychological well-being across life's domain. *Canadian Psychology, 49*(1), 14–23. doi:10.1037/0708-5591.49.1.14

Deckop, J., & Cirka, C. (2000). The Risk and Reward of a Double-Edgedsword: Effects of a Merit Payprogram on Intrinsic Motivation. *Nonprofit and Voluntary Sector Quarterly, 29*(3), 400–418. doi:10.1177/0899764000293003

del-Pino-Casado, R., Frías-Osuna, A., & Palomino-Moral, P. A. (2011). Subjective burden and cultural motives for caregiving in informal caregivers of older people. *Journal of Nursing Scholarship, 43*(3), 282–291. PMID:21884374

Department of Communities, Child Safety and Disability Services. (2012). *Ageing: Myth and reality.* Brisbane, Queensland: Queensland Government, Department of Communities, Child Safety and Disability Services.

Department of Economic and Social Affairs. (2017). *World population ageing.* New York: United Nations.

Department of Families, Housing, Community Services and Indigenous Affairs (FaHCSIA). (2009). *Footprints in Time: The Longitudinal Study of Indigenous Children – Key Summary Report from Wave 1.* Canberra: Commonwealth of Australia.

Department of Health and Human Services. (2018). *Concessions and benefits.* Melbourne, Australia: Victorian State Government.

Department of Health Australia. (2012). *Australian statistics on medicines 2010.* Canberra: Commonwealth of Australia.

Department of Health Hume Region. (2011). *Review of HACC Allied Health Services.* Melbourne: Author. Retrieved from: http://www.health.vic.gov.au/hacc/publications/downloads/hume/allied_healthreport2011.pdf

Dew, A., Veitch, C., Lincoln, M., Brentnall, J., Bulkeley, K., Gallego, G., ... Griffiths, S. (2012). The need for new models for delivery of therapy intervention to people with a disability in rural and remote areas of Australia. *Journal of Intellectual & Developmental Disability*, *37*(1), 50–53. doi:10.3109/13668250.2011.644269 PMID:22211532

Di Stefano, G. (2010). Courting the Blues: Attitudes towards depression in Australian law students and legal practitioners. *Bulletin*, *32*(4), 18.

Dickinson, H. (2017, September). Individual funding systems: What works? *Evidence Base*, *2017*(3), 1–18. doi:10.21307/eb-2017-003

Dickson, E. (2012). The assessment of students with disabilities: The Australian law as to reasonable adjustment and academic integrity. *International Journal of Law & Education*, *17*(2), 49–61.

Disability Discrimination Act, 1992 (Cwth).

Disability Standards for Education Review Team (DSERT). (2012). *Report on the Review of Disability Standards for Education 2005.* Retrieved 14 May, 2016, from https://docs.education.gov.au/system/files/doc/other/report_on_the_review_of_disability_standards_for_education_2005.pdf

Disability Standards for Education. (2005). *Attorney General.* Canberra: Author.

Distel, M. A., Willemsen, G., Ligthart, L., Derom, C. A., Martin, N. G., Neale, M. C., ... Boomsma, D. I. (2010). Genetic covariance structure of the four main features of borderline personality disorder. *Journal of Personality Disorders*, *24*(4), 427–444. doi:10.1521/pedi.2010.24.4.427 PMID:20695804

Dixon, A., Le Grand, J., Henderson, J., Murray, R., & Poteliakhoff, E. (2007). Is the British National Health Service equitable? The evidence on socioeconomic differences in utilization. *Journal of Health Services Research & Policy*, *12*(2), 104–109. doi:10.1258/135581907780279549 PMID:17407661

Dodd, S. (2013). Personalisation, individualism and the politics of disablement. *Disability & Society*, *28*(2), 260–273. doi:10.1080/09687599.2012.699283

Doel, M., Allmark, P., Conway, P., Cowburn, M., Flynn, M., Nelson, P., & Tod, A. (2010). Professional boundaries: Crossing a line or entering the shadows? *British Journal of Social Work*, *40*(6), 1866–1889. doi:10.1093/bjsw/bcp106

Doidge, N. (2015). *The Brain's Way of Healing*. London: Penguin Books Ltd.

Domes, G., Winter, B., Schnell, K., Voha, K., Fast, K., & Herpertz, S. C. (2006). The influence of emotions on inhibitory functioning in Borderline Personality Disorder. *Psychological Medicine*, *36*(08), 1163–1172. doi:10.1017/S0033291706007756 PMID:16700964

Donisch, K., Bray, C., & Gewirtz, A. (2016). Child welfare, juvenile justice, mental health, and education providers' conceptualizations of trauma-informed practice. *Child Maltreatment*, *21*(2), 125–134. doi:10.1177/1077559516633304 PMID:26957441

Donkor, S. M. K., & Wolde, Y. E. (2012). *Integrated Water Resources Management in Africa: Issues and Options. The United Nations Water Development Report.* Washington, DC: United Nations Economic Commission for Africa.

Donovan, D. M., Thomas, L. R., Sigo, R. L. W., Price, L., Lonczak, H., ... Bagley, L. (2015). Healing of the canoe: Preliminary results of a culturally grounded intervention to prevent substance abuse and promote tribal identity for native youth in two Pacific Northwest tribe. *American Indian and Alaska Native Mental Health Research*, *22*(1), 42–76. doi:10.5820/aian.2201.2015.42 PMID:25768390

Doubé, W., & Beh, J. (2012). *Typing Over Auto Complete: Cognitive Load in Website Use by Older Adults*. Melbourne, Australia: ACM Press.

Double, D. (2002). The limits of psychiatry. *British Medical Journal*, *324*(7342), 900–904. doi:10.1136/bmj.324.7342.900 PMID:11950743

Douglas, M. (1990). Risk as a forensic resource. *Daedalus*, *119*(4), 1–16.

Douglas, M. (1992). *Risk and blame: Essays in cultural theory*. London: Routledge. doi:10.4324/9780203430866

Doutrich, D., Arcus, K., Dekker, L., Spuck, J., & Pollock-Robinson, C. (2012). Cultural safety in New Zealand and the United States: Looking at a way forward together. *Journal of Transcultural Nursing*, *23*(2), 143–150. doi:10.1177/1043659611433873 PMID:22282876

Doyle, J., Skrba, Z., McDonnell, R., & Arent, B. (2010). Designing a Touch Screen Communication Device to Support Social Interaction amongst Older Adults. In *BCS '10 Proceedings of the 24th BCS Interaction Specialist Group Conference* (pp. 177-185), Swindon, UK: BCS Learning and Development Ltd.

Drescher, J. (2015). Out of DSM: Depathologizing homosexuality. *Behavioral Science*, *5*(4), 565–575. doi:10.3390/bs5040565 PMID:26690228

Drescher, J. (2015). Queer diagnoses revisited: The past and future of homosexuality and gender diagnoses in DSM and ICD. *International Review of Psychiatry (Abingdon, England)*, *27*(5), 386–395. doi:10.3109/09540261.2015.1053847 PMID:26242413

Dudgeon, P., Milroy, H., & Walker, R. (Eds.). (2014). Working together: Aboriginal and Torres Strait Islander mental health and wellbeing principles and practices. Barton, ACT: Commonwealth of Australia.

Dupre, M. E. (2013). *Social work education and disability: a multicase study of approaches to disability in core and specialized curricula in three Bachelor of Social Work programs* (Unpublished doctoral dissertation). University of Manitoba, Manitoba.

Durick, J., Robertson, T., Brereton, M., Vetere, F., & Nansen, B. (2013). *Dispelling Ageing Myths in Technology Design*. Adelaide, Australia: OzCHI.

Dykewomon, E. (2017). The caregiver and her friends. *Journal of Lesbian Studies*, 1–8. PMID:28339346

Eagleton-Pierce, M. (2016). *Neoliberalism: The key concepts*. New York: Routledge.

Early Childhood and Primary Schools: KidsMatter & KidsMatter Early Childhood. (2016). Retrieved October 08, 2017, from https://www.beyondblue.org.au/healthy-places/early-childhood-and-primary-schools

Easter, C., & Ruckman, N. (Producers). (2013). *Dr Michael Yellow Bird, Decolonizing the Mind: Healing through neurodecolonization and mindfulness* (video recording). Portland State University. Retrieved from https://vimeo.com/86995336

Edgar, P. (2013). *In Praise of Ageing*. Melbourne, Australia: Text Publishing.

Eisenberg, D., Downs, M. F., Golberstein, E., & Zivin, K. (2009). Stigma and help seeking for mental health among college students. *Medical Care Research and Review*, *66*(5), 522–541. doi:10.1177/1077558709335173 PMID:19454625

Ekeke, E. C. (2011). African traditional religion: A conceptual and philosophical analysis. *LUMINA*, 22(2). Retrieved from https://ejournals.ph/article.php?id=7341

El Ansarı, W., Stock, C., Snelgrove, T. U. K. S. H. G. S., Hu, X., Parke, S., Davies, S., ... Mabhala, A. (2011). Feeling healthy? A survey of physical and psychological wellbeing of students from seven universities in the UK. *International Journal of Environmental Research and Public Health*, *8*(5), 1308–1323. doi:10.3390/ijerph8051308 PMID:21655121

El-Fadel, M., El-Sayegh, Y., El-Fadl, K., & Khorbotly, D. (2003). The Nile River Basin: A case study in surface water conflict resolution. *Journal of Natural Resources and Life Sciences Education*, *32*, 107–117.

Elliot, A., Mcllwaine, F., Stone, N., & Proctor, K. (2015). *The Bouverie Centre's Aboriginal Family Therapy Training Program: Impact Analysis Report.* Melbourne: The Lowitja Institute.

Elpers, K., & FitzGerald, E. A. (2013). Issues and challenges in gatekeeping: A framework for implementation. *Social Work Education*, *32*(3), 286–300. doi:10.1080/02615479.2012.665867

Emanuel, E. J. (2000). Justice and managed care: Four principles for the just allocation of health care resources. *The Hastings Center Report*, *30*(3), 8–16. doi:10.2307/3528040 PMID:10862365

Embracing Carers. (2017). *Embracing the Critical Role of Caregivers Around the World.* Darmstadt, Germany: Merck GKaA.

Engel, G. L. (1977). The need for a new medical model: A challenge for biomedicine. *Science*, *8*(4286), 129–136. doi:10.1126cience.847460 PMID:847460

Ennals, P., Fossey, E., & Howie, L. (2015). Postsecondary study and mental ill-health: A meta-synthesis of qualitative research exploring students' lived experiences. *Journal of Mental Health (Abingdon, England)*, *24*(2), 111–119. doi:10 .3109/09638237.2015.1019052 PMID:25915818

Erickson, R. J. (2005). Why emotion work matters: Sex, gender, and the division of household labor. *Journal of Marriage and the Family*, *67*(2), 337–351. doi:10.1111/j.0022-2445.2005.00120.x

European Environment Agency. (2015). *Annual Report 2014.* Luxembourg: European Union.

Evans, B. R. (1999). *The cost of corruption.* Teddington, UK: Tearfund.

Fallot, R. D., & Harris, M. (2008). Trauma-informed approaches to systems of care. *Trauma Psychology Newsletter*, *3*(1), 6–7.

FAO. (2011). *The state of the world's land and water resources for food and agriculture (SOLAW): Managing systems at risk.* Earthscan.

Fawcett, B., & Plath, D. (2014). A National Disability Insurance Scheme: What social work has to offer. *British Journal of Social Work*, *44*(3), 747–762. doi:10.1093/bjsw/bcs141

Fish, J. (2006). *Heterosexism in health and social care.* Springer. doi:10.1057/9780230800731

Fleck, L. (2001). Healthcare justice and rational democratic deliberation. *The American Journal of Bioethics*, *1*(2), 20–21. doi:10.1162/152651601300168852 PMID:11951873

Fonseca-Pedrero, E., Paino, M., Lemos-Giraldez, S., Sierra-Baigrie, S., Gonzalez, M. P., Bobes, J., & Muniz, J. (2011). Borderline personality traits in nonclinical young adults. *Journal of Personality Disorders*, *25*(4), 542–556. doi:10.1521/pedi.2011.25.4.542 PMID:21838568

Forrester-Jones, R., & Barnes, A. (2008). On being a girlfriend not a patient: The quest for an acceptable identity amongst people diagnosed with a severe mental illness. *Journal of Mental Health (Abingdon, England)*, *17*(2), 153–172. doi:10.1080/09638230701498341

Foster, M. M., Mitchell, G., Haines, T., Tweedy, S., Cornwell, P., & Fleming, J. (2008). Does Enhanced Primary Care enhance primary care? Policy-induced dilemmas for allied health professionals. *The Medical Journal of Australia*, *188*(1), 29. PMID:18205560

Foucault, M. (1967). *Madness and civilization*. London: Routledge.

Francis, A. P., Pulla, V., & Goel, K. (2014). Community development and mental health promotion. In K. Goel, V. Pulla, & A. P. Francis (Eds.), *Community work: Theories, experiences & challenges* (pp. 162–180). Bangalore, India: Niruta Publications.

Frankland, R., Bamblett, M., & Lewis, P. (2011). Forever Business: A framework for maintaining and restoring cultural safety in Aboriginal Victoria. *Indigenous Law Bulletin*, *7*(24), 27–30.

Fredriksen-Goldsen, K. I., & Hooyman, N. R. (2007). Caregiving research, services, and policies in historically marginalized communities: Where do we go from here? *Journal of Gay & Lesbian Social Services*, *18*(3-4), 129–145. doi:10.1300/J041v18n03_08

Fredriksen-Goldsen, K. I., Kim, H. J., Muraco, A., & Mincer, S. (2009). Chronically ill midlife and older lesbians, gay men, and bisexuals and their informal caregivers: The impact of the social context. *Sexuality Research and Social Policy Journal of NSRC*, *6*(4), 52–64. doi:10.1525rsp.2009.6.4.52 PMID:20436796

Fried, E. J., Bockting, C., Ajard, R., Borsboom, D., Amshoff, M., Cramer, O. J., ... Carr, D. (2015). From loss to loneliness: The relationship between bereavement and depressive symptoms. *Journal of Abnormal Psychology*, *124*(2), 256–265. doi:10.1037/abn0000028 PMID:25730514

Fromene, R., & Guerin, B. (2014). Talking with Australian Indigenous Clients with a Borderline Personality Disorder Diagnosis: Finding the Context behind the Label. *The Psychological Record*, *64*(3), 569–579. doi:10.100740732-014-0058-3

Fromene, R., Guerin, B., & Krieg, A. (2014). Australian Indigenous Clients with a Borderline Personality Disorder Diagnosis: A Contextual Review of the Literature. *The Psychological Record*, *64*(3), 599.

Fulcher, G. (1989). *Disabling policies?: a comparative approach to education, policy, and disability*. New York: Falmer Press.

Fuller, M., Healey, M., Bradley, A., & Hall, T. (2004). Barriers to learning: A systematic study of the experience of disabled students in one university. *Studies in Higher Education*, *29*(3), 303–318. doi:10.1080/03075070410001682592

Garner, H. (2014). *This house of grief*. Melbourne: Text Publishing.

Garve, R., Garve, M., Türp, J. C., Fobil, J. N., & Meyer, C. G. (2017). Scarification in sub-Saharan Africa: Social skin, remedy and medical import. *Tropical Medicine & International Health*, *22*(6), 708–715. doi:10.1111/tmi.12878 PMID:28380287

Gay and Lesbian Health Victoria. (n.d.). *LGBTI Inclusive Practice*. Retrieved from https://www.glhv.org.au/lgbti-inclusive-practice

Gehrig, J., & Rogers, M. (2009). *Water and conflict: incorporating peacebuilding into water development*. Baltimore, MD: Catholic Relief Services.

Ghafoor, S. (2008). Out of harms way. *Nursing Standard (through 2013)*, *22*(43), 61-61.

Gichuki, F. (2002). Water conflicts in the Upper Ewaso Ngiro North Basin: causes, impacts and management strategies. E-conference paper.

Gill, D., & Warburton, W. (2014). An Investigation of the Biosocial Model of Borderline Personality Disorder. *Journal of Clinical Psychology*, *70*(9), 866–873. doi:10.1002/jclp.22074 PMID:24585693

Gillis, H., & Lewis, J. S. (2004). Addressing the issue of psychiatric disability in social work interns: The need for a problem-solving framework. *Journal of Social Work Education*, *40*(3), 391–402. doi:10.1080/10437797.2004.10672295

Glaesser, R. S., & Patel, B. R. (2016). Psychological Trauma and LGBT Caregivers: A Conceptual Framework to Guide Practice. *Journal of Evidence-Informed Social Work*, *13*(5), 458–468. doi:10.1080/23761407.2016.1166825 PMID:27119978

Glasby, J. a., & Littlechild, R. (2016). Direct payments and personal budgets: putting personalisation into practice (3rd ed.). Bristol, UK: Policy Press.

Glendinning, C. (2008). Increasing choice and control for older and disabled people: A critical review of new developments in England. *Social Policy and Administration*, *42*(5), 451–469. doi:10.1111/j.1467-9515.2008.00617.x

Glymour, M., Weuve, J., Martha, E., Glass, T., & Berkman, L. (2008). Social ties and cognitive recovery after stroke: Does social integration promote cognitive resilience? *Neuroepidemiology*, *31*(1), 10–20. doi:10.1159/000136646 PMID:18535395

Goffman, E. (1959). *The presentation of self in everyday life*. London: Penguin.

Goffman, E. (1963). *Stigma: notes on the management of spoiled identity*. New York: Touchstone.

Golberstein, E., Eisenberg, D., & Gollust, S. E. (2009). Perceived stigma and help-seeking behavior: Longitudinal evidence from the healthy minds study. *Psychiatric Services (Washington, D.C.)*, *60*(9), 1254–1256. doi:10.1176/ps.2009.60.9.1254 PMID:19723742

Goldney, R. D. (2012). Problems with suicide risk assessment. *The Australian and New Zealand Journal of Psychiatry*, *46*(2), 172–173. doi:10.1177/0004867411433223 PMID:22311534

Gone, J. P. (2009). A community based treatment for Native American historical trauma: Prospects for evidence-based practice. *Journal of Consulting and Clinical Psychology*, *77*(4), 751–762. doi:10.1037/a0015390 PMID:19634967

Gooding, P. (2016). From deinstitutionalisation to consumer empowerment: Mental health policy, neoliberal restructuring and the closure of the 'Big bins' in Victoria. *Health Sociology Review*, *25*(1), 33–47. doi:10.1080/14461242.2015.1134261

Graham, I. D., Logan, J., Harrison, M. B., Straus, S. E., Tetroe, J., Caswell, W., & Robinson, N. (2006). Lost in knowledge translation: Time for a map? *The Journal of Continuing Education in the Health Professions*, *26*(1), 13–24. doi:10.1002/chp.47 PMID:16557505

Graham, S., & Weiner, B. (1996). *Theories and Principles of Motivation. Cognition and Motivation*. New York: Prentice Hall.

Gratz, K. L., & Roemer, L. (2004). Multidimensional assessment of emotion regulation and dysregulation: Development, factor structure, and initial validation of the Difficulties in Emotion Regulation Scale. *Journal of Psychopathology and Behavioral Assessment*, *26*(1), 41–54. doi:10.1023/B:JOBA.0000007455.08539.94

Gratz, K. L., & Roemer, L. (2008). The relationship between emotion dysregulation and deliberate self-harm among female undergraduate students at an urban commuter university. *Cognitive Behaviour Therapy*, *37*(1), 14–25. doi:10.1080/16506070701819524 PMID:18365795

Gray, M., Coates, J., Yellow Bird, M. & Hetherington, T. (Eds.). (2013). Decolonising Social Work. Burlington, VT: Ashgate.

Gray, M., Yellow Bird, M., & Coates, J. (Eds.). (2008). Towards an understanding of Indigenous Social Work. In M. Gray, M. Yellow Bird & J. Coates (Eds.), Indigenous Social Work Around the World: Towards Culturally Relevant Education and Practice (pp. 49-58). Burlington, VT: Ashgate.

Greenberg, J. S. (1995). The Other Side of Caring: Adult Children with Mental Illness as Supports to Their-Mothers in Later Life. *Social Work*, *40*(3), 414–423. PMID:7761928

Greene, S. (1998). The shaman's needle: Development, shamanic agency, and intermedicality in Aguarana Lands, Peru. *American Ethnologist*, *25*(4), 634–658. doi:10.1525/ae.1998.25.4.634

Greenwood, N., Habibi, R., Smith, R., & Manthorpe, J. (2015). Barriers to access and minority ethnic carers' satisfaction with social care services in the community: A systematic review of qualitative and quantitative literature. *Health & Social Care in the Community*, *23*(1), 64–78. doi:10.1111/hsc.12116 PMID:25135207

Greider, T., & Garkovich, L. (1994). Landscapes: The social construction of nature and the environment. *Rural Sociology*, *59*(2), 1–24.

Grotto, J., Gerace, A., O'Kane, D., Simpson, A., Oster, C., & Muir-Cochrane, E. (2015). Risk assessment and absconding: Perceptions, understandings and responses of mental health nurses. *Journal of Clinical Nursing*, *24*(5-6), 855–865. doi:10.1111/jocn.12671 PMID:25209549

Gruskin, S., & Daniels, N. (2008). Process is the point: justice and human rights: priority setting and fair deliberative process. *American Journal of Public Health*, *98*(9), 1573–1577. doi:10.2105/AJPH.2007.123182 PMID:18633088

Gruskin, S., Mills, E. J., & Tarantola, D. (2007). History, principles, and practice of health and human rights. *Lancet*, *370*(9585), 449–455. doi:10.1016/S0140-6736(07)61200-8 PMID:17679022

Gunderson, J. G. (2006). *A BPD Brief: An introduction to Borderline Personality Disorder*. New York: Borderline Personality Disorder Resource Center.

Gunderson, J. G., Stout, R. L., McGlashan, T. H., Shea, M. T., Morey, L. C., Grilo, C. M., ... Skodol, A. E. (2011). Ten-year course of borderline personality disorder: Psychopathology and function from the Collaborative Longitudinal Personality Disorders study. *Archives of General Psychiatry*, *68*(8), 827–837. doi:10.1001/archgenpsychiatry.2011.37 PMID:21464343

Guzder, J., Paris, J., Zelkowitz, P., & Feldman, R. (1999). Psychological risk factors for borderline pathology in school-age children. *Journal of the American Academy of Child and Adolescent Psychiatry*, *38*(2), 205–212. doi:10.1097/00004583-199902000-00021 PMID:9951221

Hagay, G., Baram-Tsabari, A., Ametller, J., Cakmakci, G., Lopes, B., Moreira, A., & Pedrosa-de-Jesus, H. (2013). The Generalizability of Students' Interests in Biology across Gender, Country and Religion. *Research in Science Education*, *43*(3), 895–919. doi:10.100711165-012-9289-y

Haghiri-Vijeh, R. (2013). The Importance of Including the Needs of the LGBTIQ Community in the Millennium Development Goals and Education of Healthcare Professionals. *Journal of Global Citizenship & Equity Education*, *3*(1), 68.

Haines, T. P., Foster, M. M., Cornwell, P., Fleming, J., Tweedy, S., Hart, A., & Mitchell, G. (2010). Impact of Enhanced Primary Care on equitable access to and economic efficiency of allied health services: A qualitative investigation. *Australian Health Review*, *34*(1), 30–35. doi:10.1071/AH09732 PMID:20334753

Hallahan, L. (2015). Disability policy in Australia: A triumph of the scriptio inferior on impotence and neediness? *The Australian Journal of Social Issues*, *50*(2), 191–209. doi:10.1002/j.1839-4655.2015.tb00344.x

Hamilton, S., Tew, J., Szymczynska, P., Clewett, N., Manthorpe, J., Larsen, J., & Pinfold, V. (2016). Power, choice and control: How do personal budgets affect the experiences of people with mental health problems and their relationships with social workers and other practitioners? *British Journal of Social Work*, *46*(3), 719–736. doi:10.1093/bjsw/bcv023

Hanjra, M. A., & Qureshi, M. E. (2010). Global water crisis and future food security in an era of climate change. *Food Policy*, *35*(5), 365–377. doi:10.1016/j.foodpol.2010.05.006

Happell, B. (2007). Appreciating the importance of history: A brief historical overview of mental health, mental health nursing and education in Australia. *The International Journal of Psychiatric Nursing Research*, *12*(2), 1439–1445. PMID:17283958

Harley, D. A., Nowak, T. M., Gassaway, L. J., & Savage, T. A. (2002). Lesbian, gay, bisexual, and transgender college students with disabilities: A look at multiple cultural minorities. *Psychology in the Schools*, *39*(5), 525–538. doi:10.1002/pits.10052

Harris, K. M., & Edlund, M. J. (2005). Self-medication of mental health problems: New evidence from a national survey. *Health Services Research*, *40*(1), 117–134. doi:10.1111/j.1475-6773.2005.00345.x PMID:15663705

Harris, M., & Fallot, R. D. (2001). *Using trauma theory to design service systems*. San Francisco, CA: Jossey Bass.

Hart, L. M., Mason, R. J., Kelly, C. M., Cvetkovski, S., & Jorm, A. F. (2016). 'teen Mental Health First Aid': A description of the program an initial evaluation. *International Journal of Mental Health Systems*, *10*(3), 1–18. PMID:26788123

Harvey, A., Burnheim, C., & Brett, M. (2016). Towards a fairer chance for all: Revising the Australian student equity framework. In A. Harvey, C. Burnheim, & M. Brett (Eds.), *Student Equity in Australian Higher Education: Twenty-five Years of A Fair Chance for All*. Singapore: Springer. doi:10.1007/978-981-10-0315-8_1

Harvey, P., & Thurnwald, I. (2009). Ageing Well, Ageing Productively: The Essential Contribution of Australia's Ageing Population to the Social and Economic Prosperity of the Nation. *Health Sociology Review*, *18*(4), 379–386. doi:10.5172/hesr.2009.18.4.379

Harvey, R., Black, D. W., & Blum, N. (2010). Systems Training for Emotional Predictability and Problem Solving (STEPPS) in the United Kingdom: A Preliminary Report. *Journal of Contemporary Psychotherapy*, *40*(4), 225–232. doi:10.100710879-010-9150-4

Hash, K. M., & Netting, F. E. (2009). It takes a community: Older lesbians meeting social and care needs. *Journal of Gay & Lesbian Social Services*, *21*(4), 326–342. doi:10.1080/10538720802497910

Hay, J. (2012). Considering the spiritual dimension of human life and its relevance to social work education: Social workers', educators' and students' views. *Advances in Social Work and Welfare Education*, *14*(1), 52–66.

HeadStrong 2.0. (2017). Retrieved October 14, 2017, from https://www.blackdoginstitute.org.au/education-training/community-and-schools/free-school-resources/headstrong-2.0

Hebb, D. O. (1949). *The organization of behaviour*. New York: Wiley.

Hepworth, J. (1999). *The social construction of anorexia nervosa*. London: Sage Publications.

Herman, J. L. (1997). *Trauma and Recovery*. New York: Basic Books.

Herring, S., Spangaro, J., Lauw, M., & McNamara, L. (2013). The intersection of trauma, racism and cultural competence in effective work with Aboriginal people: Waiting for trust. *Australian Social Work*, *66*(1), 104–117. doi:10.1080/0312407X.2012.697566

Hidi, S., & Renninger, K. A. (2006). The four-phase model of interest development. *Educational Psychologist*, *41*(2), 111–127. doi:10.120715326985ep4102_4

Hill, T., Cass, B., Newton, B., & Valentine, K. (2012). *Indigenous carers*. Social Policy Research Paper No. 45.

Hillman, A., Tadd, W., Calnan, S., Calnan, M., Bayer, A., & Read, S. (2013). Risk, governance and the experience of care. *Sociology of Health & Illness*, *35*(6), 939–955. doi:10.1111/1467-9566.12017 PMID:23356787

Hinrichsen, D., & Tacio, H. (2011). *Finding the source: The coming freshwater crisis is already here*. Washington, DC: Woodrow Wilson International Center for Scholars.

Hochschild, A. R. (1979). Emotion work, feeling rules, and social structure. *American Journal of Sociology*, *85*(3), 551–575. doi:10.1086/227049

Horlick-Jones, T. (2005a). Informal logics of risk: Contingency and modes of practical reasoning. *Journal of Risk Research*, *8*(3), 253–272. doi:10.1080/1366987042000270735

Horlick-Jones, T. (2005b). On 'risk work': Professional discourse, accountability, and everyday action. *Health Risk & Society*, *7*(3), 293–307. doi:10.1080/13698570500229820

House of Representatives Standing Committee on Aboriginal and Torres Strait Islander Affairs. (2011). *Doing Time - Time for Doing: Indigenous youth in the criminal justice system*. Canberra, ACT: Commonwealth of Australia. Retrieved from: https://www.aph.gov.au/binaries/house/committee/atsia/sentencing/report/fullreport.pdf

Howe, B., & Duffy, M. (1992). *Disability Discrimination Bill, Explanatory Memorandum*. Canberra: Parliament of Australia. Retrieved 20 May, 2016, from http://www.humanrights.gov.au/disability-discrimination-bill-1992-explanatory-memorandum

Hudson, P. (2013). Improving support for family carers: Key implications for research, policy and practice. *Palliative Medicine*, *27*(7), 581–582. doi:10.1177/0269216313488855 PMID:23780618

Huggins, R., Izushi, H., Prokop, D., & Thompson, P. (2014). *The global competitiveness of regions: Regions and cities*. London, UK: Routledge.

Human Rights and Equal Opportunity Commission. (1997). *Bringing Them Home: National Inquiry into the Separation of Aboriginal and Torres Strait Islander Children from Their Families*. Sydney, NSW: Commonwealth of Australia.

Hunter and New England Local Health District v. McKenna (2014) (HCA) (Austl.).

Hunter Institute of Mental Health. (2014). *Reporting suicide and mental illness: A Mindframe resource for media professionals*. Newcastle, Australia: Hunter Institute of Mental Health.

Hunter, E., Gill, N., & Toombs, M. (2013). Mental health among Indigenous Australians. In R. Hampton & M. Toombs (Eds.), *Indigenous Australians and health: The wombat in the room* (pp. 206–224). South Melbourne: Oxford University Press.

Hunt, J., & Eisenberg, D. (2010). Mental health problems and help-seeking behavior among college students. *The Journal of Adolescent Health*, *46*(1), 3–10. doi:10.1016/j.jadohealth.2009.08.008 PMID:20123251

Hutchison, P., Lord, J., & Salisbury, B. (2006). North American approaches to individualised planning and direct funding. In J. Leece & J. Bornat (Eds.), *Developments in Direct Payments* (pp. 49–62). Bristol, UK: The Policy Press, University of Bristol. doi:10.2307/j.ctt1t898xj 8

Ianculescu, M., Lupeanu, E., Alexandru, A., Tudora, E., Coman, O. & Coman, L. (2011). Strengthening the Role of Medical Informatics in Promoting a Successful Positive Ageing. *Recent Advances in Applied & Biomedical Informatics and Computational Engineering in Systems Applications*, 305-310.

Ife, J. (2010). *Human rights from below: Achieving rights through community development.* Cambridge, UK: Cambridge University Press.

Ikenga-Metuh, E. (1985). Ritual dirt and purification rites among the Igbo. *Journal of Religion in Africa. Religion en Afrique*, *15*(1), 3–24. doi:10.1163/157006685X00020

Imison, C., Sonola, L., Honeyman, M., & Ross, S. (2014). The reconfiguration of clinical services. *What is the evidence*.

Irish Association of Social Workers (IASW). (2011). *Lesbian, Gay & Bisexual People: A Guide to Good Practice for Social Workers*. Retrieved from https://www.iasw.ie/download/4/5f24c87f-8792-4df1-a8d6-294bdbe6e851.PDF

Irlam, C. B. (2012). *LGBTI Data: developing an evidence-informed environment for LGBTI health policy*. Sydney: National LGBTI Health Alliance.

Irwin, L. (2007). Homophobia and heterosexism: Implications for nursing and nursing practice. *The Australian Journal of Advanced Nursing*, *25*(1), 70.

Izquierdo, L., Stangerhaugen, M., Castillo, D., Nixon, R., & Jimenez, G. (2010). *Water Crisis in Central Asia: Key Challenges and Opportunities*. New York: Graduate Program in International Affairs, New School University.

Jackson, H., & Burgess, P. M. (2000). Personality Disorders in the Community: A report from the Australian National Survey of Mental Health and Wellbeing. *Social Psychiatry and Psychiatric Epidemiology*, *12*(53), 1–8. PMID:11213842

Jeffrey, C., & Craig, D. (2011). Application of Environmental Conflict Resolution to Public Interest Issues in Water Disputes. International Journal of Rural Law and Policy, 1, 1-13.

Jeong, H. (2011). *The Skill of Communication in Aged Care (Master of Science)*. Aged and Community Services.

Johnson, C. V., Mimiaga, M. J., & Bradford, J. (2008). Health care issues among lesbian, gay, bisexual, transgender and intersex (LGBTI) populations in the United States: Introduction. *Journal of Homosexuality*, *54*(3), 213–224. doi:10.1080/00918360801982025 PMID:18825859

Johnstone, M. J., & Kanitsaki, O. (2009). The spectrum of 'new racism' and discrimination in hospital contexts: A reappraisal. *Collegian (Royal College of Nursing, Australia)*, *16*(2), 63–69. doi:10.1016/j.colegn.2009.03.001 PMID:19583175

Johnston, K. N., Mackintosh, S., Alcock, M., Conlon-Leard, A., & Manson, S. (2016). Reconsidering inherent requirements: A contribution to the debate from the clinical placement experience of a physiotherapy student with vision impairment. *BMC Medical Education*, *16*(1), 74. doi:10.118612909-016-0598-0 PMID:26922499

Joint Standing Commitee. (2017). *Joint Standing Committee Report on the National Disability Insurance Scheme, Provision of services under the NDIS for people with psychosocial disabilities related to a mental health condition*. Retrieved from http://www.aph.gov.au/Parliamentary_Business/Committees/Joint/National_Disability_Insurance_Scheme/MentalHealth/Report

Jones, D. K., Bradley, K. W., & Oberlander, J. (2014). Pascal's Wager: Health insurance exchanges, Obamacare, and the Republican dilemma. *Journal of Health Politics, Policy and Law*, *39*(1), 97–137. doi:10.1215/03616878-2395190 PMID:24193607

Jones, S., & Fernyhough, C. (2007). A new look at the neural diathesis stress model of schizophrenia: The primacy of social evaluative and uncontrollable situations. *Schizophrenia Bulletin*, *33*(5), 1171–1177. doi:10.1093chbulbl058 PMID:17105966

Jongerden, J. (2010). Dams and politics in Turkey: Utilizing water, developing conflict. *Middle East Policy*, *17*(1), 137–143. doi:10.1111/j.1475-4967.2010.00432.x

Jordans, M. J. D., Tol, A. W., Komproe, I. H., & de Jong, J. V. T. M. (2009). Systematic review of evidence and treatment approaches: Psychosocial and mental health care for children in war. *Child and Adolescent Mental Health*, *14*(1), 2–14. doi:10.1111/j.1475-3588.2008.00515.x

Jorm, A. F. (2011). Mental Health Literacy: Empowering the Community to Take Action for Better Mental Health. *The American Psychologist*, 1–12. PMID:22040221

Jorm, A. F., & Kelly, C. M. (2007). Improving the public's understanding and response to mental disorders. *Australian Psychologist*, *42*(2), 81–89. doi:10.1080/00050060701280565

Jorm, A. F., Kelly, C. M., & Wright, A. (2007). Improving mental health literacy as a strategy to facilitate early intervention for mental disorders. *The Medical Journal of Australia*, *187*, S26–S30. PMID:17908021

Jorm, A. F., & Wright, A. (2007). Beliefs of young people and their parents about the effectiveness of interventions for mental disorders. *The Australian and New Zealand Journal of Psychiatry*, *41*(8), 656–666. doi:10.1080/00048670701449179 PMID:17620162

Jorm, A.F., Korten, A.E., Jacomb, P.A., Christensen, H., & Rodgers, B., & Pollitt. (1997). "Mental health literacy": A survey of the public's ability to recognise mental disorders and their beliefs about the effectiveness of treatment. *The Medical Journal of Australia*, *166*, 182–186. PMID:9066546

Jowett, A., & Peel, E. (2009). Chronic illness in non-heterosexual contexts: An online survey of experiences. *Feminism & Psychology*, *19*(4), 454–474. doi:10.1177/0959353509342770

Julal, F. S. (2015). Predictors of undergraduate students' university support service use during the first year of university. *British Journal of Guidance & Counselling*, 1–11.

Jung, K. E. (2003). Chronic illness and academic accommodation: Meeting disabled students' unique needs and preserving the institutional order of the university. *Journal of Sociology and Social Welfare*, *30*, 91.

Kalanithi, P. (2017). *When breath becomes air*. London: Penguin Random House.

Kameri-Mbote, P. (2007). Water, conflict, and cooperation: Lessons from the Nile river basin 4. Washington, DC: Woodrow Wilson International Center for Scholars' Conflict Resolution and Peacebuilding Program.

Kay-Lambkin, F., Kemp, E., Stafford, K., & Hazell, T. (2007, June). Mental Health Promotion and Early Intervention in Early Childhood and Primary School Setting: A Review. *Journal of Student Wellbeing*, *1*(1), 31–56. doi:10.21913/JSW.v1i1.115

Keane, B. (1987). *Study of mental health nursing in Australia. Commonwealth department of Australia*. Canberra: Australian Government Printing Service.

Kenny, S. (2011). *Developing communities for the future* (4th ed.). South Melbourne, Australia: Thomson.

Kerns, C. M. (2013). *The influence of social norms on attitudes toward help seeking behavior of college undergraduates at a major midwestern university* (Unpublished doctoral dissertation). Ohio University, Athens, OH.

Kessler, R. C., Berglund, P., Demler, O., Jin, R., Merikangas, K., & Walters, E. (2005). Lifetime prevalence and age-of-onset distributions of DSM-IV disorders in the national comorbidity survey replication. *Archives of General Psychiatry*, *62*(6), 593–603. doi:10.1001/archpsyc.62.6.593 PMID:15939837

Kessler, R. C., Gaxiola, S. A., Alonso, J., Chatterji, S., Lee, S., Ormel, J., ... Wang, P. S. (2009). The global burden of mental disorders: An update from the WHO World Mental Health (WMH) surveys. *Epidemiologia e Psichiatria Sociale*, *18*(1), 23–33. doi:10.1017/S1121189X00001421 PMID:19378696

Kessler, R. C., Olfson, M., & Berglund, P. A. (1998). Patterns and predictors of treatment contact after first onset of psychiatric disorders. *The American Journal of Psychiatry*, *155*(1), 62–69. doi:10.1176/ajp.155.1.62 PMID:9433340

Kia, H. (2012). "I'm part of this family": How five care-giving partners of gay men story their experiences. *Journal of Gay & Lesbian Social Services*, *24*(2), 140–157. doi:10.1080/10538720.2012.669369

Kidd, S. A., Veltman, A., Gately, C., Chan, K. J., & Cohen, J. N. (2011). Lesbian, gay, and transgender persons with severe mental illness: Negotiating wellness in the context of multiple sources of stigma. *American Journal of Psychiatric Rehabilitation*, *14*(1), 13–39. doi:10.1080/15487768.2011.546277

KidsMatter. (n.d.). Retrieved 06 August, 2017, from http://www.pai.edu.au/content/kidsmatter-primary

King, P. (2017). *Effective interventions for working with individuals with borderline personality disorder* (Unpublished PhD thesis). RMIT University, Melbourne, Australia.

Kinzie, J. D. (2006). Immigrants and refugees: The Psychiatric perspective. *Transcultural Psychiatry*, *43*(4), 577–591. doi:10.1177/1363461506070782 PMID:17166947

Kittikorn, N., Street, A. F., & Blackford, J. (2006). Managing shame and stigma: Case studies of female carers of people with AIDS in Southern Thailand. *Qualitative Health Research*, *16*(9), 1286–1301. doi:10.1177/1049732306293992 PMID:17038758

Kleinman, A. (1977). Depression, Somatization and the new cross-cultural psychiatry. *Social Science & Medicine*, *11*(1), 3–9. doi:10.1016/0037-7856(77)90138-X PMID:887955

Kleinman, A. (1988). *Rethinking psychiatry: From cultural category to personal experience, cross-cultural comparison, psychiatry, psychopathology, socioeconomic factors*. New York, NY: The Free Press.

Klein, R. (1993). Dimensions of rationing: Who should do what? *BMJ (Clinical Research Ed.)*, *307*(6899), 309–311. doi:10.1136/bmj.307.6899.309 PMID:8374382

Klein, R., & Maybin, J. (2012). *Thinking about rationing*. King's Fund.

Knauer, N. J. (2016). lgbt older adults, chosen family, and caregiving. *The Journal of Law and Religion*, *31*(2), 150–168. doi:10.1017/jlr.2016.23

Knowles, S., Combs, R., Kirk, S., Griffiths, M., Patel, N., & Sanders, C. (2016). Hidden caring, hidden carers? Exploring the experience of carers for people with long-term conditions. *Health & Social Care in the Community*, *24*(2), 203–213. doi:10.1111/hsc.12207 PMID:25706665

Koerner, K., & Linehan, M. (2000). Research on dialectical behavior therapy for patients with borderline personality disorder. *The Psychiatric Clinics of North America*, *23*(1), 151–167. doi:10.1016/S0193-953X(05)70149-0 PMID:10729937

Konur, O. (2002). Assessment of disabled students in higher education: Current public policy issues. *Assessment & Evaluation in Higher Education*, *27*(2), 131–152. doi:10.1080/02602930220128715

Koons, C. R., Robins, C. J., Tweed, J. L., Lynch, T. R., Gonzalez, A. M., Morsh, J. Q., ... Bastian, L. A. (2001). Efficacy of dialectical behavior therapy in women veterans with borderline personality disorder. *Behavior Therapy*, *32*(2), 371–390. doi:10.1016/S0005-7894(01)80009-5

Koschorke, M., Padmavati, R., Kumar, S., Cohen, A., Weiss, H. A., Chatterjee, S., ... Balaji, M. (2017). Experiences of stigma and discrimination faced by family caregivers of people with schizophrenia in India. *Social Science & Medicine*, *178*, 66–77. doi:10.1016/j.socscimed.2017.01.061 PMID:28213300

KPMG. (2011). *Child FIRST and integrated family services final report: Prepared for the Department of Human Services.* Retrieved September 2016, from http://www.dhs.vic.gov.au/_data/assets/pdf_file/0008/646820/childFIRSTandintfam-servicesfullreport_09082011.pdf

Kramer, A., Wolf, A., Carius, A. & Dabelko, G. (2013). The key to managing conflict and cooperation over water. *A World of Science, 11*(1), 4-12.

Krapp, A. (2002). An Educational-Psychological Theory of Interest and its Relation to Self-Determination Theory. In E. Deci & R. Ryan (Eds.), *The Handbook of Self-determination Research* (pp. 405–427). New York: University of Rochester Press.

Krieg, A. (2009). The experience of collective trauma in Australian Indigenous communities. *Australasian Psychology*, *17*(1_suppl), 28–32. doi:10.1080/10398560902948621 PMID:19579102

Krimayer, L. J. (2006). Beyond the 'new cross-cultural psychiatry': Cultural biology, discursive psychology and the ironies of globalization. *Transcultural Psychiatry*, *43*(1), 126–144. doi:10.1177/1363461506061761 PMID:16671396

Krimayer, L. J., Gomez-Carrillo, A., & Veissiére, S. (2017). Culture and depression in global mental health: An ecosocial approach to the phenomenology of psychiatric disorders. *Social Science & Medicine*, *183*, 163–168. doi:10.1016/j.socscimed.2017.04.034 PMID:28478959

Kutcher, S., Wei, Y., & Morgan, C. (2015). Successful Application of a Canadian Mental Health Curriculum Resource by Usual Classroom Teachers in Significantly and Sustainably Improving Student Mental Health. *Canadian Journal of Psychiatry*, *60*(12), 580–586. doi:10.1177/070674371506001209 PMID:26720827

Lachman, S. (1997). Learning is a process: Toward an improved definition of learning. *The Journal of Psychology*, *131*(5), 477–480. doi:10.1080/00223989709603535

Laidlaw, A., McLellan, J., & Ozakinci, G. (2015). Understanding undergraduate student perceptions of mental health, mental well-being and help-seeking behaviour. *Studies in Higher Education*, 1–13.

Landau, J. (2010). Communities that care for families: The LINC Model for enhancing individual family, and community resilience. *The American Journal of Orthopsychiatry*, *80*(4), 516–524. doi:10.1111/j.1939-0025.2010.01054.x PMID:20950292

Lane, H., Sarkis, M., Martin, J., & Haines, T. (2017). Equity in healthcare resource allocation decision-making: A systematic review. *Social Science & Medicine*, *175*, 11–27. doi:10.1016/j.socscimed.2016.12.012 PMID:28043036

Lane, K., & Reiger, K. (2013). Regime change in Australian maternity hospitals. *Social Theory & Health*, *11*(4), 407–427. doi:10.1057th.2013.7

Laporte, L., & Guttman, H. (1996). Traumatic childhood experiences as risk factors for borderline and other personality disorders. *Journal of Personality Disorders*, *10*(3), 247–259. doi:10.1521/pedi.1996.10.3.247

Laragy, C., Sanders, F., & Brophy, L. (2015). *Implications for family carers when people with psychosocial disability have individualised funding packages - literature review*. Retrieved from Melbourne: https://www.mindaustralia.org.au/sites/default/files/publications/Implications_for_family_carers_literature_review.pdf

Laragy, C., Fisher, K. R., Purcal, C., & Jenkinson, S. (2015). Australia's individualised disability funding packages: When do they provide greater choice and opportunity? *Asian Social Work and Policy Review*, *9*(3), 282–292. doi:10.1111/aswp.12068

Laragy, C., & Ottmann, G. (2011). Towards a framework for implementing Individual Funding based on an Australian case study. *Journal of Policy and Practice in Intellectual Disabilities*, *8*(1), 18–27. doi:10.1111/j.1741-1130.2011.00283.x

Larcombe, W., Finch, S., Sore, R., Murray, C. M., Kentish, S., Mulder, R. A., & Williams, D. A. (2016). Prevalence and socio-demographic correlates of psychological distress among students at an Australian university. *Studies in Higher Education*, *41*(6), 1074–1091. doi:10.1080/03075079.2014.966072

Large, M., Kaneson, M., Myles, N., Myles, H., Gunaratne, P., & Ryan, C. (2016). Meta-analysis of longitudinal cohort studies of suicide risk assessment among psychiatric patients: Heterogeneity in results and lack of improvement over time. *PLoS One*, *11*(6), 1–17. doi:10.1371/journal.pone.0156322 PMID:27285387

Large, M., Sharma, S., Cannon, E., Ryan, C., & Nielssen, O. (2011). Risk factors for suicide within a year of discharge from psychiatric hospital: A systematic meta-analysis. *The Australian and New Zealand Journal of Psychiatry*, *45*(8), 619–628. doi:10.3109/00048674.2011.590465 PMID:21740345

Larsen, I. B., & Terkelsen, T. B. (2014). Coercion in a locked psychiatric ward: Perspectives of patients and staff. *Nursing Ethics*, *21*(4), 426–436. doi:10.1177/0969733013503601 PMID:24106262

Latour, B., & Woolgar, S. (1979). *Laboratory life: the social construction of scientific facts*. Princeton University Press.

Lavoie, J. G., Forget, E. L., Prakash, T., Dahl, M., Martens, P., & O'Neil, J. D. (2010). Have investments in on-reserve health services and initiatives promoting community control improved First Nations' health in Manitoba? *Social Science & Medicine*, *71*(4), 717–724. doi:10.1016/j.socscimed.2010.04.037 PMID:20554364

Lawn, S., & McMahon, J. (2015). Experiences of care by Australians with a diagnosis of borderline personality disorder. *Journal of Psychiatric and Mental Health Nursing*, *22*(7), 510–521. doi:10.1111/jpm.12226 PMID:26122817

Lawrence, D., Johnson, S., Hafekost, J., Boterhoven De Haan, K., Sawyer, M., Ainley, J., & … . (2015). *The Mental Health of Children and Adolescents. Report on the second Australian Child and Adolescent Survey of Mental Health and Wellbeing*. Canberra: Department of Health.

Leichsenring, F., Leibing, E., Kruse, J., New, A. S., & Leweke, F. (2011). Borderline personality disorder. *Lancet*, *377*(9759), 74–84. doi:10.1016/S0140-6736(10)61422-5 PMID:21195251

Leonard, W., Lyons, A., & Bariola, E. (2015). *A Closer Look at Private Lives 2*. Retrieved from https://www.glhv.org.au/sites/default/files/Closer_Look_Private_Lives2.pdf

Leonard, W., Marshall, D., Hillier, L., Mitchell, A., & Ward, R. (2010). *Beyond homophobia: meeting the needs of same sex attracted and gender questioning (SSAGQ) young people in Victoria. A policy blueprint* (Doctoral dissertation). William Buckland Foundation.

Leonard, W. (2002). *What's the difference? Health issues of major concern to gay lesbian bisexual transgender and intersex (GLBTI) Victorians. Ministerial Advisory Committee on Gay and Lesbian Health (MACGLH)*. Melbourne: Department of Human Services.

Leonard, W., Pitts, M., Mitchell, A., Lyons, A., Smith, A., Patel, S., & Barrett, A. (2012). *Private Lives 2: The second national survey of the health and wellbeing of gay, lesbian, bisexual and transgender (GLBT)*. Australians.

Lesser, I. O., Nardulli, B. R., & Arghavan, L. A. (1998). Sources of conflict in the Greater Middle East. In *Sources of conflict in the 21st century: Regional futures and U. S. strategy*. Santa Monica, CA: RAND.

Levinger, G. (1964). Task and social behaviour in marriage. *Sociometry*, *27*(4), 433–448. doi:10.2307/2785657

Lightman, E., Vick, A., Herd, D., & Mitchell, A. (2009). 'Not disabled enough': Episodic disabilities and the Ontario Disability Support Program. *Disability Studies Quarterly*, *29*(3). doi:10.18061/dsq.v29i3.932

Lim, F. A., Brown, D. V. Jr, & Jones, H. (2013). Lesbian, gay, bisexual, and transgender health: Fundamentals for nursing education. *The Journal of Nursing Education*, *52*(4), 198–203. doi:10.3928/01484834-20130311-02 PMID:23471873

Linehan, M. (1993). *Cognitive–behavioral treatment of borderline personality disorder*. New York: Guilford Press.

Linehan, M. M. (2000). The empirical basis of Dialectical Behavior Therapy: Development of new treatments versus evaluation of existing treatments. *Clinical Psychology: Science and Practice*, *7*(1), 113–119. doi:10.1093/clipsy.7.1.113

Linehan, M. M., Armstrong, H. E., Suarez, A., Allmon, D., & Heard, H. L. (1991). Cognitive- behavioral treatment of chronically parasuicidal borderline patients. *Annals of General Psychiatry*, *48*(12), 1060–1064. doi:10.1001/archpsyc.1991.01810360024003 PMID:1845222

Linehan, M. M., Schmidt, H., Dimeff, L. A., Craft, J. C., Kanter, J., & Comtois, K. A. (1999). Dialectical behavior therapy for patients with borderline personality disorder and drug dependence. *The American Journal on Addictions*, *8*(4), 279–292. doi:10.1080/105504999305686 PMID:10598211

Linehan, M. M., Wilks, M., & Chelsey, R. (2015). The Course and Evolution of Dialectical Behavior Therapy. *American Journal of Psychotherapy*, *69*(2), 97–110. doi:10.1176/appi.psychotherapy.2015.69.2.97 PMID:26160617

Link, P. M., Piontek, F., Scheffran, J., & Schilling, J. (2012). *On foes and flows: Water conflict and cooperation in the Nile River Basin in times of climate change*. Hamburg, Germany: CLISEC, University of Hamburg.

Livesley, W. J., Schroeder, M. L., Jackson, D. N., & Jang, K. L. (1994). Categorical Distinctions in the Study of Personality Disorder—Implications for Classification. *Journal of Abnormal Psychology*, *103*(1), 6–17. doi:10.1037/0021-843X.103.1.6 PMID:8040482

Lloyd, L. (2003). Caring Relationships: Looking Beyond Welfare Categories of Carers' and Service Users'. *Research Highlights in Social Work,* 37-55.

Lo, S., & Horton, R. (2016). Transgender health: An opportunity for global health equity. *Lancet*, *388*(10042), 316–318. doi:10.1016/S0140-6736(16)30675-4 PMID:27323923

Loucks, D. P., & van Beek, E. (2005). *Water resources systems planning and management: Facts about water*. Paris, France: UNESCO Publishing Company.

Lupton, D. (2013). Risk and emotion: Towards an alternative theoretical perspective. *Health Risk & Society*, *15*(8), 634–647. doi:10.1080/13698575.2013.848847

Lustig, S., Madon, T., Hyun, J. K., & Quinn, B. C. (2006). Graduate student mental health: Needs assessment and utilization of counseling services. *Journal of College Student Development*, *47*(3), 247–266. doi:10.1353/csd.2006.0030

Lymbery, M. (2014). Understanding personalisation: Implications for social work. *Journal of Social Work*, *14*(3), 295–312. doi:10.1177/1468017313477326

Lynch, T. R., Morse, J. Q., Mendelson, T., & Robins, C. J. (2003). A randomized trial of dialectical behavior therapy for depressed older adults: Post-treatment and six month follow- up. *The American Journal of Geriatric Psychiatry*, *11*(1), 33–45. doi:10.1097/00019442-200301000-00006 PMID:12527538

Manuel, J., & Crowe, M. (2014). Clinical responsibility, accountability, and risk aversion in mental health nursing: A descriptive, qualitative study. *International Journal of Mental Health Nursing*, *23*(4), 336–343. doi:10.1111/inm.12063 PMID:24548741

Marginson, S. (2006). Dynamics of national and global competition in higher education. *Higher Education*, *52*(1), 1–39. doi:10.100710734-004-7649-x

Markoulakis, R. (2014). *The social relations of accessibility: Explicating the work of accommodation for students with mental health problems in university* (Unpublished doctoral dissertation). University of Toronto, Toronto, Canada.

Marmot, M., Friel, S., Bell, R., Houweling, T. A., Taylor, S., & Health, C. (2008). Closing the gap in a generation: Health equity through action on the social determinants of health. *Lancet*, *372*(9650), 1661–1669. doi:10.1016/S0140-6736(08)61690-6 PMID:18994664

Martin, J. (2015). *Conflict Management.* Ginninderra Press.

Martin, J. M. (2010). Stigma and student mental health in higher education. *Higher Education Research & Development*, *29*(3), 259–274. doi:10.1080/07294360903470969

Martin, S. S. (2009). Illness of the mind or illness of the spirit? Mental health-related conceptualization of and practices of older Iranian immigrants. *Health & Social Work*, *34*(2), 117–126. doi:10.1093/hsw/34.2.117 PMID:19425341

Martyr, P. (2010). Behaving wildly: Diagnoses of lunacy among Indigenous persons in western Australia, 1870-1914. *Social History of Medicine*, *24*(2), 316–333. doi:10.1093hm/hkq046

Mason, S. J., & Blank, D. (2013). *Mediating Water Use Conflicts in Peace Processes.* Zurich, Switzerland: Center for Security Studies, Swiss Federal Institute of Technology, ETH Zurich.

Matthew, R. A., Halle, M., & Switzer, J. (2002). *Conserving the peace: Resources, livelihoods and security.* Winnipeg, Canada: International Institute for Sustainable Development.

Mavromaras, K., Moskos, M., & Mahutea, S. (2016). *Evaluation of the NDIS Intermediate Report.* Retrieved from National Institute of Labour Studies (NILS) Flinders University Adelaide: https://www.dss.gov.au/sites/default/files/documents/11_2016/final_intermediate_report_wcag_compliant_24_nov_2016.pdf

Maylea, C. (2016). A rejection of involuntary treatment in mental health social work. *Ethics & Social Welfare*, *1*(1), 1–17.

Mazrui, A. A. (1986). *The Africans: A triple heritage.* London, UK: Little Brown.

Mazza, E. T. (2015). Working with students with psychiatric disabilities or other emotional problems. *Journal of Teaching in Social Work*, *35*(4), 425–448. doi:10.1080/08841233.2015.1066916

Mbiti, J. S. (1989). *African religions and philosophy* (2nd ed.). Johannesburg, SA: Heinemann.

McAllister, M., Wynaden, D., Happell, B., Flynn, T., Walters, V., Duggan, R., ... Gaskin, C. (2014). Staff experiences of providing support to students who are managing mental health challenges: A qualitative study from two Australian universities. *Advances in Mental Health*, *12*(3), 192–201. doi:10.1080/18374905.2014.11081897

McCann, E., Lee, R., & Brown, M. (2016). The experiences and support needs of people with intellectual disabilities who identify as LGBT: A review of the literature. *Research in Developmental Disabilities*, *57*, 39–53. doi:10.1016/j.ridd.2016.06.013 PMID:27372882

McCarthy, D. (2007). Teaching self-advocacy to students with disabilities. *About Campus: Enriching the Student Learning Experience, 12*(5), 10–16. doi:10.1002/abc.225

McEldowney, R., & Connor, M. (2011). Cultural safety as an ethics of care: A praxiological process. *Journal of Transcultural Nursing, 22*(4), 342–349. doi:10.1177/1043659611414139 PMID:21844246

McGorry, P., & Matthew, H. (2016). Stepwise expansion of evidence-based care is needed for mental health reform. *The Medical Journal of Australia, 204*(9), 351–353. doi:10.5694/mja16.00120 PMID:27169969

McGorry, P., Purcell, R., Hickie, I., & Jorm, A. (2007). Investing in youth mental health is a best buy. *The Medical Journal of Australia, 187*(suppl. 7), S5–S7.

McGough, S., Wynaden, D., & Wright, M. (2018). Experience of providing cultural safety in mental health to Aboriginal patients: A grounded theory study. *International Journal of Mental Health Nursing, 27*(1), 204–213. doi:10.1111/inm.12310 PMID:28165178

McKay, B. (2011). Lesbian, gay, bisexual, and transgender health issues, disparities, and information resources. *Medical Reference Services Quarterly, 30*(4), 393–401. doi:10.1080/02763869.2011.608971 PMID:22040245

McLean, K. (2008). Inside, outside, nowhere: Bisexual men and women in the gay and lesbian community. *Journal of Bisexuality, 8*(1-2), 63–80. doi:10.1080/15299710802143174

Mcluckie, A., Kutcher, S., Wei, Y., & Weaver, C. (2014). Sustained improvements in students' mental health literacy with use of a mental health curriculum in Canadian schools. *BMC Public Health, 14*, 379. PMID:25551789

McNair, R. P., & Hegarty, K. (2010). Guidelines for the primary care of lesbian, gay, and bisexual people: A systematic review. *Annals of Family Medicine, 8*(6), 533–541. doi:10.1370/afm.1173 PMID:21060124

McNaught, K. (2013). The potential impacts of 'Inherent Requirements' and 'Mandatory Professional Reporting'on students, particularly those with mental health concerns, registering with university disability support/equity services. *Journal of the Australia and New Zealand Students Services Association, 42*, 25–29.

McWhinney, E. (2017). The Declaration on the Granting of Independence to Colonial Powers and Peoples. New York: United Nations.

Meacham, M., Tandy, C., Giddings, M., Vodde, R., Curington, A., Morris, B., & Holliman, D. (2004). The thorny dilemma of gatekeeping versus inclusion for students with disabilities. *Journal of Social Work in Disability & Rehabilitation, 3*(4), 69–88. doi:10.1300/J198v03n04_05

Meaney-Tavares, R., & Hasking, P. (2013). Coping and Regulating Emotions: A Pilot Study of a Modified Dialectical Behavior Therapy Group Delivered in a College Counseling Service. *Journal of American College Health, 61*(5), 303–309. doi:10.1080/07448481.2013.791827 PMID:23768227

Meekosha, H., & Dowse, L. (2007). Integrating critical disability studies into social work education and practice: An Australian perspective. *Practice, 19*(3), 169–183. doi:10.1080/09503150701574267

Mehl, L. E. (1988). Modern shamanism: integration of biomedicine with traditional world views. In Shaman's path (pp. 127-138). Boston: Shambhala.

Mehta, L., Veldwisch, G. J., & Franco, J. (2012). Introduction to the Special Issue: Water grabbing? Focus on the (re) appropriation of finite water resources. *Water Alternatives, 5*(2), 193–207.

Mejia-Canales, D., & Leonard, W. (2016). *Something for them.* Retrieved from https://www.glhv.org.au/sites/default/files/2016-09/somethingforthem.pdf

Mental Health Australia. (2016). *Letter to Disability Reform Council on 2017 Productivity Commission review on the NDIS*. Author.

Mental Health Coordinating Council. (2017). *Reimagine, mental health, my recovery and the NDIS*. Retrieved from http://reimagine.today/

Midelfort, H. C. E. (1992). *Madness and civilization in early modern Europe: a reappraisal of Michel Foucault. In Critical thought series: 2, critical essays on Michel Foucault*. Scolar Press.

Miller, P., & Hayward, D. (2017). Social policy 'generosity' at a time of fiscal austerity: The strange case of Australia's National Disability Insurance Scheme. *Critical Social Policy*, *37*(1), 128–147. doi:10.1177/0261018316664463

MindMatters. (n.d.). Retrieved 06 August, 2017, from http://www.pai.edu.au/content/mindmatters

Mission Australia and Black Dog Institute. (2016). *Youth mental health report: Youth Survey 2012-16*. Sydney: Mission Australia.

Mitchell, P., Bruxner, A., & Brophy, L. (2014). *People making choices: The support needs and preferences of people with psychosocial disability*. Retrieved from http://dro.deakin.edu.au/view/DU:30079593

Mitchell, J., Kaplan, I., & Crowe, L. (2007). Two cultures: One life. *Community Development Journal: An International Forum*, *42*(3), 282–298. doi:10.1093/cdj/bsl016

Mizielińska, J., & Stasińska, A. (2017). "There Is Nothing Like a Family": Discourses on Families of Choice in Poland. *Journal of Homosexuality*, *64*(13), 1793–1815. doi:10.1080/00918369.2016.1267460 PMID:27918870

Moleiro, C., & Pinto, N. (2015). Sexual orientation and gender identity: Review of concepts, controversies and their relation to psychopathology classification systems. *Frontiers in Psychology*, *6*, 1511. doi:10.3389/fpsyg.2015.01511 PMID:26483748

Mollie, F. (2009). River basin planning and management: The social life of a concept. *Geoforum*, *40*(3), 484–494. doi:10.1016/j.geoforum.2009.03.004

Molyneaux, V., Butchard, S., Simpson, J., & Murray, C. (2011). Reconsidering the term 'carer': A critique of the universal adoption of the term 'carer'. *Ageing and Society*, *31*(3), 422–437. doi:10.1017/S0144686X10001066

Morgan, R. (2016). *Over 400,000 Australians intend to retire in the next 12 months, increasing burden on government funding*. Melbourne, Australia: Roy Morgan Research.

Morrisette, J. J., & Borer, D. A. (2004). Where Oil and Water Do Mix: Environmental Scarcity and Future Conflict in the Middle East and North Africa. *Parameters*, *34*, 94–96.

Moscati, I. (2016). Retrospectives: How economists came to accept expected utility theory: The case of Samuelson and Savage. *The Journal of Economic Perspectives*, *30*(2), 219–236. doi:10.1257/jep.30.2.219

Mullen, A., Drinkwater, V., & Lewin, T. J. (2014). Care zoning in a psychiatric intensive care unit: Strengthening ongoing clinical risk assessment. *Journal of Clinical Nursing*, *23*(5-6), 731–743. doi:10.1111/jocn.12493 PMID:24329872

Mungai, N. W. (2014). Ubuntu approaches to working with immigrant communities. In K. Goel, V. Pulla & A.P. Francis (Eds.), Community work: Theories, experiences & challenges (pp. 214-235). Bangalore, India: Niruta Publications.

Mungai, N. W. (2017). Community development: Is it coming back? *New Community*, *15*(1-2), 57–58.

Muraco, A., & Fredriksen-Goldsen, K. I. (2014). The highs and lows of caregiving for chronically ill lesbian, gay, and bisexual elders. *Journal of Gerontological Social Work*, *57*(2-4), 251–272. doi:10.1080/01634372.2013.860652 PMID:24224896

Murphy, B. (2011). *Final report of the Koori Youth Alcohol and Drug Healing Service: YSAS & Ngwala*. Melbourne: Youth Research Centre, University of Melbourne.

Mustafa, D., Akhter, M., & Nasrallah, N. (2013). *Understanding Pakistan's water-security nexus. Peaceworks, No. 88.* Washington, DC: United States Institute of Peace.

Nadal, K. L., Whitman, C. N., Davis, L. S., Erazo, T., & Davidoff, K. C. (2016). Microaggressions toward lesbian, gay, bisexual, transgender, queer, and genderqueer people: A review of the literature. *Journal of Sex Research*, *53*(4-5), 488–508. doi:10.1080/00224499.2016.1142495 PMID:26966779

National Disability Insurance Agency (NDIA). (2015). *2015 – 2019 Corporate Plan*. Retrieved from https://www.ndis.gov.au/html/sites/default/files/NDIA Corporate Plan 2015 -19 FINAL_0.pdf

National Disability Insurance Agency. (2017). *Quarterly Report to COAG Disability Reform Council, 2016-17 Quarter 4, 30 June 2017.* Retrieved from https://www.ndis.gov.au/medias/documents/hac/h30/8803440066590/COAG-DRC-Report-2016-17-Q4.pdf

National LGBTI Health Alliance. (2016). *The Statistics at a Glance: The Mental Health of Lesbian, Gay, Bisexual, Transgender and Intersex People in Australia.* Retrieved 28th August, 2017 from http://lgbtihealth.org.au/statistics/

National Mental Health Commission. (2014). *The national review of mental health programmes and services*. Sydney: National Mental Health Commission.

Nicholas, A., & Reifels, L. (2014). *Mental health and the NDIS: A literature review*. Melbourne: Centre for Mental Health, University of Melbourne.

Nickell, A. D., Waudby, C. J., & Trull, T. J. (2002). Attachment, parental bonding and borderline personality disorder features in young adults. *Journal of Personality Disorders*, *16*(2), 148–159. doi:10.1521/pedi.16.2.148.22544 PMID:12004491

Niemiec, C., & Ryan, R. (2009). Autonomy, Competence and Relatedness in the Classroom: Applying Self-Determination Theory to Educational Practice. *Theory and Research in Education*, *7*(2), 133–144.

Nimrod, G. (2010). Seniors' online communities: A quantitative content analysis. *The Gerontologist*, *50*(3), 382–392. doi:10.1093/geront/gnp141 PMID:19917645

Noels, K., Pelletier, L., Clement, R., & Vallerand, R. (2000). Why are you learning a second language? Motivational orientations and Self-Determination Theory. *Journal of Research in Language Studies*, *50*(1), 57–85.

Norrie, J., Davidson, K., Tata, P., & Gumley, A. (2013). Influence of therapist competence and quantity of cognitive behavioural therapy on suicidal behaviour and inpatient hospitalisation in a randomised controlled trial in borderline personality disorder: Further analyses of treatment effects in the BOSCOT st. *Psychology and Psychotherapy: Theory, Research and Practice*, *86*(3), 280–293. doi:10.1111/papt.12004 PMID:23420622

O'Donovan, L. J. (2000). A profession of trust: Reflections on a fundamental virtue. In D. C. Thomasma & J. L. Kissell (Eds.), *The health care professional a friend and healer: Building on the work of Edmund D. Pellegrino* (pp. 1–10). Washington, DC: Georgetown University Press.

O'Halloran, P. (2014). *About psychosocial disability and the NDIS, introduction to the concept of holistic psychosocial disability support*. Canberra, Australia: National Disability Insurance Agency. Retrieved from https://www.ndis.gov.au/html/sites/default/files/O'Halloran paper.pdf

O'Leary, P., Tsui, M., & Ruch, G. (2013). The boundaries of the social work relationship revisited: Towards a connected, inclusive and dynamic conceptualisation. *British Journal of Social Work*, *43*(1), 135–153. doi:10.1093/bjsw/bcr181

Offredy, M. (1998). The application of decision making concepts by nurse practitioners in general practice. *Journal of Advanced Nursing*, *28*(5), 988–1000. doi:10.1046/j.1365-2648.1998.00823.x PMID:9840870

Ohlsson, V. L. (1999). Water scarcity and conflict. *International Security Challenges in a Changing World*, *3*, 211.

Ohlsson, V. L. (2000). Water conflicts and social resource scarcity. *Physics and Chemistry of the Earth. Part B: Hydrology, Oceans and Atmosphere*, *25*(3), 213–220. doi:10.1016/S1464-1909(00)00006-X

Olenchek, C. (2008). Dialectical Behavior Therapy — Treating Borderline Personality Disorder. *Socialwork Today*, *8*(6), 22.

Olfson, M., Kessler, R. C., Berglund, P. A., & Lin, E. (1998). Psychiatric disorder onset and first treatment contact in the United States and Ontario. *The American Journal of Psychiatry*, *155*(10), 1415–1422. doi:10.1176/ajp.155.10.1415 PMID:9766774

Ong, K. S., Kelaher, M., Anderson, I., & Carter, R. (2009). A cost-based equity weight for use in the economic evaluation of primary health care interventions: Case study of the Australian Indigenous population. *International Journal for Equity in Health*, *8*(1), 34. doi:10.1186/1475-9276-8-34 PMID:19807930

Orel, N. A., & Coon, D. W. (2016). The Challenges of Change: How Can We Meet the Care Needs of the Ever-Evolving LGBT Family? *Generations (San Francisco, Calif.)*, *40*(2), 41–45.

Organisation for Economic Co-operation and Development. (2015). *Ageing in Cities*. Paris, France: OECD Publishing.

Organisation for Economic Co-operation and Development. (2018). *Definition of elderly population*. Retrieved from: https://data.oecd.org/pop/elderly-population.htm

Ortman, J. M., Velkoff, V. A., & Hogan, H. (2014). *An aging nation: the older population in the United States*. United States Census Bureau, Economics and Statistics Administration, US Department of Commerce.

Orygen Youth Health. Anxiety & Young People. (2008). Retrieved September 24, 2017, from http://oyh.org.au/sites/oyh.org.au/files/factsheets/oyh_fs_anx.pdf

Ottmann, G., Laragy, C., & Haddon, M. (2009). Experiences of disability consumer-directed care users in Australia: Results from a longitudinal qualitative study. *Health & Social Care in the Community*, *17*(5), 466–475. doi:10.1111/j.1365-2524.2009.00851.x PMID:19689678

Oyebode, J. (2003). Assessment of carers' psychological needs. *Advances in Psychiatric Treatment*, *9*(1), 45–53. doi:10.1192/apt.9.1.45

Pacific Institute. (2015). *Water conflict: The world's water*. Retrieved from: http://worldwater.org/water-conflict/

Pallotta-Chiarolli, M., & Rajkhowa, A. (2017). Systemic Invisibilities, Institutional Culpabilities and Multicultural-Multifaith LGBTIQ Resistances. *Journal of Intercultural Studies (Melbourne, Vic.)*, *38*(4), 429–442. doi:10.1080/07256868.2017.1341013

Parker, R., & Milroy, H. (2014). Mental Illness in Aboriginal and Torres Strait Islander Peoples. In Working together: Aboriginal and Torres Strait Islander mental health and wellbeing principles and practices (pp. 113-124). Barton, ACT: Commonwealth of Australia.

Parslow, O., & Hegarty, P. (2013). Who cares? UK lesbian caregivers in a heterosexual world. *Women's Studies International Forum*, *40*, 78–86. doi:10.1016/j.wsif.2013.03.003

Parsons, W. (2002). From muddling through to muddling up-evidence based policy making and the modernisation of British Government. *Public Policy and Administration, 17*(3), 43-60.

Pawar, M., & Anscombe, B. (2015). Reflective social work practice: Thinking, doing and being. Sydney, Australia: Cambridge.

Pearson, M., & Polden, M. (2011). *The journalist's guide to media law.* NSW: Allen & Unwin.

Peer Support Australia. Who We Are. (2014). Retrieved September 29, 2017, from http://peersupport.edu.au/about-peer-support-australia/who-we-are/

Peeters, L., Hamann, S., & Kelly, K. (2014). The Maramuli Program: Healing for Stolen Generations. In Working together: Aboriginal and Torres Strait Islander mental health and wellbeing principles and practices (pp. 493-508). Barton, ACT: Commonwealth of Australia.

Perlin, M. L. (1999). Half-wracked prejudice leaped forth: Sanism, pretextuality, and why and how mental disability law developed as it did. *Journal of Contemporary Legal Issues, 10*(3).

Perrier, E. (2015). *Positive disruption: Healthcare, ageing and participation in the age of technology.* Sydney, NSW: McKell Institute.

Perry, J. C., Herman, J. L., Van der Kolk, B. A., & Hoke, L. (1990). Psychotherapy and psychological trauma in borderline personality disorder. *Psychiatric Annals, 26*(1), 33–43. doi:10.3928/0048-5713-19900101-08

Peterson, S., Buchanan, A., & Falkmer, T. (2014). The impact of services that offer individualised funds, shared management, person-centred relationships, and self-direction on the lived experiences of consumers with mental illness. *International Journal of Mental Health Systems, 8*(1), 1–14. doi:10.1186/1752-4458-8-20 PMID:24944564

Phiriyapokan, T. (2011). *Is a Big Button Interface Enough for Elderly Users? Towards User Interface Guidelines for Elderly Users* (Master's thesis). Eskilstuna, Sweden: Malardalen University.

Pimentel, D., Berger, B., Filiberto, D., Newton, M., Wolfe, B., Karabinakis, E., ... Nandagopal, S. (2004). Water resources: Agricultural and environmental issues. *Bioscience, 54*(10), 909–918. doi:10.1641/0006-3568(2004)054[0909:WRAAEI]2.0.CO;2

Piwowarczyk, L., Bishop, H., Yusuf, A., Mudymba, F., & Raj, A. (2014). Congolese and Somali beliefs about mental health services. *The Journal of Nervous and Mental Disease, 202*(3), 209–216. doi:10.1097/NMD.0000000000000087 PMID:24566506

Pollack, S. (2010). Labelling clients 'risky': Social Work and the neo-liberal welfare state. *British Journal of Social Work, 40*(4), 1263–1278. doi:10.1093/bjsw/bcn079

Poole, J., Jivraj, T., Arslanian, A., Bellows, K., Chiasson, S., Hakimy, H., ... Reid, J. (2012). Sanism,'mental health'and social work/education: A review and call to action. *Intersectionalities: A Global Journal of Social Work Analysis. Research, Polity, and Practice, 1*(1), 20–36.

Popa, T. (2017). Righting Wrongs: Lawyers' reflections on the amendments to the Wrongs Act 1958 (Vic) on medical negligence and mental harm claims.(Australia). *Torts Law Journal, 24*(1), 64–82.

Porter, R. (1987). *A social history of madness: stories of the insane.* London: Phoenix Giants.

Porter, R. (2002). *Madness: a brief history.* New York: Oxford University Press.

Posnett, J. (2002). Are bigger hospitals better. *Hospitals in a changing. Europe,* 100–118.

Postel, S. L., & Wolf, A. T. (2001). Dehydrating conflict. *Foreign Policy*, *126*(126), 60–67. doi:10.2307/3183260

Preiss, B. (2013). RMIT students slam 'invasive' mental health test. *The Age*. http://www.theage.com.au/national/tertiary-education/rmit-students-slam-invasive-mental-health-test-20130624-2osy1.html

Price, E. (2011). Caring for mum and dad: Lesbian women negotiating family and navigating care. *British Journal of Social Work*, *41*(7), 1288–1303. doi:10.1093/bjsw/bcr015

Price, E. (2012). Gay and lesbian carers: Ageing in the shadow of dementia. *Ageing and Society*, *32*(3), 516–532. doi:10.1017/S0144686X11000560

Price, E. G. (2006). *Hip-Hop culture*. Santa Barbara, CA: ABC-CLIO.

Price, M. (2011). *Mad at School: Rhetorics of Mental Disability and Academic Life*. Ann Arbor, MI: University of Michigan Press. doi:10.3998/mpub.1612837

Priebe, S., Sandhu, S., Dias, S., Gaddini, A., Greacen, T., & Loannidis, E. … Bogic, M. (2011). Good practice in health care for migrants: Views and experiences of care professionals in 16 European countries. *BMC Public Health*, *11*(187). Retrieved October 20, 2017 from https://www.ncbi.nlm.nih.gov/pmc/articles/PMC3071322/

Probert, B. (2015). *The Quality of Australia's Higher Education System: How it Might be Defined, Improved and Assured*. Canberra: Office for Learning and Teaching.

Probst, B. (2013). "Walking the tight rope": Clinical social workers' use of diagnostic and environmental perspectives. *Clinical Social Work Journal*, *41*(2), 184–191. doi:10.100710615-012-0394-1

Productivity Commission. (2017). *National Disability Insurance Scheme (NDIS) Costs, Study Report*. Retrieved from http://www.pc.gov.au/inquiries/completed/ndis-costs/report/ndis-costs.pdf

Purcal, C., Fisher, K. R., & Laragy, C. (2014). Analysing choice in Australian individual funding disability policies. *Australian Journal of Public Administration*, *73*(1), 88–102. doi:10.1111/1467-8500.12063

Quan-Haase, A., Guang, Y., & Wellman, B. (2018). Connected seniors: How older adults in East York exchange social support online and offline. *Information Communication and Society*, *20*(7), 967–983. doi:10.1080/1369118X.2017.1305428

Quinn, N., Wilson, A., MacIntyre, G., & Tinklin, T. (2009). 'People look at you differently': Students' experience of mental health support within higher education. *British Journal of Guidance & Counselling*, *37*(4), 405–418. doi:10.1080/03069880903161385

Ramsden, I. (1995). *Cultural Safety: Implunmting the Concept*. Paper presented at The Social Force of Nursing and Midwifery Conference, Wellington, New Zealand.

Ramsden, I. M. (2002). *Cultural safety and nursing education in Aoteraroa and Te Waipounamu* (Unpublished doctoral thesis). Victoria University of Wellington.

Ramsden, I. (1990). Cultural Safety. *The New Zealand Nursing Journal. Kai Tiaki*, *83*(11), 18–19. PMID:2267106

Ramsden, I. (1993). Cultural safety in nursing education in Aotearoa (New Zealand). *Nursing Praxis in New Zealand Inc*, *8*(3), 4–10. PMID:8298296

Ravnborg, H. M. (2004). *Water and conflict: Conflict prevention and mitigation in water resources management. DIIS REPoRT 2004:2*. Copenhagen: Danish Institute for International Studies.

Rawls, J. (2009). *A theory of justice*. Harvard University Press.

Reading, R., & Rubin, L. R. (2011). Advocacy and empowerment: Group therapy for LGBT asylum seekers. *Traumatology, 17*(2), 86–98. doi:10.1177/1534765610395622

Reamer, F. G. (2001). *Tangled relationships: Managing boundary issues in human services.* New York, NY: Columbia University Press. doi:10.7312/ream12116

Reamer, F. G. (2003). Boundary issues in social work: Managing Dual relationships. *Social Work, 48*(1), 121–133. doi:10.1093w/48.1.121 PMID:12564713

Reavley, N. J., & Jorm, A. F. (2011). *National Survey of Mental Health Literacy and Stigma.* Canberra: Department of Health and Ageing.

Reczek, C., & Umberson, D. (2016). Greedy spouse, needy parent: The marital dynamics of gay, lesbian, and heterosexual intergenerational caregivers. *Journal of Marriage and the Family, 78*(4), 957–974. doi:10.1111/jomf.12318 PMID:27672229

Redmond, M., & Bright, E. (2007). Gatekeeping in the academy: lessons for Canadian social work educators from Young v. Bella. *Canadian Social Work Review/Revue canadienne de service social*, 167-181.

Regehr, C., Stalker, C. A., Jacobs, M., & Pelech, W. (2001). The Gatekeeper and the Wounded Healer. *The Clinical Supervisor, 20*(1), 127–143. doi:10.1300/J001v20n01_10

Reid, J., & Poole, J. (2013). Mad students in the social work classroom? Notes from the beginnings of an inquiry. *Journal of Progressive Human Services, 24*(3), 209–222. doi:10.1080/10428232.2013.835185

Reisner, S. L., Poteat, T., Keatley, J., Cabral, M., Mothopeng, T., Dunham, E., ... Baral, S. D. (2016). Global health burden and needs of transgender populations: A review. *Lancet, 388*(10042), 412–436. doi:10.1016/S0140-6736(16)00684-X PMID:27323919

Renninger, K. A., & Su, S. (2012). *Interest and Its Development. In Handbook of Human Motivation.* Oxford University Press.

Response Ability. (2012). Retrieved October 22, 2017, from http://www.responseability.org/home

Reygan, F. (2016). Black lesbian (non) representation in 'gay'media in Cape Town: Constructing a globalized white, male, affluent, gay consumer. *African Identities, 14*(1), 85–98. doi:10.1080/14725843.2015.1100105

Richardson, J., Sinha, K., Iezzi, A., & Maxwell, A. (2012). Maximising health versus sharing: Measuring preferences for the allocation of the health budget. *Social Science & Medicine, 75*(8), 1351–1361. doi:10.1016/j.socscimed.2012.05.036 PMID:22795915

Rickwood, D., Deane, F. P., Wilson, C. J., & Ciarrochi, J. (2005). Young people's help-seeking for mental health problems. *Australian e-Journal for the Advancement of Mental Health, 4*(3), 218–251. doi:10.5172/jamh.4.3.218

Ridani, R., Shand, F. L., Christensen, H., McKay, K., Tighe, J., Burns, J., & Hunter, E. (2015). Suicide prevention in Australian Aboriginal communities: A review of past and present programs. *Suicide & Life-Threatening Behavior, 45*(1), 111–140. doi:10.1111ltb.12121 PMID:25227155

Rine, C. M. (2013). Therapeutic uses of rap and hip-hop. *Health & Social Work, 38*(1), 59–62. doi:10.1093/hsw/hls061

Ripa, Y. (1990). *Women and madness: the incarceration of women in nineteenth century France.* Cambridge, UK: Polity Press.

Robert Wood Johnson Foundation (RWJF). (2010). *Developing and implementing self-direction programs and policies: A handbook.* Retrieved from USA: https://www.bc.edu/content/dam/files/schools/gssw_sites/nrcpds/cc-full.pdf

Robert, G., Harlock, J., & Williams, I. (2014). Disentangling rhetoric and reality: An international Delphi study of factors and processes that facilitate the successful implementation of decisions to decommission healthcare services. *Implementation Science; IS*, *9*(1), 123. doi:10.118613012-014-0123-y PMID:25204900

Rogers, H., & Barnes, M. (2003). Caring voices: Carers' participation in policy and practice. *Research Highlights in Social Work*, 117-136.

Rogers, B., & Dunne, E. (2013). A Qualitative Study on the Use of the Care Programme Approach with Individuals with Borderline Personality Disorder. *Journal of Psychosocial Nursing and Mental Health Services*, *51*(10), 38–45. doi:10.3928/02793695-20130628-03 PMID:23855437

Rogers, R. W. (1975). A protection motivation theory of fear appeals and attitude change. *The Journal of Psychology*, *91*(1), 93–114. doi:10.1080/00223980.1975.9915803 PMID:28136248

Rosenstreich, G. (2011). LGBTI people mental health and suicide. *National LGBTI Health Alliance*, 1-12.

Rosenstreich, G. (2013). *LGBTI People Mental Health and Suicide* (2nd ed.). Sydney: National LGBTI Health Alliance.

Rosenthal, B., & Wilson, W. C. (2008). Mental health services: Use and disparity among diverse college students. *Journal of American College Health*, *57*(1), 61–68. doi:10.3200/JACH.57.1.61-68 PMID:18682347

Ross, M. (2003). The legal framework of caring. *Research Highlights in Social Work*, 177-194.

Ross, L. E., Dobinson, C., & Eady, A. (2010). Perceived determinants of mental health for bisexual people: A qualitative examination. *American Journal of Public Health*, *100*(3), 496–502. doi:10.2105/AJPH.2008.156307 PMID:20075326

Rossman, K., Salamanca, P., & Macapagal, K. (2017). A qualitative study examining young adults' experiences of disclosure and non-disclosure of LGBTQ identity to healthcare providers. *Journal of Homosexuality*. (accepted for publication)

Ruger, J. P. (2004). Health and social justice. *Lancet*, *364*(9439), 1075–1080. doi:10.1016/S0140-6736(04)17064-5 PMID:15380968

Russell, D. (1995). *Women, madness & medicine*. Cambridge, UK: Polity Press.

Rutherford, K., McIntyre, J., Daley, A., & Ross, L. E. (2012). Development of expertise in mental health service provision for lesbian, gay, bisexual and transgender communities. *Medical Education*, *46*(9), 903–913. doi:10.1111/j.1365-2923.2012.04272.x PMID:22891911

Ryan, C. J., Callaghan, S., & Large, M. (2015). The importance of least restrictive care: The clinical implications of a recent High Court decision on negligence. *Australasian Psychiatry*, *23*(4), 415–417. doi:10.1177/1039856215590025 PMID:26104773

Ryan, C., Nielssen, O., Paton, M., & Large, M. (2010). Clinical decisions in psychiatry should not be based on risk assessment. *Australasian Psychiatry*, *18*(5), 398–403. doi:10.3109/10398562.2010.507816 PMID:20863176

Ryan, R., & Deci, E. (2000). Intrinsic and Extrinsic Motivations: Classic Definitions and New Directions. *Contemporary Educational Psychology*, *25*(1), 54–67. doi:10.1006/ceps.1999.1020 PMID:10620381

Ryle, A., & Kerr, I. B. (2002). *Introducing Cognitive Analytic Therapy. Principles and Practices*. Retrieved from http://www.ucl.ac.uk/clinical-psychology/competency-maps/pd- framework/Specific psychological interventions/Cognitive Analytic Therapy for webpage.pdf

Sabik, L. M., & Lie, R. K. (2008). Priority setting in health care: Lessons from the experiences of eight countries. *International Journal for Equity in Health*, *7*(1), 4. doi:10.1186/1475-9276-7-4 PMID:18208617

Sackett, S., & Richardson, R. (2006). Evidence-based practice. *Found Evidence-Based Social Work Pract, 35.*

Safer, D. L., Telch, C. F., & Agras, W. S. (2011). Dialectical behavior therapy for bulimia nervosa. *The American Journal of Psychiatry, 158*(4), 632–634. doi:10.1176/appi.ajp.158.4.632 PMID:11282700

Sajadi, S. F., Arshadi, N., Zargar, Y., Mehrabizade Honarmand, M., & Haijari, Z. (2015). Borderline Personality Features in Students: The Predicting Role of Schema, Emotion Regulation, Dissociative Experience and Suicidal Ideation. *International Journal of High Risk Behaviors & Addiction, 4*(2). doi:10.5812/ijhrba.20021v2 PMID:26401490

Sander, M., Oxlund, B., Jespersen, A., Krasnik, A., Mortensen, E., Westendorp, R., & Rasmussen, L. (2015). The challenges of human population ageing. *Age and Ageing, 44*(2), 185–187. doi:10.1093/ageing/afu189 PMID:25452294

Satariano, W., Scharlach, A., & Lindeman, D. (2014). Aging, place, and technology: Toward improving access and wellness in older populations. *Journal of Aging and Health, 26*(8), 1373–1389. doi:10.1177/0898264314543470 PMID:25502245

Sawyer, M. G., Arney, F. M., Baghurst, P. A., Clark, J. J., Graetz, B. W., Kosky, R. J., & ... . (2000). *Child and adolescent component of the national survey of mental health and well-being.* Canberra: Mental Health and Special Programs Branch of the Commonwealth Department of Health and Aged Care.

Sayago, S., & Blat, J. (2011). An Ethnographical Study of the Accessibility Barriers in the Everyday Interactions of Older People with the Web. *Universal Access in the InfoPrmation Society, 10*(4), 359–371. doi:10.100710209-011-0221-4

Scheyett, A. (2005). The mark of madness: Stigma, serious mental illnesses, and social work. *Social Work in Mental Health, 3*(4), 79–97. doi:10.1300/J200v03n04_05

Schiele, J. H. (1996). Afrocentricity: An emerging paradigm in social work practice. *Social Work, 41*(3), 284–294. PMID:8936084

Schiele, J. H. (2000). *Human services and the Afrocentric paradigm.* New York, NY: Haworth Press.

Schofield, H., Bloch, S., Herman, H., Murphy, B., Nankervis, J., & Singh, B. (1998). *Family Caregivers: Disability, Illness and Ageing.* St Leonards, N.S.W: Allen & Unwin in association with the Victorian Health Promotion Foundation (VicHealth).

Schore, A. N. (1994). *Affect regulation and the origin of the self: The neurobiology of emotional development.* Hillsdale, NJ: Lawrence Erlbaum and Associates.

Schulz, S. L. (2018). The Informed Consent Model of Transgender Care: An Alternative to the Diagnosis of Gender Dysphoria. *Journal of Humanistic Psychology, 58*(1), 72–92. doi:10.1177/0022167817745217

Schwartz, A. J. (2006). Are college students more disturbed today? Stability in the acuity and qualitative character of psychopathology of college counseling center clients: 1992-1993 through 2001-2002. *Journal of American College Health, 54*(6), 327–337. doi:10.3200/JACH.54.6.327-337 PMID:16789648

Scottish Executive National Health System. (2006). *Allied Health Professions: Workload Measurement and Management.* Retrieved from http://www.sehd.scot.nhs.uk/ahp/_documents/ ahpworkloadmeasureandmanage.pdf

Scottish Parliament. (2013). Social Care (Self-directed Support)(Scotland) Act 2013. *Scottish Parliament.*

Scott, R. (2006). Hunter Area Health Services v Presland: Liability of Mental Health Services for Failing to Admit or Detain a Patient With Mental Illness. *Psychiatry, Psychology and Law, 13*(1), 49–59. doi:10.1375/pplt.13.1.49

Scott, S. D., Pringle, A., & Lumsdaine, C. (2004). *Sexual Exclusion–Homophobia and health inequalities: a review.* London: Health First.

Scull, A. (2015). *Madness in civilization: a cultural history of insanity, from the bible to Freud, from the madhouse to modern medicine*. Princeton University Press. doi:10.1515/9781400865710

Secondary schools program. (2016). Retrieved September 24, 2017, from https://www.beyondblue.org.au/healthy-places/secondary-schools-and-tertiary/secondary-schools-program

Secretariat of National Aboriginal and Islander Child Care. (2013). *Whose voice counts: Aboriginal and Torres Strait Islander participation in child protection decision-making*. Melbourne: SNAICC.

Sen, A. (2002). Why health equity? *Health Economics*, *11*(8), 659–666. doi:10.1002/hec.762 PMID:12457367

SenseAbility. (2016). Retrieved September 24, 2017, from https://www.beyondblue.org.au/healthy-places/secondary-schools-and-tertiary/senseability/download-sensibility

Shakespeare, T. (2014). *Disability rights and wrongs revisited*. Abingdon, UK: Routledge.

Shamir, Y. & Kutner, R. (2003). *Alternative dispute resolution approaches and their application*. PCCP, UNESCO-IHP, Series 7, 1-43.

Shapin, S. (1982). History of science and its sociological reconstructions. *History of Science*, *20*(3), 157–211. doi:10.1177/007327538202000301

Sheehan, M., Cahill, H., Rowling, L., Marshall, B., Wynn, J., & Holdsworth. (2002). Establishing A Role for Schools in Mental Health Promotion: The MindMatters Project. In G. Martin, L. Rowling & L. Walker (Eds.), *Mental Health Promotion: Concepts and Practice Young People* (pp. 111 - 127). Sydney: McGraw-Hill Australia Pty Limited.

Sheldon, K., & Krieger, L. (2007). Understanding the negative effects of legal education on law students: A longitudinal test of Self-Determination Theory. *Personality and Social Psychology Bulletin*, *33*(6), 883–897. doi:10.1177/0146167207301014 PMID:17483395

Shen, C., Smyer, M., Mahoney, K. J., Simon-Rusinowitz, L., Shinogle, J., Norstrand, J., ... del Vecchio, P. (2008). Consumer-directed care for beneficiaries with mental illness: Lessons from New Jersey's Cash and Counseling program. *Psychiatric Services (Washington, D.C.)*, *59*(11), 1299–1306. doi:10.1176/ps.2008.59.11.1299 PubMed

Sheppard, E. (1872). On some of the teachings of insanity. *The Journal of Mental Science*, *17*(80), 499–514. doi:10.1192/bjp.17.80.499

Shiu, C., Muraco, A., & Fredriksen-Goldsen, K. (2016). Invisible care: Friend and partner care among older lesbian, gay, bisexual, and transgender (LGBT) adults. *Journal of the Society for Social Work and Research*, *7*(3), 527–546. doi:10.1086/687325 PMID:28367277

Shlonsky, A., Parolini, A., Tan, W. W., Ma, J., Mildon, R., Albers, B., & Tinkler, M. (2016). *The Family Matters report: measuring trends to turn the tide on Aboriginal and Torres Strait Islander child safety and removal*. Melbourne: University of Melbourne, SNAICC & Save the Children. Retrieved from https://nacchocommunique.files.wordpress.com/2016/11/family_matters_report_2016.pdf

Showalter, E. (1985). *The female malady: women, madness, and English culture, 1830-1980*. London: Virago.

Showalter, E. (1987). *The female malady: Women, madness and English culture, 1830-1980*. London: Virago.

Shuval, H. I. (1992). Approaches to resolving the water conflicts between Israel and her neighbors: A regional water-for-peace plan. *Water International*, *17*(3), 133–143. doi:10.1080/02508069208686133

Sibbald, S. L., Singer, P. A., Upshur, R., & Martin, D. K. (2009). Priority setting: What constitutes success? A conceptual framework for successful priority setting. *BMC Health Services Research*, *9*(1), 43. doi:10.1186/1472-6963-9-43 PMID:19265518

Siever, L. J., & Koenigsberg, H. W. (2000). *The frustrating no-mans-land of borderline personality disorder. Cerebrum*. New York: The Dana Forum on Brain Science.

Sifris, A. (2014). *Gay and lesbian parenting: The legislative response*. Retrieved from https://aifs.gov.au/publications/families-policy-and-law/10-gay-and-lesbian-parenting-legislative-response

Silburn, S., Robinson, G., Leckning, B., Henry, D., Cox, A., & Kickitt, D. (2014). Preventing suicide among Aboriginal Australians. In Working together: Aboriginal and Torres Strait Islander mental health and wellbeing principles and practices (pp. 145-164). Barton, ACT: Commonwealth of Australia.

Silvia, P. J. (2006). *Exploring the psychology of interest*. Melbourne, Australia: Oxford University Press. doi:10.1093/acprof:oso/9780195158557.001.0001

Simon-Rusinowitz, L., Croft, B., Loughlin, D., & Mahoney, K. (2013). *An environmental scan of self-direction in behavioral health: A review of the literature*. Chestnut Hill, MA: Human Services Research Institute and The National Resource Center for Participant-Directed Services.

Skodol, A. E., Gunderson, J. G., Pfohl, B., Widigier, T. A., Livesley, W. J., & Siever, L. J. (2002). The borderline diagnosis I: Psychopathology, comorbidity, and personality structure. *Biological Psychiatry*, *51*(12), 936–960. doi:10.1016/S0006-3223(02)01324-0 PMID:12062877

Skre, I., Friborg, O., Breivik, C., Johnsen, L. I., Arnesen, Y., & Wang, C. E. A. (2013). A school intervention for mental health literacy in adolescents: Effects of a non-randomized cluster controlled trial. *BMC Public Health*, *13*, 873.

Slade, M., & Longden, E. (2015). *The empirical evidence about mental health and recovery: how likely, how long, what helps*. Melbourne: MI Fellowship.

Slemon, A., Jenkins, E., & Bungay, V. (2017). Safety in psychiatric inpatient care: The impact of risk management culture on mental health nursing practice. *Nursing Inquiry*, *24*(4).

Smith, N. G., & Ingram, K. M. (2004). Workplace Heterosexism and Adjustment Among Lesbian, Gay, and Bisexual Individuals: The Role of Unsupportive Social Interactions. *Journal of Counseling Psychology*, *51*(1), 57–67. doi:10.1037/0022-0167.51.1.57

Smye, V., & Browne, A. (2002). Cultural safety and the analysis of health policy affecting Aboriginal people. *Nurse Researcher*, *9*(3), 42–56. doi:10.7748/nr2002.04.9.3.42.c6188 PMID:11985147

Soares, M. O. (2012). Is the QALY blind, deaf and dumb to equity? NICE's considerations over equity. *British Medical Bulletin*, *101*(1), 17–31. doi:10.1093/bmb/lds003 PMID:22331197

Solomon, A. (2001). *The noonday demon: An anatomy of depression*. London, UK: Chatto & Windus.

Solomon, A. (2015). Notes on an exorcism. In C. Burns & A. Gopnik (Eds.), *The moth: This is a true story* (pp. 34–42). London, UK: Serpent's Tail.

Sowbel, L. R. (2012). Gatekeeping: Why shouldn't we be ambivalent? *Journal of Social Work Education*, *48*(1), 27–44. doi:10.5175/JSWE.2012.201000027

Spandler, H., & Vick, N. (2006). Opportunities for independent living using direct payments in mental health. *Health & Social Care in the Community*, *14*(2), 107–115. doi:10.1111/j.1365-2524.2006.00598.x PMID:16460360

Stacey, D., Murray, M. A., Legare, F., Sandy, D., Menard, P., & O'connor, A. (2008). Decision coaching to support shared decision making: A framework, evidence, and implications for nursing practice, education, and policy. *Worldviews on Evidence-Based Nursing*, *5*(1), 25–35. doi:10.1111/j.1741-6787.2007.00108.x PMID:18266768

Stalker, K. (2003). Chapter One. In G. Grant & P. Ramcharan (Eds.), *Reconceptualising Work with 'carers': New Directions for Policy and Practice*. Jessica Kingsley Publishers.

Stallman, H. M. (2010). Psychological distress in university students: A comparison with general population data. *Australian Psychologist*, *45*(4), 249–257. doi:10.1080/00050067.2010.482109

Standage, M., Duda, J., & Ntoumanis, N. (2005). A test of self-determination theory in school physical education. *The British Journal of Educational Psychology*, *75*(3), 411–433. doi:10.1348/000709904X22359 PMID:16238874

Stansfeld, S., Smuk, M., Onwumere, J., Clark, C., Pike, C., McManus, S., ... Bebbington, P. (2014). Stressors and common mental disorder in informal carers–An analysis of the English Adult Psychiatric Morbidity Survey 2007. *Social Science & Medicine*, *120*, 190–198. doi:10.1016/j.socscimed.2014.09.025 PMID:25259657

State of Victoria Department of Health. (2013). *National Practice Standards for the mental health workforce*. Retrieved 04 December 2017 from http://www.health.gov.au/internet/main/publishing.nsf/Content/5D7909E82304E6D2CA257C430004E877/$File/wkstd13.pdf

Stern, B., & Yeomans, F. (2015). *Transference-Focused Psychotherapy (TFP)*. New York: The Center for Transference-Focused Psychotherapy.

Stoffers, J. M., Völlm, B. A., Rücker, G., Timmer, A., Huband, N., & Lieb, K. (2012). Psychological therapies for people with borderline personality disorder. *The Cochrane Database Of Systematic Reviews*, (8).

Stone, K. (n.d.). What the new DSM-V says about post-partum depression and psychosis. *Post-partum Progress*. Retrieved from: http://www.postpartumprogress.com/what-the-new-dsm-v-says-about-postpartum-depression-psychosis

Stone, G. (2011). *Self-orientation and relational-orientation in suicidal risk: Possible facilitative and protective aspects*. ProQuest Dissertations Publishing.

Stone, L. (1982). *Madness. In Critical thought series: 2, critical essays on Michel Foucault*. Scolar Press.

Stuart, H. L., Arboleda-Flórez, J., & Sartorius, N. (2012). *Paradigms lost: fighting stigma and the lessons learned*. New York: Oxford University Press. doi:10.1093/med/9780199797639.001.0001

Substance Abuse & Mental Health Administration. (2014). *SAMHSA's Concept of Trauma and Guidance for a Trauma-Informed Approach*. Rockville, MD: Author.

Suls, J., & Rothman, A. (2004). Evolution of the biopsychosocial model: Prospects and challenges for health psychology. *Health Psychology*, *27*(2), 119–125. doi:10.1037/0278-6133.23.2.119 PMID:15008654

Summers, N. (2010). *Managing social service staff for excellence: Five keys to exceptional supervision*. Hoboken, NJ: John Wiley & Sons. doi:10.1002/9781118270004

Szasz, T. (2007). *The medicalization of everyday life: selected essays*. New York: Syracuse University Press.

Szmukler, G., & Rose, N. (2013). Risk assessment in mental health care: Values and costs. *Behavioral Sciences & the Law*, *31*(1), 125–140. doi:10.1002/bsl.2046 PMID:23296543

Tam, D., & Coleman, H. (2009). Defining criteria on professional suitability for social work practice. *The Journal of Baccalaureate Social Work*, *14*(2), 105–121.

Tanner, F. (2000). Conflict prevention and conflict resolution: Limits of multilateralism. *Revue Internationale de la Croix-Rouge. International Review of the Red Cross, 82*(839), 541–559. doi:10.1017/S1560775500184615

Taylor, K., & Guerin, P. (2010). *Health care and Indigenous Australians: Cultural Safety in Practice* (2nd ed.). South Yarra: Palgrave Macmillan.

teen MHFA Course Information. (2017). Retrieved September 30, 2017, from https://mhfa.com.au/cms/teen-mhfa-course-information

Tew, J., Ramon, S., Slade, M., Bird, V., Melton, J., & Le Boutillier, C. (2011). Social factors and recovery from mental health difficulties: A Review of the evidence. *British Journal of Social Work, 42*(3), 443–460. doi:10.1093/bjsw/bcr076

The beyondblue Mental Health in Education program. (2016). Retrieved September 30 September, 2017, from https://www.beyondblue.org.au/about-us/about-our-work/childhood-and-education-program/the-i-beyondblue-i-mental-health-in-education-program

The Bouverie Centre. (2016). *The Bouverie Centre Aboriginal Family Therapy Training Program Evidence Brief August 2015*. Brunswick, VIC: The Bouverie Centre.

The Joint Commission. (2011). *Advancing effective communication, cultural competence, and patient-and family-centered care for the lesbian, gay, bisexual, and transgender (LGBT) community: A field guide*. Retrieved from https://www.jointcommission.org/lgbt/

thedesk. (2016). Retrieved October 15, 2017, from https://www.beyondblue.org.au/healthy-places/secondary-schools-and-tertiary/thedesk

Theed, R., Eccles, F., & Simpson, J. (2017). Experiences of caring for a family member with Parkinson's disease: A meta-synthesis. *Aging & Mental Health, 21*(10), 1007–1016. doi:10.1080/13607863.2016.1247414 PMID:27802771

Thomas, L. Y. (2015). *Faculty on the frontline: Faculty attitudes toward mental illness in 2-year college students* (Unpublished doctoral dissertation). Mercer University, Atlanta.

Thomas, R., Pega, F., Khosla, R., Verster, A., Hana, T., & Say, L. (2017). Ensuring an inclusive global health agenda for transgender people. *Bulletin of the World Health Organization, 95*(2), 154–156. doi:10.2471/BLT.16.183913 PMID:28250518

Thomasson, F. (2004). *Water and local conflict: A brief review of the academic literature and other sources*. Stockholm, Sweden: Conflict and Water Group, Swedish Waterhouse.

Thomas, W. J. (1993). The Oregon Medicaid Proposal: Ethical Paralysis, Tragic Democracy, and the Fate of a Utilitarian Health Care Program. *Oregon Law Review, 72*, 47.

Thompson, A., Hunt, C., & Issakidis, C. (2004). Why wait? Reasons for delay and prompts to seek help for mental health problems in an Australian clinical sample. *Social Psychiatry and Psychiatric Epidemiology, 39*(10), 810–817. doi:10.100700127-004-0816-7 PMID:15669662

Timmerman, L. C., & Mulvihill, T. M. (2015). Accommodations in the college setting: The perspectives of students living with disabilities. *Qualitative Report, 20*(10), 1609.

Tinney, J., Dow, B., Maude, P., Purchase, R., Whyte, C., & Barrett, C. (2015). Mental health issues and discrimination among older LGBTI people. *International Psychogeriatrics, 27*(9), 1411–1416. doi:10.1017/S1041610214002671 PMID:26223452

Tin, T. B. (2013). Exploring the Development of 'Interest' in Learning English as a Foreign/Second Language. *RELC Journal*, *44*(2), 129–146. doi:10.1177/0033688213488388

Tong, H. C., Haig, A. J., Nelson, V. S., Yamakawa, K. S. J., Kandala, G., & Shin, K. Y. (2003). Low back pain in adult female caregivers of children with physical disabilities. *Archives of Pediatrics & Adolescent Medicine*, *157*(11), 1128–1133. doi:10.1001/archpedi.157.11.1128 PMID:14609905

Towle, A., Godolphin, W., Greenhalgh, T., & Gambrill, J. (1999). Framework for teaching and learning informed shared decision making. *BMJ: British Medical Journal*, *319*(7212), 766–771. doi:10.1136/bmj.319.7212.766 PMID:10488010

Transparency International. (2008). *Global corruption report 2008: Corruption in the water sector*. New York: Cambridge University Press.

Trull, T. J., Useda, J. D., Conforti, K., & Doan, B.-T. (1997). Borderline Personality Disorder Features in Nonclinical Young Adults: 2. Two Year Outcome. *Journal of Abnormal Psychology*, *106*(2), 307–314. doi:10.1037/0021-843X.106.2.307 PMID:9131850

Tsuchiya, A., & Dolan, P. (2009). Equality of what in health? Distinguishing between outcome egalitarianism and gain egalitarianism. *Health Economics*, *18*(2), 147–159. doi:10.1002/hec.1355 PMID:18484571

Tuck, E., & Yang, K. (2012). Decolonisation is not a metaphor. Indigeneity. *Education and Society*, *1*(1), 1–40.

Turnbull, C., Grimmer-Somers, K., Kumar, S., May, E., Law, D., & Ashworth, E. (2009). Allied, scientific and complementary health professionals: A new model for Australian allied health. *Australian Health Review*, *33*(1), 27–37. doi:10.1071/AH090027 PMID:19203331

Tyson, E. H. (2011). Hip-Hop healing: Rap music in grief therapy with an African American adolescent male. In S. Hadley & G. Yancy (Eds.), *Therapeutic uses of rap and hip hop* (pp. 293–306). New York, NY: Routledge.

UN General Assembly. (2007). *Convention on the Rights of Persons with Disabilities: resolution adopted by the General Assembly, 24 January 2007, A/RES/61/106*. Retrieved from http://www.refworld.org/docid/45f973632.html

Undrill, G. (2011). Calling time on risk assessments. *Journal of Psychiatric Intensive Care*, *7*(2), 67–72. doi:10.1017/S1742646411000045

United Nations Development Program. (2006a). *Human development report 2002: Deepening democracy in a fragmented world*. New York: Oxford University Press.

United Nations Development Program. (2006b). *Annual report 2006: Global partnership for development*. New York: UNDP.

United Nations Educational, Scientific and Cultural Organization. (2015). *The United Nations World Water Development Report 2015*. Paris: UNESCO Publishing.

United Nations Educational, Scientific, and Cultural Organization. (2013). Water for people, water for life (The United Nations World Water Development Report). Paris, France: UNESCO Publishing and Berghahn Books.

United Nations Sustainable Development Goals. (2016). *244 million international migrants living abroad worldwide, new UN statistics reveal*. Retrieved October 20, 2017 from http://www.un.org/sustainabledevelopment/blog/2016/01/244-million-international-migrants-living-abroad-worldwide-new-un-statistics-reveal/

United States Agency for International Development. (2014). *The Conflict Early Warning and Response Mechanism (CEWARN)*. Washington, DC: USAID.

Urbis. (2015). *Report on the Review of Disability Standards for Education 2005*. Retrieved 16 May, 2016 from http://auspeld.org.au/wp-content/uploads/2012/08/Report_on_the_Review_of_DSE.pdf

Uren, D. (2017). *A super fail: 80pc retire on pension benefits. The Australian. 12.00am, August 26*. Canberra, Australia: News Corp Australia.

Uribe, R., & Gunter, B. (2007). Are "sensational" news stories more likely to trigger viewers' emotions than non-sensational news stories? *European Journal of Communication, 22*(2), 207–228. doi:10.1177/0267323107076770

Urwin, C. A., Soest, D. V., & Kretzschmar, J. A. (2006). Key principles for developing gatekeeping standards for working with students with problems. *Journal of Teaching in Social Work, 26*(1-2), 163–180. doi:10.1300/J067v26n01_10

Ussher, J. (1991). *Women's madness: misogyny or mental illness?* Boston: University of Massachusetts Press.

Valenti, K., & Katz, A. (2014). Needs and perceptions of LGBTQ caregivers: The challenges of services and support. *Journal of Gay & Lesbian Social Services, 26*(1), 70–90. doi:10.1080/10538720.2013.865575

Van der Kolk, B. A. (1987). *Psychological trauma*. Washington, DC: American Psychiatric Press.

Van der Kolk, B. A. (1988). Trauma spectrum: The interaction of biological and social events in the genesis of the trauma response. *Journal of Traumatic Stress, 1*(3), 273–290. doi:10.1002/jts.2490010302

Varnham, S., & Kamvounias, P. (2009). Unfair, unlawful, or just unhappy: Issues surrounding complaints of discrimination made by students against their universities in Australia. *International Journal of Law & Education, 14*(5).

Veltre, V. J., & Hardley, S. (2011). Hip-Hop: A Hip-Hop feminist approach to music therapy with adolescent females. In S. Hadley & G. Yancy (Eds.), *Therapeutic uses of rap and hip hop* (pp. 79–98). New York, NY: Routledge.

Victoria State Government. (2017). *Clinical risk management*. Retrieved October 3, from https://www2.health.vic.gov.au/hospitals-and-health-services/quality-safety-service/clinical-risk-management

Victoria State Government. (n.d.). *Allied health therapy and science disciplines: Position Paper*. Melbourne: Health and Human Services. Retrieved from https://www2.health.vic.gov.au/about/publications/policiesandguidelines/allied-health-categories-position-paper

Victorian Aboriginal Child Care Agency. (2018). *VACCA*. Retrieved from: https://www.vacca.org/

Victorian Government Solicitor's Office. (2015). *High Court decision- Stuart v Kirkland-Veenstra [2009] HCA 15*. Retrieved October 2, 2017, from http://vgso.vic.gov.au/content/high-court-decision-stuart-v-kirkland-veenstra-2009-hca-15

Villiers, M. D. (2000). *Water: The fate of our most precious resource*. New York: Mariner Books.

Voumard, S. (2016). *The media and the massacre: port arthur 1996-2016*. Melbourne: Transit Lounge Publishing.

Vuković, M. (2008). The identification of water conflict and its resolution. *FACTA UNIVERSITATIS, Series Philosophy, Sociology. Psychology and History, 7*(1), 81–93.

Wade, D. T., & Halligan, P. W. (2017). The biopsychosocial model of illness: A model whose time has come. *Clinical Rehabilitation, 31*(8), 995–1004. doi:10.1177/0269215517709890 PMID:28730890

Waldeck, E., & Guthrie, R. (2004). *Disability Discrimination in Education and the Defence of Unjustifiable Hardship*. School of Business Law, Curtin University of Technology.

Wallensteen, P. (2002). *Understanding Conflict Resolution, War, Peace and the Global System*. London: Sage Publications.

Walters, K. L., & Old Person, R. L. (2008). Lesbians, gays, bisexuals, and transgender people of color: Reconciling divided selves and communities. *Social Work Practice with Lesbian, Gay, Bisexual, and Transgender people*, 41-68.

Wand, T. (2011). Investigating the Evidence for the Effectiveness of risk assessment in mental health care. *Issues in Mental Health Nursing*, *33*(1), 2–7. doi:10.3109/01612840.2011.616984 PMID:22224960

Wand, T., Isobel, S., & Derrick, K. (2015). Surveying clinician perceptions of risk assessment and management practices in mental health service provision. *Australasian Psychiatry*, *23*(2), 147–153. doi:10.1177/1039856214568227 PMID:25688130

Wang, P. S., Berglund, P. A., Olfson, M., & Kessler, R. C. (2004). Delays in initial treatment contact after first onset of a mental disorder. *Health Services Research*, *39*(2), 393–416. doi:10.1111/j.1475-6773.2004.00234.x PMID:15032961

Ward, D. (2000). Ageism and the abuse of older people in health and social care. *British Journal of Nursing (Mark Allen Publishing)*, *9*(9), 560–563. doi:10.12968/bjon.2000.9.9.6292 PMID:11904891

Warr, D., Dickinson, H., Olney, S., Hargrave, J., Karanikolas, A., Kasidis, V., & Wheeler, J. (2017). *Choice, control and the NDIS: Service users' perspectives on having choice and control in the new National Disability Insurance Scheme.* Melbourne: Social Equity Institute, University of Melbourne.

Washington, K. T., McElroy, J., Albright, D., Oliver, D. P., Lewis, A., Meadows, S., & Elliott, S. (2015). Experiences of sexual and gender minorities caring for adults with non-AIDS-related chronic illnesses. *Social Work Research*, *39*(2), 71–81. doi:10.1093wrvu030

Watkinson, A. M., & Chalmers, D. (2008). Disability, professional unsuitability and the profession of social work: A case study. *Social Work Education*, *27*(5), 504–518. doi:10.1080/02615470701379974

Watts R. (2016). *Public Universities, Managerialism and the Value of the University.* Palgrave-McMillan.

Watts, O., Stickels, C., Fraser, C., Carroll, R., Stewart, N., & Radloff, A. (2000). *Guidelines and Procedures to assist Universities to Examine the Inherent Requirements of their Courses.* Curtin University of Technology. Retrieved 28 April, 2016, from http://www.adcet.edu.au/download/attachment/5200%E2%80%901/

Wayne, R. H. (2004). Legal guidelines for dismissing students because of poor performance in the field. *Journal of Social Work Education*, *40*(3), 403–414. doi:10.1080/10437797.2004.10672296

Weare, K. & Nind, M. (2011). Mental health promotion and problem prevention in schools: what does the evidence say? *Health Promotion International, 26*(S1), i29-i69.

Webber, M., Treacy, S., Carr, S., Clark, M., & Parker, G. (2014). The effectiveness of personal budgets for people with mental health problems: A systematic review. *Journal of Mental Health (Abingdon, England)*, *23*(3), 146–155. doi:10.3109/09638237.2014.910642 PMID:24803221

Wehmeier, S. (2000). *Oxford Advanced Learner's Dictionary of Current English* (6th ed.). New York: Oxford University Press.

Weinthal, E. (2006). Water Conflict and Cooperation in Central Asia. *Human Development Report Occasional Paper, 32*, 1-36.

Weiss, R. (2015). *Confronting cultural challenges for migrant healthcare in Switzerland. Independent Study Project (ISP) Collection, PAPER 2104*. Retrieved October 20, 2017 from http://digitalcollections.sit.edu/isp_collection/2104

Wetzelaer, P., Farrell, J., Evers, S. M., Jacob, G. A., Lee, C. W., Brand, O., ... Arntz, A. (2014). Design of an international multicentre RCT on group schema therapy for borderline personality disorder. *BMC Psychiatry*, *18*(14), 319. doi:10.118612888-014-0319-3 PMID:25407009

What is MindMatters? (n.d.). Retrieved October 09, 2017, from https://www.mindmatters.edu.au/about-mindmatters/what-is-mindmatters

Whitehead, J., Shaver, J., & Stephenson, R. (2016). Outness, stigma, and primary health care utilization among rural LGBT populations. *PLoS One*, *11*(1), e0146139. doi:10.1371/journal.pone.0146139 PMID:26731405

Whitehead, M. (1991). The concepts and principles of equity and health. *Health Promotion International*, *3*(6), 217–228. doi:10.1093/heapro/6.3.217

Why it is needed? (n.d.). Retrieved October 21, 2017, from https://www.kidsmatter.edu.au/primary/about-kidsmatter-primary/why-it-needed-0

Williams, C. (2018). Revisiting cross-cultural practice. In M. Connolly, L. Harms & J. Maidment (Eds.), Social work: Contexts and practice (pp. 64-80). South Melbourne, Australia: Oxford.

Williams, J. (2013). *The international implications of China's water policies*. Bristol, UK: E-International Relations (E-IR). Retrieved from: http://www.e-ir.info/2013/02/15/chinas-water-policies-and-their-international-implications/

Williams, C. (2007). "Permission to speak": A carer's experience. *Australian Health Review*, *31*(2), 167–171. doi:10.1071/AH070167 PMID:17470035

Williams, C. (2012). Chronic illness and informal carers: 'Non-persons' in the health system, neither carers, workers or citizens. *Health Sociology Review*, *21*(1), 58–68. doi:10.5172/hesr.2012.21.1.58

Williams, G., & Deci, E. (1996). Internalization of biopsychosocial values by medical students: A test of Self-Determination Theory. *Journal of Personality and Social Psychology*, *70*(4), 767–779. doi:10.1037/0022-3514.70.4.767 PMID:8636897

Williams, R. (1999). Cultural safety: What does it mean for our work practice? *Australian and New Zealand Journal of Public Health*, *23*(2), 212. doi:10.1111/j.1467-842X.1999.tb01240.x PMID:10330743

Williams, T., & Smith, G. (2014). Can the National Disability Insurance Scheme work for mental health? *The Australian and New Zealand Journal of Psychiatry*, *48*(5), 391–394. doi:10.1177/0004867414530007 PMID:24671233

Willis, P., Ward, N., & Fish, J. (2011). Searching for LGBT carers: Mapping a research agenda in social work and social care. *British Journal of Social Work*, *41*(7), 1304–1320. doi:10.1093/bjsw/bcr114

Wilson, W. A. W., & Yellowbird, M. (Eds.). (2005). For Indigenous eyes only: A decolonisation handbook. Santa Fe, NM: School of American Research.

Wilson, C. (2011). *Neuroandragogy: Making the Case for a Link with Andragogy and Brain-Based Learning. In Midwest Research-to-Practice Conference in Adult, Continuing, Community and Extension Education* (pp. 21–23). St. Charles, MO: Lindenwood University, September.

Wilson, R. D., Lewis, S. A., & Murray, P. K. (2009). Trends in the Rehabilitation Therapist Workforce in Underserved Areas: 1980-2000. *The Journal of Rural Health*, *25*(1), 26–32. doi:10.1111/j.1748-0361.2009.00195.x PMID:19166558

Winsper, C., Marwaha, S., Lereya, S. T., Thompson, A., Eyden, J., & Singh, S. P. (2015). Clinical and psychosocial outcomes of borderline personality disorder in childhood and adolescence: A systematic review. *Psychological Medicine*, *45*(11), 2237–2251. doi:10.1017/S0033291715000318 PMID:25800970

Wintrob, R. (2010, January). Cross-cultural psychiatry: Introduction. *The Psychiatric Times*.

Wolf, A. T., Kramer, A., Carius, A., & Dabelko, G. D. (2005). Managing water conflict and cooperation: State of the world 2005. In Redefining global security (pp. 80-95). Washington, DC: The World Watch Institute.

Wolf, A., Yoffe, S. & Giordano, M. (2003). *International waters: Indicators for identifying basins at risk*. PCCP, UNESCO-IHP, 1-24.

Wolf, A. T. (1998). Conflict and cooperation along international waterways. *Water Policy*, *1*(2), 251–265. doi:10.1016/S1366-7017(98)00019-1

Wondemaghen, M. (2013). Depressed but not legally mentally impaired. *International Journal of Law and Psychiatry*, *37*(2), 160–167. doi:10.1016/j.ijlp.2013.11.010 PMID:24268825

World Commission on Dams. (2000). *Dams and development: A new framework for decision-making*. London: Earthscan.

World Economic Forum. (2017). *Life expectancy*. Washington, DC: The World Bank.

World Health Organisation (WHO). (2013). *Mental health Action Plan*. Retrieved October 20, 2017 from http://www.who.int/mental_health/action_plan_2013/bw_version.pdf?ua=1

World Health Organisation (WHO). (2017). *Mental health: A state of well-being*. Retrieved October 20, 2017 from http://www.who.int/features/factfiles/mental_health/en/

World Health Organisation. (2013). *Depression: factsheet no. 369*. Available at http://www.who.int/medicalcentre/factsheets/fs369/en/index.html

World Health Organisation. (2013). *Mental Health action plan 2013-2020*. Geneva, Switzerland: World Health Organisation.

World Health Organisational Regional Office for Europe. (1994). *Promoting the Health of Young People in Europe: Health Education in Schools: A Training Manual for Teachers and Others Working with Young People*. Edinburgh, UK: Health Education Board for Scotland.

World Health Organization. (2013). *Addressing the causes of disparities in health service access and utilization for lesbian, gay, bisexual and trans (LGBT) persons*. 52nd Directing Council. 65th Session of the Regional Committee. Concept Paper, 30.

World Health Organization. (2015). *The ICD-10 Classification of Mental and Behavioural Disorders*. Retrieved from http://www.who.int/classifications/icd/en/bluebook.pdf

Wreford, J. (2005). Missing each other: Problems and potential for collaborative efforts between biomedicine and traditional healers in South Africa in the time of AIDS. *Social Dynamics*, *31*(2), 55–89. doi:10.1080/02533950508628708

Wright, M., & O'Connell, M. (2015). Negotiating the right path: Working together to effect change in healthcare service provision to Aboriginal peoples. *Action Learning and Action Research Journal*, *21*, 108–123.

Wright, N., & Owen, S. (2001). Feminist conceptualizations of women's madness: A review of the literature. *Journal of Advanced Nursing*, *36*(1), 143–150. doi:10.1046/j.1365-2648.2001.01951.x PMID:11555058

Wrongs Act. 1958. (Vic) (Austl.)

Wyden, R. G. (2007). *Administrative perceptions of mental health trends and college counseling services* (Unpublished doctoral dissertation). University of North Florida, Jacksonville, FL.

Yancey, A. K., Cole, B. L., & McCarthy, W. J. (2010). A graphical, computer-based decision-support tool to help decision makers evaluate policy options relating to physical activity. *American Journal of Preventive Medicine*, *39*(3), 273–279. doi:10.1016/j.amepre.2010.05.013 PMID:20709260

Yancy, G., & Hadley, S. (2011). Introduction: Give 'em just one mic: Therapeutic agency of rap and hip hop. In S. Hadley & G. Yancy (Eds.), *Therapeutic uses of rap and hip hop (pp. xxiii-xlii)*. New York, NY: Routledge.

Yañez, A. M. (2014). *"Think with your feet": The cultural politics of Native Dance* (Unpublished doctoral dissertation). University of California, San Diego, CA

Yeandle, S., & Ungerson, C. (2007). Conceptualizing cash for care: The origins of contemporary debates. In C. Ungerson (Ed.), *Cash for Care in Developed Welfare States* (pp. 1–11). Basingstoke, UK: Palgrave Macmillan.

Yoffe, S., Wolfe, A. T., & Giordano, M. (2001). *Conflict and cooperation over international freshwater resources: Indicators and findings of the Basins at Risk project*. Retrieved from: http://transboundarywaters.science.oregonstate.edu/sites/transboundarywaters.science.oregonstate.edu/filesDatabase/ResearchProjects/BAR/BAR_chapter4.pdf

Youth Research Centre and Centre for Social Health. (1996). *Mental Health Education in Australian Secondary Schools*. Canberra: Australian Government Publishing Service.

Zanarini, M. C. (2000). Childhood experiences associated with the development of borderline personality disorder. *The Psychiatric Clinics of North America*, *23*(1), 89–101. doi:10.1016/S0193-953X(05)70145-3 PMID:10729933

Zanarini, M. C., & Frankenburg, F. R. (1997). Pathways to the development of borderline personality disorder. *Journal of Personality Disorders*, *11*(1), 93–104. doi:10.1521/pedi.1997.11.1.93 PMID:9113824

Zimmerman, M., Chelminski, I., & Young, D. (2008). The frequency of personality disorders in psychiatric patients. *The Psychiatric Clinics of North America*, *31*(3), 405–420. doi:10.1016/j.psc.2008.03.015 PMID:18638643

Zimmerman, M., Rothschild, L., & Chelminski, I. (2005). The prevalence of DSM-IV personality disorders in psychiatric outpatients. *The American Journal of Psychiatry*, *162*(10), 1911–1918. doi:10.1176/appi.ajp.162.10.1911 PMID:16199838

Zubrick, J., Holland, C., Kelly, K., Calma, T., & Walker, R. (2014). The evolving policy context in mental health and wellbeing. In Working together: Aboriginal and Torres Strait Islander mental health and wellbeing principles and practices (pp. 69-90). Barton, ACT: Commonwealth of Australia.

About the Contributors

Jennifer Martin is well experienced in the field of mental health as a social work researcher, educator and practitioner. Current research is focused on inter-disciplinary collaboration across health disciplines to improve communication skills and client outcomes. This includes effective use of technology to enhance inter-disciplinary collaboration. Her research into workforce development in social work, mental health and aged care focuses on issues of access and equity highlighting the importance of evidence-based research to inform practice outcomes and the importance of communicating this in reputable peer reviewed publications as well as to policy makers and in practice forums. Jennifer is regarded as an expert in the fields of education, mental health and social work. She currently holds invited appointments with TEQSA as an expert panel member, membership of the Board of Studies at Charles Sturt University and is a past academic advisor at the University of Malaysia-Sarawak, and past Chair of the RMIT University Appeals Committee. Jennifer is an invited university sector representative on the executive of the Victorian Department of Health and Human Services Allied Health Therapy Research Network and is a founding member of the NHMRC funded: Evidence Translation in Allied Health (EviTAH).

***

(Isobel) Ruth Bailey has a background in psychotherapy and social work, spanning over 30 years of clinical and academic engagement. She is a Lecturer in the School of Humanities and Social Sciences at Charles Sturt University, in New South Wales, Australia, where she teaches in mental health, counselling and ethical practice. Her interest is in relationship-based therapeutic practices and their intersection with structural/societal contexts and their preventative force in relation to mental health matters across the globe. Ruth has published on narcissism, on the importance of a courageous analysis of ego-defences, and on peer consultation as an avenue for restoring meaning to clinical supervision in the age of supervision-as-surveillance.

Jeanie Beh is a PhD student within Swinburne's Department of Communication and Digital Media Design. She has completed a Masters of Multimedia from Swinburne University of Technology and worked in the industry as a multimedia developer, web designer, user experience designer and software tester. Currently, Jeanie is working as a research associate in Swinburne's Future Self and Design Living Lab. She is passionately interested in overturning the perception that older adults are unable or disinterested in developing skills in using technology. Her research focuses on ways to engage older adults with mobile touch screen technologies through the role of human interest which is also the theme of her soon to be submitted PhD.

Fatih Bodzemir is PhD candidate in the School of Global, Urban and Social Studies at RMIT University, and has a background in management of water resources, environment and conflicts. Currently, he is working as chief technical advisor to the Food and Agriculture Organization of the United Nations. His research interest mainly cover basin-level private water conflicts in environmentally degrading regions of the world. He is advocating sustainable land and water resources management in these regions through affiliations with the Turkish Ministry of Agriculture and the United Nations in avoiding water-induced conflicts. Climate change is also his expertise, and he is promoting risk management instead of management of crises in the context of climate change. His research subject is expected to draw the attention of policy makers in these parts of the world in strengthening the regulations that will create a working together environment.

Steve Boucher is a student rights officer from the RMIT University Student Union. Steve has a background in social work and is a strong advocate for students with mental health issues. He is particularly concerned about fair and equitable policies and decision-making processes that are transparent and not unduly complicated or open to misinterpretation. He is a passionate advocate for students with disabilities ensuring their human rights upheld and in particular access to education in a supportive environment that enables them to perform well. He is particularly concerned about Fitness to Study initiatives in universities that could result in discrimination against people with mental health issues when applying to study and during their studies. Steve is concerned students may not disclose issues and seek help in fear of discrimination and possible termination of their studies if they are "deemed unfit". He is also concerned about protecting student's privacy in terms of university access to students' medical reports.

Matthew Dale is currently employed by Mind Australia Ltd. as a Community Mental Health Practitioner in their Family & Carer services program. He is also a sessional teacher at Holmesglen TAFE in their Certificate IV and Diploma mental health courses. He has worked in the Mental Health sector for over sixteen years for several different organisations in various positions, including roles in Mental Health Promotion, Peer Work, Outreach Support, Respite and Mental Health Education. His passion and interest is in Mental Health Promotion and Early Intervention/Prevention. He also volunteers as a Peer Ambassador for SANE Australia and is a committee member of the organisation Bipolar Life. He was drawn to working in the Mental Health sector due to his own experience of mental ill-health and recovery. He believes in empowering individuals who have a mental illness to develop self-belief, confidence and hope for a meaningful life despite their mental health challenges.

Christina David is an Early Career Researcher and lecturer in social work at RMIT University, Australia. Christina researches and publishes in the areas of disability, applied human rights, social inclusion, and consumer directed policy and practice reforms. She is particularly interested in the implications of contemporary policy moves and service markets for diverse and marginalised groups, for practitioners, and for social justice and change. Christina is engaged in a range of funded and applied social research projects addressing questions related to social inclusion and community development and using participatory research methodologies.

Kellie Grant is a PhD candidate at Monash University and a sessional academic at RMIT University. Her research explores how the concept of risk influences the decision making of health professionals. She is very interested in understanding how concepts such as risk can shape the relationships between care providers and the people with whom they work. Kellie is a social worker; most recently she has worked in hospital social work, in maternity, paediatrics and oncology. Prior to this she held positions in a range of community services, including in mental health, pregnancy options counselling, youth work, and disability. Kellie has over 10 years of experience working in the health and community sectors. She completed her honours thesis on the challenges arising for feminist practitioners in the neoliberal context and graduated with first class honours. Kellie is a member of the NHMRC funded Evidence Translation in Allied Health (EviTAH) investigative team. Outside of work, she is an avid nature lover and an amateur harpist.

Emily Greenwood is a research assistant at Swinburne University and has expertise in conducting systematic literature reviews using Covidence software and conducting quality assessments of articles. She is also experienced in online survey design. Emily is a graduate of Biomedicine at Melbourne University and is particularly interested in health and wellbeing and the intersection of human rights and social justice issues on a person's access to services and health outcomes. Research projects Emily has worked on include substance abuse and misuse for adolescents and evidence-based models of service delivery. She has also researched trauma-informed, culturally safe models of service delivery and was a member of a research team that developed a *Framework for Culturally Safe, Trauma-Informed Organisations for Aboriginal People* acknowledging the impacts of colonisation, and ongoing transgenerational trauma arising from the Stolen Generations for application with government, health organisations and the community.

Terrence Haines is Head of School of Primary and Allied Health Care Monash University. Previous appointments are Director of Research, Southern Physiotherapy Clinical School and Director of the Allied Health Research Unit, Monash Health. He is a distinguished researcher in health and has received two fellowships; NHMRC Career Development Fellowship Level 1 (2010-2013), NHMRC Career Development Fellowship Level 2 (2014-2017). He has been a chief investigator on four NHMRC project grants (CIA, CIC, CIB, CIB), three NHMRC partnership grants (CID, CIE, CIA), two ARC linkage grants (CID, CII), and multiple grants and research tenders from nationally competitive funding bodies. In total, he has received over $18 million in competitive research funding from national and international sources with over $14 million coming in the past 5 years. Since 2010 he has had a total of 141 full, peer reviewed publications.

Zac Haussegger is a research assistant at Swinburne University, having worked primarily on projects concerning the health and wellbeing of Aboriginal adolescents in out-of-home-care. He has helped his research team develop the Framework for Culturally Safe, Trauma-Informed Organisations for Aboriginal People, as well as a developing a feasibility study for the implementation of Dialectical Behaviour Therapy within Aboriginal adolescents in residential care. He is a graduate of Biomedicine at the University of Melbourne with a major in Neuroscience, and has a particular interest in the importance of service design that is responsive to individual and community needs. He has expertise as an editorial assistant, having worked on various projects within the Social Work Department at Swinburne University. In his spare time, he plays and loves the guitar, and has recently formed a rock-and-roll band that plays shows at different pubs across Melbourne.

Elizabeth Hudson is a PhD candidate and former Research Manager at a large not-for-profit Human Services Organisation. As Research Manager, she was responsible for a small team whose role was to explore national and international best practice within the disability, community service and mental health industries through partnered research with Australian universities and other community organisations. Elizabeth is also the former CEO of a specialized mental health employment service and has 15+ years' experience in management roles in the Australian community/employment sector. She left the sector briefly to work in Human Resources Management in a law firm for 5 years. Liz has a teaching background and Master of Education. Her research interests include: Community mental health, person-centred practices, mental health recovery orientated practice, disability rights and social inclusion. Liz's PhD research topic is: Gateways and Gatekeepers: An exploration of the issues facing people with episodic mental illness during transition to the National Disability Insurance Scheme.

Peter King is a qualified mental health nurse, psychotherapist, educator and clinical supervisor who started a professional career in the mental health sector in 1994 working as psychiatric services officer whilst completing a Bachelor of Nursing degree at university. He has also worked in an emergency department and on a crisis assessment treatment team (CATT). His current professional roles include Executive Director at the Centre for Mental Health Education, owner of the Essentia Health & Wellbeing Centres, accreditation as a Somatic Trauma Therapy & Dialectical Behaviour Therapy educator and one of only three supervisors to accredit somatic trauma therapists internationally with treatment developer Babette Rothschild. He has recently completed his doctoral thesis entitled: *Effective interventions for working with individuals with borderline personality disorder*.

Haylee Lane is currently completing her PhD at Monash University, Frankston, Australia. Her research interest and expertise explore issues regarding decision making and equity within healthcare resource allocation decisions, specifically within allied health. Haylee has worked as an Occupational Therapist in a range of settings including community health, inpatient rehabilitation and paediatrics across both the public and private sectors. Recent publications on this topic emanating from her PhD are: Lane, H. et al. (2018). How do allied health professionals define and apply equity when making resource allocation decisions? *International Journal of Health Services*, 48(2), 349-368; Lane et al. (2017). What Factors do Allied Health Take into Account When Making Resource Allocation Decisions? *International Journal of Health Policy and Management*, 6(x), 1-9 and Lane et al. (2017). Equity in healthcare resource allocation decision-making: A systematic review. *Social Science and Medicine*, 175: 11-27.

Bruno Mascitelli is an Associate Professor in International Studies at Swinburne University of Technology in Melbourne Australia. Prior to joining academia he was employed for 17 years by the Australian Consulate in Milan, Italy. His teaching has been in the area of expatriate voting and European political economy and his research interests cover a wide array of themes. He is a Jean Monnet Chair in Australia which was awarded 2016-2019. He has published 19 books and many journal articles and book chapters. He is President of the European Studies Association of Australia.

Ndungi wa Mungai is a senior lecturer in social work at Charles Sturt University. Since 2010 Ndungi has taught a range of social work subjects including human rights, social work theory and practice and social work research methods. Ndungi has also worked in Australia in various fields including homelessness, asylum seekers, torture, trauma counselling and relationship counselling. Research interests include mental health, human rights, ageing, food security, refugee settlement and social and ecological sustainability. Ndungi has contributed about 20 refereed book chapters and journal articles. Most recent publications include: Transcultural issues in regional settlement of refugees (with Ignatius Chida), (2018); Early career researcher's peer support group (2018); and Community Development: Is it coming back? (2017).

Jeanette Ninnis is a social work practitioner who has specialised for twenty years in mental health clinical therapy and counselling. As a clinician for people with serious mental illness, Jeanette facilitated programs for: young people and families impacted by first episode psychosis; women with life threatening self-harm behaviours, and; children of parents with mental illness. Jeanette also worked as a sexual assault counsellor. For the last seven years, she has been working as a torture and trauma counsellor for Service for the Treatment and Rehabilitation of Torture and Trauma Survivors (STARTTS). Jeanette also teaches social work at Charles Sturt University, Australia. Jeanette has recently completed her Master's dissertation, focusing on the development of a cross-cultural trauma counselling model from a literature review of what women from Congo report assists their psychological wellbeing after conflict related sexual violence.

Sonja Pedell is Director of Swinburne's Future Self and Design Living Lab, where her research contributes extensive knowledge of human-computer interaction (HCI) and research methods to the teaching of digital media and communication design. Alongside this role, she is also Department Research Director for Swinburne's Department of Communication and Digital Media Design. Sonja's research interests include user-centred design methods, scenario-based and mobile design, domestic technology development, and the design of engaging novel technologies for various user groups, in particular for the ageing population. Prior to taking up these roles at Swinburne, Sonja completed a Masters of Psychology from the Technical University of Berlin and was employed as an Interaction Designer, Usability Consultant and Product Manager in industry for several years.

Susan Roberts, with a major in sociology, is a Liaison Librarian with a responsibility to students who are studying online, such as Open Universities Australia and Transnational programs. Having worked in a variety of special and academic libraries she has amassed a broad range of experience in all areas of librarianship. Her particular interests lie in the area of equitable provision of reference and liaison services to students who study online, including the development of information literacy programs for off campus students and also the accessibility of library services for students with disabilities. Susan has written and presented several peer reviewed conference papers and two academic articles on her favourite topics.

Peter Robertson is senior lecturer in History and Sociology at Swinburne University of Technology, Melbourne. His first book, The Changing World of Gay Men (Palgrave Macmillan, 2008) examined the lives of three generations of Australian men, aged 20–79 and won The Australian Sociological Association (TASA) inaugural Raewyn Connell prize in 2010. His research interests include ageing, sexuality, social justice, and work. His second book, Gay Men's Relationships Across the Life Course analysed the life stories of a diverse sample of 97 gay men from nine international cities. Published by Palgrave

Macmillan in 2013 it includes a Foreword by the Hon. Michael Kirby, AC CMG. In 2017 Palgrave Macmillan published his third book, Gay Men's Working Lives, Retirement and Old Age with a Foreword by Humphrey McQueen. In 2016 he became co-editor of Nexus, TASA's quarterly magazine.

Samuel Teague is a post-graduate student at Swinburne University of Technology, Melbourne. He is enrolled in a PhD and is researching Australian journalists' use of principal mental health narratives when telling their stories about the mentally ill. In 2014, his Honours thesis investigated Australian journalists' contribution to mental health stigma, and he graduated with first class Honours. Samuel is the sole convener, lecturer, and tutor of a Pathways and Vocational Education (PAVE) unit, SOC10011 Sociology in Context, as well as tutor in Higher Education units, including SOC20005 Sport and Australian Society, SOC30010 Sociology of Health, and SOC10004 Sociological Foundations.

Jenni White is an occupational therapist with over with 25 years of experience. Her vision is to lead research that informs evidence towards the provision of patient centred care that reduces distress experienced by health care recipients. She is currently a Research Fellow at Monash University researching evidence-based resource allocation in health settings. Prior to this she was a Research Fellow at the Tom Baker Cancer Centre, Calgary. She has an internationally recognised track record in qualitative and quantitative research, with 33 publications. Jenni has expertise in research design, data collection, analysis and manuscript preparation. She has made a significant contribution towards knowledge and management of the chronic disease, especially stroke, and interventions that may ameliorate distress and poor quality of life. Jenni has supervised many research students to completion exploring a range of stroke interventions and health system processes.

Index

N

O

P

Q

R

S

T

U

V

W

Y

www.ingramcontent.com/pod-product-compliance
Lightning Source LLC
LaVergne TN
LVHW062142300926
849161LV00010B/2599